Peripheral Vascular Ultrasound

To Wendy, Tony and June

For Elsevier:

Associate Development Editor: Dinah Thom
Development Editor: Kerry McGechie
Project Manager: Ailsa Laing
Designer: Judith Wright
Illustration Manager: Bruce Hogarth

Peripheral Vascular Ultrasound

HOW, WHY AND WHEN

SECOND EDITION

Abigail Thrush MSc

Medical Physicist, Department of Clinical Physics,
St Bartholomew's Hospital, Bart's and the London NHS Trust, London, UK

Timothy Hartshorne

Vascular Technologist, Department of Surgery,
Leicester Royal Infirmary, University Hospitals of Leicester NHS Trust, Leicester, UK

ELSEVIER
CHURCHILL
LIVINGSTONE

EDINBURGH   LONDON   NEW YORK   OXFORD   PHILADELPHIA   ST LOUIS   SYDNEY   TORONTO   2005

ELSEVIER
CHURCHILL
LIVINGSTONE

First published 1999
Second edition 2005, 2006

ISBN 0 443 07283 3

British Library Cataloguing in Publication Data
A catalogue record for this book is available from the British Library.

Library of Congress Cataloging in Publication Data
A catalog record for this book is available from the Library of Congress.

Notice
Knowledge and best practice in this field are constantly changing. As new research and experience broaden our knowledge, changes in practice, treatment and drug therapy may become necessary or appropriate. Readers are advised to check the most current information provided (i) on procedures featured or (ii) by the manufacturer of each product to be administered, to verify the recommended dose or formula, the method and duration of administration, and contraindications. It is the responsibility of the practitioner, relying on their own experience and knowledge of the patient, to make diagnoses, to determine dosages and the best treatment for each individual patient, and to take all appropriate safety precautions. To the fullest extent of the law, neither the Publisher nor the author assumes any liability for any injury and/or damage.

The Publisher

ELSEVIER
your source for books,
journals and multimedia
in the health sciences
www.elsevierhealth.com

Working together to grow
libraries in developing countries
www.elsevier.com | www.bookaid.org | www.sabre.org

ELSEVIER   BOOK AID International   Sabre Foundation

The
Publisher's
policy is to use
**paper manufactured
from sustainable forests**

Printed in China

Contents

Acknowledgments vi
Preface vii

1. Introduction 1

2. Ultrasound and imaging 5

3. Doppler ultrasound 23

4. Creation of a color flow image 35

5. Blood flow and its appearance on color flow imaging 49

6. Factors that influence the Doppler spectrum 63

7. Optimizing the scan 75

8. Ultrasound assessment of the extracranial cerebral circulation 85

9. Duplex assessment of lower limb arterial disease 111

10. Duplex assessment of upper extremity arterial disease 133

11. Duplex assessment of aneurysms 145

12. Anatomy of the lower limb venous system and assessment of venous insufficiency 163

13. Duplex assessment of deep venous thrombosis and upper limb venous disorders 189

14. Graft surveillance and preoperative vein mapping for bypass surgery 207

Appendix A: Decibel scale 225
Appendix B: Sensitivity and specificity 227

Index 229

Acknowledgments

We would like to thank David Evans, Hayley Handford, Pouran Khodabakhsh, Nick London, Salvatore Luca, May Naylor, Ross Naylor, Yvonne Sensier, and Jo Walker for their help and support in the preparation of this book.

Preface

Vascular ultrasound is a speciality in its own right and vascular surgeons are becoming increasingly dependent on the skills of vascular sonographers for the investigation of patients suffering from peripheral vascular disease. This book aims to provide an understanding of the principles and practice of vascular ultrasound.

An introduction to some of the basic theory behind the science and technology of ultrasound is included. This will help sonographers to understand the function of scanner controls and enable them to obtain optimal images and Doppler recordings. B-mode imaging, color flow and spectral Doppler images are all prone to artefacts, and it is essential that their presence be recognized. The potential sources of errors in any measurements made by ultrasound should be understood. Specific disorders of the arterial and venous systems are covered, and the techniques for diagnosing these problems are described. Examples of normal and abnormal images and Doppler recordings are included and the interpretation of these discussed. British readers please note that the publishers have used American spelling in this edition.

We hope this book will serve as a useful reference to sonographers new to this field.

London, 2005   Abigail Thrush
Leicester, 2005   Timothy Hartshorne

Chapter 1

Introduction

Since the first edition of this book there have been significant developments in ultrasound technology, magnetic resonance imaging (MRI) and magnetic resonance angiography (MRA), computed tomographic (CT) scanning and vascular and endovascular surgical procedures. The latest generation of duplex systems produce clearer images, especially with the use of techniques such as harmonic imaging and compound imaging. Scanners are more sensitive to detecting flow in the arterial and venous systems. The images produced by MRA can be visually stunning, and it has been suggested that MRA and spiral CT may replace duplex investigations in the future. However, duplex scanning still has many advantages. Apart from improvements in image resolution, it is the ability to visualize flow in real time, make quantitative measurements of blood velocity and detect flow direction that will ensure duplex scanning will remain an important imaging technique for the foreseeable future. Cost and resource implications also are important factors. For instance, it is not cost-effective to screen patients for carotid disease or aortic aneurysm with MRI. However, MRI or CT scanning is essential for planning endovascular repair of an aortic aneurysm. Therefore, each modality has its part to play in the management of patients with vascular disorders. In many centers, diagnostic angiography and venography have been largely replaced by the use of duplex ultrasound investigations. This has the advantage of allowing surgeons and physicians to select patients for surgical treatment or conservative management without the need for invasive investigations. In addition, vascular radiologists can spend more time performing therapeutic procedures, such as angioplasty, rather than diagnostic angiograms.

Vascular ultrasound examinations rely on the use of ultrasound to produce a black and white anatomical image that can demonstrate the presence of disease along an arterial wall or the presence of thrombus in a vein. Doppler ultrasound can provide a functional map in the form of a color flow image, which displays the blood flow in arteries and veins. Spectral Doppler analysis enables Doppler waveforms to be recorded from vessels. It is then possible to visualize changes in flow patterns in vessels and calculate velocity measurements, enabling the sonographer to grade the severity of the vascular disease (Fig. 1.1).

Arterial disease is one of the major causes of morbidity and mortality in the developed world. There are many risk factors associated with the development of arterial disease, but it is widely accepted that tobacco smoking is one of the primary causes. Atherosclerotic plaques develop over time, leading to arterial obstruction or embolization. Radiologists and surgeons are able to perform a variety of procedures to treat arterial disorders. Angioplasty involves the use of a balloon mounted on the end of a

catheter which is guided, using angiography, to the area of stenosis (narrowing) or occlusion (blockage). The balloon is then positioned across the stenosis or occlusion and inflated for a short period of time, to

Figure 1.1 An example of a carotid ultrasound scan showing how B-mode imaging, color flow imaging and spectral Doppler are used to investigate a stenosis.

Figure 1.2 A: An angiogram demonstrating a significant stenosis in the right common iliac artery (arrow). B: The stenosis has been dilated by percutaneous balloon angioplasty.

dilate the lesion, increasing the diameter of the flow lumen (Fig. 1.2). Surgical bypass or endarterectomy can be performed when angioplasty is not possible or is not suitable to treat specific problems. Endovascular or minimally invasive procedures can now be used to treat a range of vascular disorders, including the repair of aortic aneurysms, and are less traumatic for the patient. The long-term outcome of endovascular procedures is still unknown, but duplex scanning has a role to play in the follow-up of patients who have undergone these techniques.

Ultrasound has also had a significant impact on the investigation of venous disorders. Ultrasound allows the detection of deep vein thrombosis, which can lead to fatal pulmonary embolism. The investigation of venous insufficiency in the superficial and deep veins has proved extremely useful for assessing patients with varicose veins and venous ulcers. This enables surgeons to select patients for venous surgery or nonsurgical treatments, such as compression dressings.

It is recommended that the reader obtain an overview of other imaging modalities in order to have an understanding of the role of vascular ultrasound in relation to these other techniques for investigating vascular disorders. In addition, it is important to know about the different radiological and surgical techniques used to treat peripheral vascular disease.

Chapter 2

Ultrasound and imaging

CHAPTER CONTENTS

Introduction 5
Nature of ultrasound 5
  Wavelength and frequency 6
  Speed of ultrasound 6
Generation of ultrasound waves 7
  Pulsed ultrasound 7
  Frequency content of pulses 8
  Beam shape 9
Interaction of ultrasound with surfaces 9
Loss of ultrasound energy in tissue 11
Producing an ultrasound image 12
Amplification of received ultrasound
  echoes 13
Dynamic range, compression curves and
  gray-scale maps 14
Transducer designs and beam forming 15
Focusing the beam 18
Image resolution 19
Tissue harmonic imaging 21

INTRODUCTION

It is important to understand how ultrasound interacts with tissue to be able to interpret ultrasound images and to identify artifacts. Knowledge of how an image is produced allows optimal use of the scanner controls. The aim of this and the next two chapters is to give a simple explanation of the process involved in producing images and blood flow measurements.

NATURE OF ULTRASOUND

Ultrasound, as the name implies, is high-frequency sound. Sound waves travel through a medium by causing local displacement of particles within the medium; however, there is no overall movement of the medium. Unlike light, sound cannot travel through a vacuum as sound waves need a supporting medium. Consider a piece of string held at both ends: with one end briefly shaken, the vibration caused will travel along the string and in so doing transmit energy from one end of the string to the other. This is known as a transverse wave, as the movement of the string is at right angles to the direction in which the wave has moved. Ultrasound is a longitudinal wave, as the displacement of the particles within the medium is in the same direction as that in which the wave is travelling. Figure 2.1 shows a medium with particles distributed evenly within it. The position of the particles within the medium will change as a sound wave passes through it, causing local periodic displacement of these particles (Fig. 2.1B). The size, or amplitude,

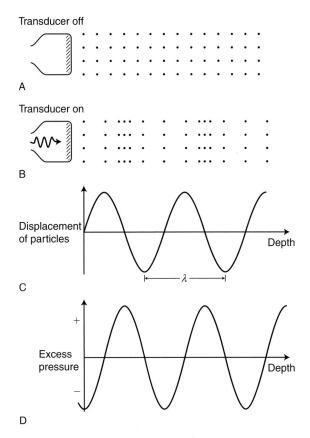

Transducer off

A

Transducer on

B

Displacement of particles

Depth

C

Excess pressure

Depth

D

Figure 2.1 A: A medium consisting of evenly distributed particles. B: The positions of the particles change (shown here at a given point in time) as the ultrasound wave passes through the medium. C: The amplitude of the particle displacement. D: Excess pressure.

Table 2.1	Speed of sound in different tissues
Medium	Speed of sound (m/s)
Air	330
Water (20° C)	1480
Fat	1450
Blood	1570
Muscle	1580
Bone	3500
Soft tissue (average)	1540

taken for the wave to move forwards through the medium by one wavelength is known as the period (τ). The frequency, f, is the number of cycles of displacements passing through a point in the medium during 1 second (s) and is given by:

$$f = \frac{1}{\tau} \qquad (2.1)$$

The unit of frequency is the hertz (Hz), with 1 Hz being one complete cycle per second. Audible sound waves are in the range of 20 Hz to 20 kHz, whereas medical ultrasound scanners typically use high frequencies of between 2 and 15 MHz (i.e., between 2 000 000 and 15 000 000 Hz).

Speed of ultrasound

Sound travels through different media at different speeds (e.g., sound travels faster through water than it does through air). The speed of a sound wave, c, is given by the distance travelled by the disturbance during a given time and is constant in any specific material. The speed can be found by multiplying the frequency by the wavelength and is usually measured in meters per second (m/s):

$$c = \lambda f \qquad (2.2)$$

The speed of sound through a material depends on both the density and the compressibility of the material. The more dense and the more compressible the material, the slower the wave will travel through it. The speed of sound is different for the various tissues in the body (Table 2.1). Knowledge of the speed of sound is needed to determine how far an ultrasound wave has travelled. This is required in both imaging and pulsed Doppler (as

of these displacements is shown in Figure 2.1C. As the particles move within the medium, local increases and decreases in pressure are generated (Fig. 2.1D).

Wavelength and frequency

Ultrasound is usually described by its frequency, which is related to the length of the wave produced. The wavelength of a sound wave is the distance between consecutive points where the size and direction of the displacement are identical and the direction in which the particles are travelling is the same. The wavelength is represented by the symbol λ and is shown in Figure 2.1C. The time will be seen later), but ultrasound systems usually make an estimate by assuming that the speed of sound is the same in all tissues: 1540 m/s. This can lead to small errors in the estimated distance travelled because of the variations in the speed of sound in different tissues.

GENERATION OF ULTRASOUND WAVES

The term transducer simply means a device that converts one form of energy into another. In the case of an ultrasound transducer, this conversion is from electrical energy to mechanical vibration. The piezoelectric effect is the method by which most medical ultrasound is generated. Piezoelectric materials will vibrate mechanically when a varying voltage is applied across them. The frequency of the voltage applied will affect the frequency with which the material vibrates. The thickness of the piezoelectric element will determine the frequency at which the element will vibrate most efficiently; this is known as the resonant frequency of the transducer. The speed of sound within the element will depend on the material from which it is made. A resonant frequency occurs when the thickness of the element is half the wavelength of the sound wave generated within it. At this frequency, the reflected waves from the front and back faces of the element act to reinforce each other, so increasing the size of the vibration produced. When an appropriate coupling medium is used (e.g., ultrasound gel), this vibration will be transmitted into a surrounding medium, such as the body. The named frequency of a transducer is its resonant frequency. This is not to say that the transducer will not function at a different frequency, but that it will be much less efficient at those frequencies. Many modern imaging transducers are designed as broad-band transducers, meaning that they will function efficiently over a wide range of frequencies, and these are usually labelled with the frequency range over which they operate (e.g., 4–7 MHz). Figure 2.2 shows how the transducer output of narrow-band and broad-band transducers varies with the frequency of the excitation voltage. A broad-band transducer is more efficient over a wider range of frequencies than a narrow-band transducer. Ultrasound transducers also use

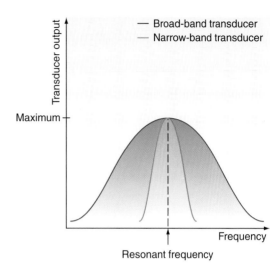

Figure 2.2   Plot of transducer output versus frequency for a broad-band and a narrow-band transducer. A broad-band transducer will be more efficient over a wider range of frequencies than a narrow-band transducer.

the piezoelectric effect to convert the returning ultrasound vibrations back into electrical signals. These signals can then be amplified, analyzed and displayed to provide both anatomical images and flow information.

Pulsed ultrasound

Simple Doppler systems operate with a continuous single-frequency excitation voltage, but all imaging systems and pulsed Doppler systems use pulsed excitation signals. If ultrasound is continuously transmitted along a particular path, the energy will also be continuously reflected back from any boundary in the path of the beam, and it will not be possible to predict where the returning echoes have come from. However, when a pulse of ultrasound is transmitted it is possible to predict the distance (d) of a reflecting surface from the transducer if the time (t) between transmission and reception of the pulse is measured and the velocity (c) of the ultrasound along the path is known, as follows:

$$d = \frac{tc}{2} \tag{2.3}$$

The factor 2 arises from the fact that the pulse travels along the path twice, once on transmission and once on its return. This can be used to predict

Figure 2.3 A signal is made up of, or can be broken down into, sine waves of different frequencies, different amplitudes and phases. (From Fish 1990, with permission.)

Figure 2.4 Four different signals (amplitude plotted against time) and their corresponding frequency spectra (power plotted against frequency). A, B: For a continuous single frequency. C, D: Signal shown in Figure 2.3. E, F: A long pulse. G, H: A short pulse. The shorter the pulse, the greater the range of frequencies within the pulse. (After Fish 1990, with permission.)

where returning echoes have originated from within the body.

Frequency content of pulses

Typically, the pulses used in imaging ultrasound are very short and will only contain 1 to 3 cycles in order that reflections from boundaries that are close together can be easily separated. Pulsed Doppler signals are longer and contain several cycles. In fact, a pulse is made up not of a single frequency but of a range of frequencies of different amplitudes. Different shaped pulses will have different frequency contents. Figure 2.3 illustrates how a

signal can be made up of the sum of several different frequencies. The frequency content of a signal can be displayed on a graph, such as those shown in Figure 2.4 (right panels). This is known as a frequency spectrum and displays the frequencies present within the signal against the relative amplitudes of these frequencies. Figure 2.4A provides an example of a continuous signal consisting of a single frequency. As only one frequency is present in the signal, the frequency spectrum displays a single line at that frequency (Fig. 2.4B). Figure 2.4C, E and G give examples of three differently shaped signals along with their frequency spectra (Fig. 2.4D, F and H), showing the range of frequencies present in each of the different signals. As ultrasound imaging uses pulsed ultrasound, the transducer is not transmitting a single frequency but a range of frequencies.

Beam shape

The shape of the ultrasound beam produced by a transducer will depend on the shape of the element(s), on the transmitted frequency and on whether the beam is focused. The shape of the beam will affect the region of tissue that will be insonated and from which returning echoes will be received. Multi-element array transducers use several elements to produce the beam, as discussed later in this chapter.

INTERACTION OF ULTRASOUND WITH SURFACES

The creation of an ultrasound image depends on the way in which ultrasound energy interacts with the tissue as it passes through the body. When an ultrasound wave meets a large smooth interface between two different media, some of the energy will be reflected back, and this is known as specular reflection. The relative proportions of the energy reflected and transmitted depend on the change in the acoustic impedance between the two materials (Fig. 2.5). The acoustic impedance of a medium is the impedance (similar to resistance) the material offers against the passage of the sound wave through it and depends on the density and compressibility of the medium. The greater the change in the acoustic impedance, the greater the proportion of the ultrasound that is reflected. There is, for example, a large difference in acoustic impedance between soft tissue and bone, or between soft tissue and air, and such interfaces will produce large reflections. This is the reason why ultrasound cannot be used to image beyond lung

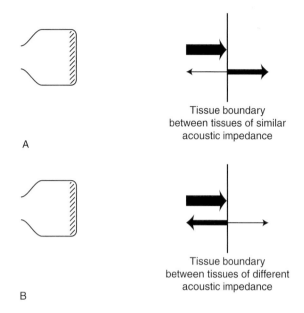

A

B

Figure 2.5 When the ultrasound beam meets a boundary between two media, some of the ultrasound will be transmitted and some will be reflected. A: When the two media have similar acoustic impedances, the majority of the ultrasound will be transmitted across the boundary. B: When the two media have different acoustic impedances, most of the ultrasound will be reflected.

Table 2.2 The ratio of reflected to incident wave amplitude for an ultrasound beam perpendicular to different reflecting interfaces (after McDicken 1981, with permission)

Reflecting interface	Ratio of reflected to incident wave amplitude
Muscle/blood	0.03
Soft tissue/water	0.05
Fat/muscle	0.10
Bone/muscle	0.64
Soft tissue/air	0.9995

or bone, except in limited situations, as only a small proportion of the ultrasound is transmitted. It is also the reason for the loss of both imaging and Doppler information beyond calcified arterial walls (Fig. 8.26), bone (Fig. 10.12) and bowel gas, leading to an acoustic shadow beyond. Table 2.2 shows the ratio of the reflected to incident wave amplitude for a range of reflecting interfaces.

The path along which the reflected ultrasound travels will also affect the amplitude of the signal detected by the transducer. If the beam is perpendicular to the interface, the reflected ultrasound will travel back along the same path to the transducer. If, however, the beam intercepts the interface at an angle of less than 90°, then the beam will be reflected along a different path. Figure 2.6 shows that the angle of incidence (θ_i) is the same as the angle of reflection (θ_r) measured from a line perpendicular to the interface. This means that when the beam is at 90° to the interface, all the

reflected ultrasound will travel back towards the transducer, but as the angle of incidence becomes smaller, the beam will be reflected away from the transducer and therefore the transducer will receive less of the reflected ultrasound. The best image of an interface will be obtained when the interface is at right angles to the beam, and likewise the poorest image will be obtained when the interface is parallel to the beam. Thus, when an artery is imaged in transverse section, the anterior and posterior walls can be seen more clearly than the side, or lateral, walls which are parallel to the beam (Fig. 8.5).

If the ultrasound beam is not perpendicular to the interface and there is a change in the speed of sound in the media on either side of the interface, the path of the beam will be bent. This is known as refraction and is illustrated in Figure 2.7. Refraction causes the beam to change its direction of travel and can lead to artifacts whereby the signal detected by the transducer has originated from a different point in the tissue than that displayed on the image. This is most important where there are large changes in the velocity of sound between media, such as the interface between the uterus and amniotic fluid. It is not usually a major problem

$\theta_i = \theta_r = 0°$

Tissue boundary

A

$\theta_i = \theta_r$

Transmitted

Reflected

Tissue boundary

B

Figure 2.6 A: When an ultrasound beam is perpendicular to an interface, the reflected ultrasound will return by the same path. B: If the interface is not perpendicular to the beam then the reflected ultrasound will travel along a different path. The angle of incidence of the beam (θ_i) is equal to the angle of reflection (θ_r).

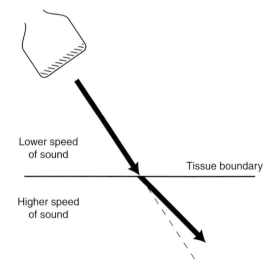

Lower speed of sound

Tissue boundary

Higher speed of sound

Figure 2.7 Refraction. When a beam is transmitted through an interface between two media in which the sound travels at different speeds and the beam is not perpendicular to the interface, the path of the beam will be bent.

in vascular ultrasound, with the exception of the presence of the skull bone in the path of a transcranial Doppler beam.

Although specular reflection occurs at large, smooth boundaries, the majority of signals returning from tissue are made up of ultrasound energy that has been back-scattered from rough surfaces or small structures within the tissue. When the ultrasound beam interacts with a rough surface or small structure it will be scattered in all directions rather than reflected back along one path. Figure 2.8 shows the difference between specular reflection and scattering from rough surfaces and small structures. Scattering occurs when the small structures are of a similar size to or smaller than the wavelength of the ultrasound and will result in less of the ultrasound returning to the transducer along the original beam path. The amount of energy lost from the beam by scattering is highly dependent on the frequency [proportional to the fourth power of

the frequency (i.e., f^4) for structures that are much smaller than the wavelength of the ultrasound]. In the case of peripheral vascular ultrasound, specular reflection will occur at the vessel walls, which are often perpendicular to the beam, leading to large reflected signals. However, ultrasound will be scattered by groups of red blood cells within the lumen, leading to much smaller returning signals, which will not normally be visible on an image.

LOSS OF ULTRASOUND ENERGY IN TISSUE

Attenuation is the loss of energy from the ultrasound beam as it passes through tissue. The more the ultrasound energy is attenuated by the tissue, the less energy will be available to return to the transducer or to penetrate deeper into the tissue. Attenuation is caused by several different processes. These include absorption, scattering, reflection and beam divergence. Absorption causes ultrasound energy to be converted into heat as the beam passes through the tissue. The rate of absorption varies in different types of tissue. Ultrasound energy can also be lost by scattering from small structures within the tissue or reflection from large boundaries that are not perpendicular to the beam, preventing the ultrasound from returning to the transducer. The attenuation coefficients of various tissues are presented in Table 2.3, from which it can be seen that muscle attenuates the ultrasound more quickly than fat. The units of the coefficient of attenuation are in $dB\,MHz^{-1}\,cm^{-1}$, showing that the rate of attenuation depends on frequency of ultrasound, with higher frequencies being

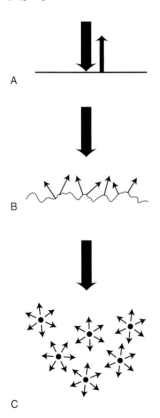

Figure 2.8 Specular reflections occur at large smooth interfaces (A), whereas ultrasound is scattered by rough surfaces (B) and small structures (C).

Table 2.3 Attenuation coefficients of different tissues

Medium	Attenuation coefficient at 1 MHz (dB cm^{-1})
Water (20° C)	0.2
Fat	60
Blood	20
Muscle	150
Bone	1000
Soft tissue (average)	70

Figure 2.9   If consecutive ultrasound pulses are sent along the same path and the returning echoes are displayed as adjacent scan lines, a motion mode, or M-mode, image (A) is produced that can be used to image movement, such as heart valve motion (B).

attenuated more quickly than lower frequencies. This is why higher ultrasound frequencies penetrate tissue less effectively than lower ultrasound frequencies and can only be used for imaging superficial structures. This is similar to the situation in which you can hear your neighbor's hi-fi bass through the partition wall better than the treble.

PRODUCING AN ULTRASOUND IMAGE

Ultrasound imaging uses information contained in reflected and scattered signals received by the transducer. If it is assumed that the speed of the ultrasound through the tissue is constant, it is possible to predict the distance from a reflective boundary or scattering particle to the transducer. When an ultrasound pulse returns to the transducer, it will cause the transducer to vibrate, and this will generate a voltage across the piezoelectric element. The amplitude of the returning pulse will depend on the proportion of the ultrasound reflected or back-scattered to the transducer and the amount by which the signal has been attenuated along its path. The amplitude of the pulse received back at the transducer can be displayed against time. This display can be calibrated such

that the time delay of the returning pulse represents the distance of the boundary from the transducer, thus showing the depth of the boundary in the tissue. The varying amplitude of the signal can be displayed as a spot of varying brightness that travels across the display with time. This type of display is known as a B scan (B-mode) or brightness scan. If a second pulse is sent into the tissue along the same path, the B scan generated by the second pulse can be displayed next to that of the first, as shown in Figure 2.9A. This display now shows the time of travel of the pulses converted into distance along the vertical axis and the time between consecutive pulses along the horizontal axis, with the amplitude of the received signal represented by the brightness of the spot on the screen. This type of scan is known as M-mode (or motion mode), and Figure 2.9A displays the motion of the mitral valve, obtained by placing a transducer over the heart (Fig. 2.9B).

If the transducer is moved slightly so that the beam now passes through the tissue along a path that is adjacent to the first, and the returning signal is displayed next to that from the first pulse, a B-mode image can be produced, as shown diagrammatically in Figure 2.10A. In this display the

Figure 2.10   If consecutive ultrasound pulses are transmitted along adjacent paths (A) and displayed in brightness mode in adjacent scan lines, a B–mode image (B) is produced.

distance travelled by the pulse is shown along the vertical axis and the distance between adjacent pulses is shown along the horizontal axis, with the amplitude of the received signal represented by the brightness on the screen. An example of a B-mode image showing a bifurcating artery is presented in Figure 2.10B.

In fact, modern scanners use electronic transducers, which typically comprise 128 piezoelectric elements that are capable of producing many adjacent beams, or scan lines, without the need to move the transducer itself. The quality of the image will obviously depend on the distance between adjacent beam paths, known as the line density. The more closely the scan lines are arranged, the more time it will take to produce an image of a given size, which will affect the rate at which the image is updated. This would not be important if a stationary object was being imaged, but most structures in the body are in motion due to cardiac and respiratory movements. The rate at which complete images are produced per second is known as the frame rate and is affected by the number of scan lines and by the width and depth of the region of tissue being imaged. The deeper the tissue being interrogated, the longer it will take for the returning signal to reach the transducer before the next pulse can be transmitted. In B-mode imaging, it is rarely a problem to produce images with a high enough line density and frame rate.

AMPLIFICATION OF RECEIVED ULTRASOUND ECHOES

There are two methods of increasing the amplitude of the returning signal: increasing the output power and increasing the receiver gain. Increasing the voltage of the excitation pulse across the transducer will cause the transducer to transmit a larger amplitude ultrasound pulse, thus increasing the amplitude of reflections. However, increasing the output power causes the patient to be exposed to more ultrasound energy. The alternative is to amplify the received signal, but there is a limit at which the amplitude of the received signal is no greater than the background noise, and at which

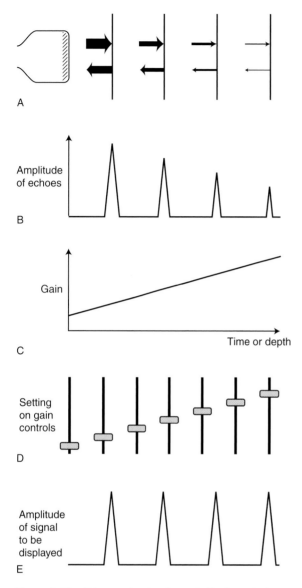

Figure 2.11   Echoes returning from similar boundaries at different depths (A) will be of different amplitudes (B) due to attenuation. The receiver gain of the scanner can be increased during the time that the echoes are received (C) using the gain controls (D) to produce signals of similar amplitude (E).

no amount of amplification will assist in differentiating the signal from the noise. For a given frequency of transducer, the depth at which the reflected or back-scattered signals are no longer greater than the noise is known as the penetration depth. Increasing the overall gain of the received signal will increase both the high-amplitude signals detected near the transducer and the lower amplitude signals detected from deeper in the tissue, which have been attenuated to a greater extent.

It is useful to be able to image the reflections from similar boundaries that lie at different depths at a similar brightness on the image. Equally, it is useful to image the back-scattered signals from tissues at different depths at a similar level of gray on the B-mode image. Figure 2.11A and B show signals returning from four identical boundaries at different depths in an attenuating medium. It can be seen that the echoes received from the deeper boundaries have been attenuated more than those from the shallower boundaries. If the gain of the receiver amplifier is increased over the time during which the pulse is returning to the transducer (Fig. 2.11C), it is possible to use greater amplification for the signal received from the deeper boundaries. By changing the gain over time, the returning echoes from the four boundaries can now be displayed at a similar brightness (Fig. 2.11E). When the next pulse is transmitted, the gain would return to the baseline value and increase with time as before. This method of varying gain over time is known as time gain compensation (TGC) or depth gain compensation (DGC). The TGC control can usually be altered by a set of sliding knobs or paddles to allow different gains to be set for signals returning from different depths, as shown in Figure 2.11D.

DYNAMIC RANGE, COMPRESSION CURVES AND GRAY-SCALE MAPS

Echoes reflected from tissue–air or tissue–bone interfaces are large compared with the low-amplitude back-scattered signals from small structures within the tissue. The larger signal amplitudes are of an order of 100 000 times greater than the smallest signal detected, just above the noise level of the scanner. This large range of signal amplitudes can best be described using the decibel scale (see Appendix A) as 100 dB. The range of signals that can be displayed by the scanner monitor is much less than 100 dB, typically about 20 dB, and therefore the range of signal amplitudes needs to be reduced in order to be displayed. This can be achieved either by selecting not to display the

A

B

C

Figure 2.12   A: An example of a compression curve, showing how the amplitude of the signal to be displayed relates to the amplitude of the input signal. This compression curve accentuates the differences in the lower to mid-range amplitude signal. B and C show the same carotid plaque imaged using two different compression curves.

lowest or the highest signals present or by compressing the signal. The signal can be compressed using a nonlinear amplifier. This applies more gain to lower amplitude signals than higher amplitude signals, so reducing the dynamic range of the signal to be displayed. Figure 2.12A gives an example of a compression curve, showing how the amplitude

of the signal to be displayed relates to the amplitude of the input signal. The input signal is the received signal, which has already been amplified by the TGC. This compression curve accentuates the differences in lower to mid-range amplitude signals. The choice of compression curve used depends on what aspect of the image is important in a given application—for example, the fine detail of backscatter from tissue or the presence of large boundaries, such as vessel walls. There are usually a range of compression curves available on modern scanners, which are often selected automatically by the system, depending on the selected application (e.g., vascular or abdominal). Figure 2.12B and C shows the same carotid plaque imaged using two different compression curves. The dynamic range of signals arriving at the transducer that can be displayed is defined as the ratio of the largest echo amplitude that does not cause saturation, resulting in peak white, to the smallest echo that can be differentiated from noise. Some modern scanners claim to have a dynamic range of 150 dB.

Finally, the scanner uses a gray-scale map to assign a level of gray dependent on the amplitude of amplified signal, to produce the gray-scale image. Some systems have a choice of gray-scale maps, used in different applications, and these will affect the appearance of the image. It is helpful for the sonographer to refer to the scanner operator manual and to explore the effect of the compression curves and gray-scale maps used on the image obtained.

TRANSDUCER DESIGNS AND BEAM FORMING

In order to produce a two-dimensional (2D) image, the ultrasound beam has to pass through adjacent areas of the tissue. This can be done by physically moving the transducer, and in early real-time scanners this was performed by rocking or rotating the transducer element. Many modern electronic imaging transducers are typically made up of 128 elements arranged in a row (Fig. 2.13A), often about 4 cm long. These are known as linear array transducers. If a group of elements are all excited simultaneously (Fig. 2.14A), the wavelets will interfere to produce a beam that is perpendicular to the transducer face. The groups of elements within the array that are excited can be varied to

A

B

C

Figure 2.13 A: Linear array transducer. This is typically made up of 128 elements in a row and produces a rectangular field of view. B: Curvilinear array transducer. This produces a sector image, with a field of view that diverges with depth. C: Phased array transducer. This uses a smaller array of elements and electronically steers the beam to produce a sector image.

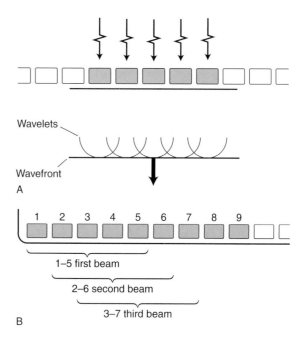

A

B

Figure 2.14 A: A group of elements within an array can be excited simultaneously, and the resulting wavelets will interfere to produce a wavefront perpendicular to the transducer face. B: The group of elements excited within an array can be varied to produce beams following parallel adjacent paths.

same at depth as it is close to the transducer (Fig. 12.13A).

A sector image can be produced by arranging the elements in a curvilinear array (Fig. 2.13B). As the beam paths diverge, the image fans out and therefore the scan lines run more closely in the portion of the image near to the transducer and become more spread out at depth. This leads to some loss of image quality at depth but allows a larger field of view compared with that produced by a linear array transducer. Curvilinear arrays are mainly used for abdominal imaging.

Using several elements to form the ultrasound beam enables the beam shape to be manipulated. If the elements used to form the beam are excited at slightly different times, the wavefronts produced by the elements will interfere differently than they would if they were all excited at the same time. For example, if the element on the far right in the array (Fig. 2.15A) is excited first, with the next element excited after a very short delay, and so forth, the

produce ultrasound beams that follow parallel adjacent paths (Fig. 2.14B)—e.g., elements 1–5 produce the first beam, 2–6 the second, 3–7 the third and so on. A linear array transducer produces a rectangular image in which the field of view is the

Figure 2.16 Compound scanning sums several images obtained with the ultrasound beam steered at slightly different angles, to improve imaging of boundaries that are perpendicular to the transducer face and to reduce noise and speckle.

Figure 2.15 A: Introducing a time delay between exciting consecutive elements within the array causes the wavelets to interfere in such a way that the beam is steered away from the path perpendicular to the transducer face (e.g., steered left or right). B: Delays between excitation of the elements in the array can be used to focus the beam.

wavefronts produced will interfere in such a way that the beam is no longer perpendicular to the front of the transducer. The angle at which the beam is produced will depend on the delay between the excitation pulses of the different elements. By changing the delay between each set of excitation pulses, it is possible to steer the beam through a range of angles from left to right.

Phased array transducers use a smaller array of elements and electronically steer the beam in this way to produce a sector image (Fig. 2.13C). This type of transducer produces a large field of view compared with the size of the transducer face, also known as the transducer footprint. Phased array transducers are used, in particular, in cardiac ultrasound, as the heart can only be imaged through small spaces between the ribs, thus requiring a transducer with a small footprint to image a large field of view at depth. Beam steering is also used in linear array transducers when a beam that is not perpendicular to the transducer face is required, such as in Doppler ultrasound (see Chs 3 and 4) and in compound imaging. In compound imaging, the target is insonated several times with the beam steered at several different angles (Fig. 2.16). The returning echoes from these different imaging beams are combined to produce a single image. This gives improved imaging of interfaces that are not parallel to the transducer face, such as the lateral walls of a vessel, and reduces noise and speckle. Figure 2.17 shows the improvement in the image that can be provided when imaging a carotid plaque with compound imaging compared to conventional imaging.

A

B

Figure 2.17 Images showing the improvement that can be provided by compound imaging of a carotid artery plaque (B) compared to conventional imaging (A).

FOCUSING THE BEAM

The ultrasound beam can be focused to improve the image quality within the focal zone. By using several elements, excited with a range of delays, it is possible to focus the beam. Figure 2.15B shows how, if the elements at each end of the group of active elements are excited first, with the next two elements being excited after a short delay, and so forth, the wavelets will interfere to produce a concave wavefront causing the beam to converge at the focal point. The distance of the focal point from the front of the transducer is governed by the

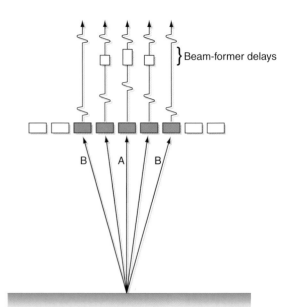

Figure 2.18 Introducing delays before summing the signals received at different elements allows dynamic focusing of the received beam. In this case, dynamic focusing allows the signals that have travelled farther along path B to be added to the signal that has travelled along path A by delaying the signal received by the middle element before summing it with the signals received by the outer elements.

length of the delays, with longer delays producing a shorter focal length.

Many modern scanners use multiple zone focusing whereby the image will be created in zones, using different focal lengths for different depths. The upper portion of the image, near to the transducer, will be produced using a short focal length, a second set of scan lines with a longer focal length will be used for the next zone of the image, and so on. The advantage is that image quality is improved throughout the image; however, the disadvantage is that the frame rate is reduced by a factor of 1/(number of focal zones).

The focus of the beam can also be altered during reception. This is known as dynamic focusing. In this case, delays are introduced between consecutive elements on reception, rather than transmission, before the received signals are summed together. With regard to Figure 2.18, dynamic focusing allows the signals that have travelled farther along

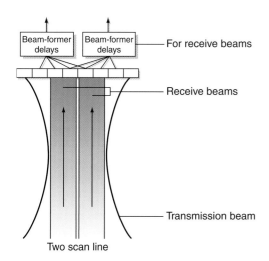

Figure 2.19 Parallel beam forming of two or more received beams from a single wide transmitted beam permits improvements in imaging frame rate. (After Whittingham 2003, with permission.)

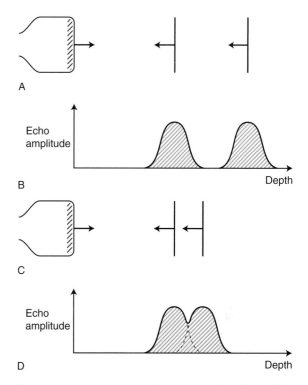

Figure 2.20 Echoes returning from two boundaries (A) can be resolved (B). However, if the boundaries are close together (C), they can no longer be seen as different echoes (D).

path B to be added to the signal that has travelled along path A by delaying the signal received by the middle element before summing it with the signals received by the outer elements. The focal point of the received signal again depends on the lengths of the delays introduced. As the delay can be varied while the signal is being received from different depths, the focal length can be optimized through the image without a reduction in frame rate.

A technique known as parallel beam forming may be used to improve the frame rate (i.e., the number of images produced per second). This uses a wide, weakly focused transmitted beam. The received signal produced from this transmitted beam can then be processed using different sets of delays in order to form two or more different received beams, simultaneously, as shown in Figure 2.19 (Whittingham 2003). This allows two or more received signals, producing two or more scan lines, for each transmitted pulse, so enabling higher frame rates.

IMAGE RESOLUTION

The resolution of a system is defined as its ability to distinguish between two adjacent objects. Figure 2.20 demonstrates how the echoes from two reflecting surfaces can be resolved and also how they can no longer be distinguished from each other if the two objects are moved closer together.

The resolution of an ultrasound image can be described in three planes—axial (along the beam), lateral (across the image) and slice thickness—as shown in Figure 2.21. Axial resolution depends on the length of the excitation pulse, which in turn depends on the operating frequency of the transducer. The higher the frequency, the better the resolution. There is, however, a compromise, as the higher the frequency, the greater the attenuation and therefore the poorer the penetration. The lateral resolution depends on factors such as the density of the scan lines and the focusing of the beam. Lateral resolution is poorer than axial resolution.

The out-of-imaging plane beam thickness, or slice thickness, will affect the region perpendicular to the scan plane over which returning echoes will be obtained. Ideally, the slice thickness should be as thin as possible to maintain image quality, so focusing is often used in this plane as well as in the imaging plane. This can be done either by

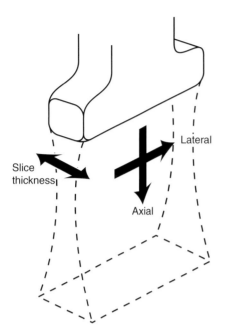

Figure 2.21 Resolution of a transducer can be described in different planes—axial and lateral. The slice thickness of the beam relates to the width of the beam in the non-imaging plane and governs the thickness of the slice of tissue being imaged.

incorporating a fixed lens into the front face of the transducer or by electronic focusing using a 2D array of elements, which allows focusing in both the imaging plane and the plane at right angles to the image. These 2D arrays are often called 1½D arrays as there are relatively few elements along the width of the array compared with the length.

Resolution of an ultrasound system can be assessed using a test object consisting of fine wires embedded in a tissue-mimicking material. The groups of six wires are positioned so the wires are at different distances apart, allowing the user to assess what is the smallest separation at which the wires can still be resolved. The tissue-mimicking material is designed to have similar attenuation to tissue and to produce a similar back-scattered signal. Figure 2.22A is a schematic diagram of the wires in the test object and in Figure 2.22B and C the images are obtained from the test object with 2.25 MHz phased array and 10 MHz linear array transducers, respectively. It can be seen that the 10 MHz transducer gives better axial resolution, as all six wires are seen, whereas the 2.25 MHz transducer provides

Figure 2.22 Assessing ultrasound axial resolution. A: Schematic diagram of a group of six unevenly spaced wires in a test object. B, C: Images of the test object in (A) obtained with 2.25 and 10 MHz transducers, respectively. The 10 MHz transducer gives better axial resolution and the 2.25 MHz transducer provides better penetration.

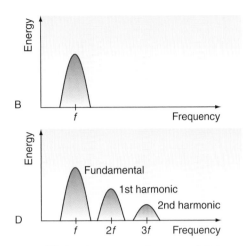

Figure 2.23 A: An undistorted pulse with its frequency spectra (B) showing a center frequency *f*. C: Large-amplitude signals become progressively distorted as they pass through tissue. D: The distorted pulse contains harmonics (*2f*, *3f*, etc.) of the fundamental frequency *f*. (After Whittingham T A 1999 Tissue harmonic imaging. European Radiology 9(Suppl 3): S323–S326. © Springer-Verlag, with permission.)

better penetration, to 12 cm depth compared with 3 cm for the 10 MHz transducer. Choosing the frequency of transducer to use for a given examination depends on a compromise between the depth of the region to be imaged and the axial resolution that can be obtained. It is preferable to select the highest frequency transducer that will provide adequate penetration. The ability to visualize objects within an image also depends on the appropriate use of imaging controls, such as gain settings.

TISSUE HARMONIC IMAGING

Tissue harmonic imaging (THI) can improve the image quality in difficult subjects; however, in good subjects poorer images may be obtained than with conventional imaging. THI utilizes the fact that high-amplitude ultrasound pulses undergo nonlinear propagation, whereby the pulse becomes progressively distorted as it passes through tissue (Fig. 2.23A and B (Whittingham 1999)). This distortion of the pulse results in the frequency content of the returning pulse being significantly different to that of the transmitted pulse. Figure 2.23D shows how the energy spectrum of the distorted pulse will contain harmonic frequencies (*2f*, *3f*, etc.) that are multiples of the original transmitted frequency, *f*. In THI mode, the receiver is tuned to a center frequency that is twice the center frequency of the transmitted pulse, as seen in Figure 2.24. Usually the transmitted pulse

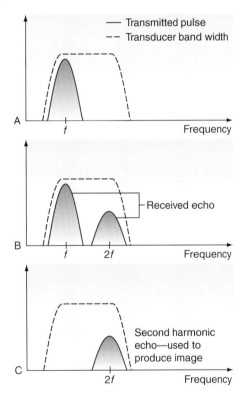

Figure 2.24 Tissue harmonic imaging. Wide transducer bandwidths enable pulses of center frequency *f* to be transmitted and use only the received harmonic frequencies, center frequency *2f*, to produce the image. (After Whittingham T A 1999 Tissue harmonic imaging. European Radiology 9(Suppl 3): S323–S326. © Springer-Verlag, with permission.)

Figure 2.25 Tissue harmonic imaging can provide improved image quality as seen by comparing conventional imaging (A) with tissue harmonic imaging (B) of an aorta.

used in THI is a lower frequency than that used in conventional imaging. For example, in an abdominal application, a center frequency of 3.5 MHz would typically be used in conventional imaging whereas a center frequency of 1.75 MHz would be used for THI, producing a second harmonic at 3.5 MHz. Improvements in transducer sensitivity over the years have enabled the production of broad-band transducers with large bandwidths, allowing the transducer to transmit ultrasound with a center frequency f and selectively receive the returning harmonics with center frequency $2f$. As nonlinear propagation only occurs in high-amplitude pulses, harmonics are not present in lower amplitude echoes produced, for example, by multiply reflected pulses, reverberations, grating lobes or side lobes. In conventional imaging it is these spurious echoes that produce noisy images. With THI these spurious echoes will contain little or no harmonics and therefore will not be detected. Figure 2.25 shows the improvement when imaging an aorta using harmonic imaging compared to conventional imaging.

References

Fish P 1990 Physics and instrumentation of diagnostic medical ultrasound. Wiley, Chichester

McDicken W N 1981 Diagnostic ultrasonics: principles and use of instruments, 2nd edn. Wiley, New York

Whittingham T A 1999 Tissue harmonic imaging. European Radiology 9(Suppl 3): S323–S326

Whittingham T A 2003 Transducers and beam-forming. In: Hoskins P R, Thrush A, Martin K, Whittingham T A (eds) Diagnostic ultrasound: physics and equipment. Greenwich Medical Media Ltd, London, pp 23–48

Further reading

Hendrick W R, Hykes D L, Starchman D E 1995 Ultrasound: physics and instrumentation. Mosby, St Louis

Kremkau F W 1998 Diagnostic ultrasound—principles and instruments, 5th edn. WB Saunders, Philadelphia

Whittingham T A 1997 New and future developments in ultrasound imaging. British Journal of Radiology 70: S119–S132

Whittingham T A 1999 Section I: New transducers. European Radiology 9(Suppl 3): S298–S303

Whittingham T A 1999 Section II: Digital technology. European Radiology 9(Suppl 3): S307–S311

Chapter 3

Doppler ultrasound

CHAPTER CONTENTS

The Doppler effect   23
  History behind the discovery of the Doppler
    effect   24
Doppler effect applied to vascular
  ultrasound   24
  Back-scatter from blood   26
Extracting the Doppler signal   26
Analysis of the Doppler signal   27
  Continuous wave (CW) Doppler   29
  Pulsed Doppler   29
  Limitations of CW versus pulsed Doppler   33
Duplex ultrasound   33
  Velocity measurements using duplex
    ultrasound   33

THE DOPPLER EFFECT

The detection and quantification of vascular disease using ultrasound depends very heavily on the use of the Doppler effect. The Doppler effect is the change in the observed frequency due to the relative motion of the source and the observer. This effect can be heard when the pitch of a police car's siren changes as the car travels towards you and then away from you. Figure 3.1 helps to explain the effect more thoroughly. In Figure 3.1A the source of the sound and the observer are both stationary, so the observed sound has the same frequency as the transmitted sound. In Figure 3.1B the source is stationary and the observer is moving toward it, causing the observer to cross the wavefronts of the emitted wave more quickly than when stationary, so that the observer witnesses a higher frequency wave than that emitted. If, however, the observer is moving away from the source (Fig. 3.1C), the wavefronts will be crossed less often and the frequency witnessed will be lower than that emitted. Figure 3.1D shows the opposite case, in which the source is moving toward a stationary observer. The source will move a short distance toward the observer between the emission of each wave, and in so doing shorten the wavelength, so the observer will therefore witness a higher frequency. Similarly, if the source is moving away from the observer, the wavelength will be increased, leading to observation of a lower frequency (Fig. 3.1E). The resulting change in the observed frequency is known as the Doppler shift, and the magnitude of the Doppler shift frequency is

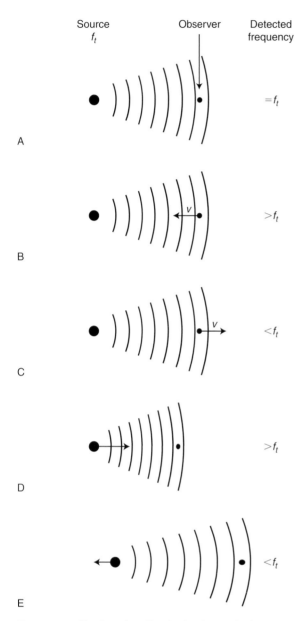

|| Source f_t || Observer || Detected frequency ||

Figure 3.1 The Doppler effect is the change in the observed frequency due to motion between the source and the observer. A: The source of the sound and the observer are both stationary, so the observed sound has the same frequency as that transmitted. B: The source is stationary and the observer is moving toward the source (with velocity v), so that the observer witnesses a higher frequency than that emitted. C: The observer is moving away from the source, so the frequency detected is lower than that emitted. D: The source is moving toward a stationary observer, so the detected frequency is increased. E: The source is moving away from the observer, thus decreasing the frequency observed.

proportional to the relative velocities of the source and the observer.

History behind the discovery of the Doppler effect

This effect was first described by an Austrian physicist named Christian Doppler in 1842. He used the Doppler effect to explain the 'color of double stars'. A rival Dutch scientist working at the same time tried to prove Doppler's theory wrong by hiring a train and two trumpeters. One trumpeter stood on the train while the other stood by the track, and an observer compared the pitch of the trumpeter who passed by on the train with that of the stationary trumpeter. This experiment actually verified Doppler's theory, although Doppler's use of this effect to explain the 'color of double stars' was actually incorrect. The Doppler effect is very important in modern cosmology, as it is used to estimate the velocity of stars, which shows that the universe is expanding.

DOPPLER EFFECT APPLIED TO VASCULAR ULTRASOUND

In the case of vascular ultrasound, the Doppler effect is used to study blood flow. The simplest Doppler ultrasound instruments use transducers consisting of two piezoelectric elements, one to transmit ultrasound beams and the other to receive the returning echoes back-scattered from the moving blood cells (Fig. 3.2). In this situation, the Doppler effect occurs twice. First, the transducer is a stationary source while the blood cells are moving receivers of the ultrasound waves (Fig. 3.1B). The ultrasound is then back-scattered from the blood cells, which now act as a moving source, with the transducer acting as a stationary observer (Fig. 3.1D). The Doppler shift observed depends on the frequency of the ultrasound originally transmitted by the transducer and the velocity of the blood cells from which the ultrasound is back-scattered. The observed frequency also depends on the angle from which the movement of the blood is observed (i.e., the angle between the ultrasound beam and the direction of the blood flow). The Doppler shift frequency, f_d (i.e., the difference

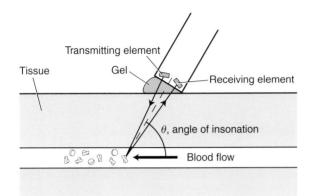

Figure 3.2 Simple Doppler ultrasound instruments use transducers consisting of two piezoelectric elements, one to transmit ultrasound and the other to receive the returning echoes back-scattered from the moving blood cells.

Table 3.1 Variation of the $\cos \theta$ term of the Doppler equation with the angle of insonation

θ (°)	$\cos \theta$
0	1
30	0.87
45	0.71
60	0.5
75	0.26
90	0

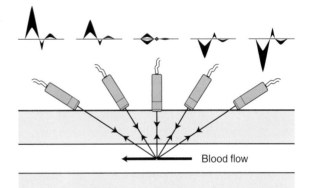

Figure 3.3 The detected Doppler shift frequency changes as the angle of insonation changes.

between the transmitted frequency, f_t, and received frequency, f_r) is given by:

$$f_d = f_r - f_t = \frac{2vf_t \cos \theta}{c} \quad (3.1)$$

where v is the velocity of the blood, θ is the angle between the ultrasound beam and the direction of blood flow (also known as the angle of insonation) and c is the speed of sound in tissue. The factor of 2 is present in the Doppler equation as the Doppler effect has occurred twice, as explained above.

Consider, for example, a 5 MHz transducer used to interrogate a blood vessel with a flow velocity of 50 cm/s using an angle of insonation of 60°. Taking the speed of sound in tissue to be 1540 m/s, the Doppler equation can be used to estimate that the Doppler shift frequency produced will be 1.6 kHz. In fact, it is a useful coincidence that the typical values of blood velocity found in the body and the transmitted frequencies used in medical ultrasound result in Doppler shift frequencies that are in the audible range (from 20 Hz to 20 kHz). The simplest Doppler systems can extract the Doppler shift frequency and output it to a loudspeaker, enabling the operator to listen to the Doppler shifts produced from the blood flow.

The Doppler equation shows that the detected Doppler shift depends on the angle of insonation,

θ, through the term '$\cos \theta$'. Table 3.1 shows how the $\cos \theta$ term varies between 0 and 1 as the angle changes from 0° to 90°. When the angle of insonation is 90°, the $\cos \theta$ term is 0, so virtually no Doppler shift is detected. When the angle of insonation is 0° (i.e., the Doppler beam is parallel to the direction of flow), the $\cos \theta$ term is 1, giving the maximum detectable Doppler shift frequency for a given velocity of blood and transmitted frequency. Figure 3.3 shows how the detected Doppler shift frequencies change as the Doppler angle changes. When the transducer is pointing toward the flow, a positive frequency shift is seen, but once the transducer is pointing away from the direction of flow, a negative frequency shift is seen. The smaller the angle of insonation, the larger the frequency shift detected, but as the angle of insonation approaches a right angle, very small frequency shifts are detected.

Back-scatter from blood

Blood is made up of red blood cells (erythrocytes), white blood cells (leukocytes) and platelets suspended in plasma. Red blood cells occupy between 36% and 54% of the total blood volume. They have a biconcave disc shape and a diameter of $7\,\mu m$, which is much smaller than the wavelength of ultrasound used to study blood flow. This means that groups of red blood cells act as scatterers of the ultrasound (see Fig. 2.8).

The back-scattered signal from blood received at the transducer is small, partly due to the back-scattered energy being radiated in all directions, unlike specular reflections, and partly because the effective cross-section of the blood cells is small compared with the width of the beam. The back-scattered power is proportional to the fourth power of the frequency (i.e., f^4), and therefore as the transmitted frequency selected to detect flow is increased, there is an increase in back-scattered power. However, this is offset by the increase in attenuation of the overlying tissue with the increase in frequency. Ultrasound systems will often use a lower transmitted frequency for Doppler than for B-mode imaging, and the imaging and Doppler transmitted frequencies are usually indicated on the image. In situations in which blood velocity is low or blood cells are stationary, such as aneurysms or venous flow, the cells may aggregate into clumps, which can sometimes produce sufficiently high-amplitude back-scattered echoes to be displayed on the B-mode image (see Fig. 12.19).

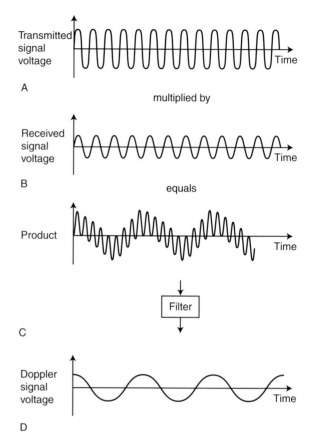

Figure 3.4 Demodulation. This is used to extract the Doppler frequency, in this case by multiplying the transmitted signal (A) by the received signal (B) and filtering out the high-frequency component (C) to leave the Doppler signal (D). (After Fish 1990, with permission.)

EXTRACTING THE DOPPLER SIGNAL

The simplest Doppler systems consist of a transducer with two piezoelectric elements (Fig. 3.2), one continuously transmitting ultrasound and the other continuously receiving back-scattered signals from both stationary tissue and flowing blood. This received signal therefore consists of both the transmitted frequency reflected by stationary objects and the Doppler-shifted frequencies back-scattered from moving blood cells. As the returning echoes are of low amplitude, first they must be amplified. The Doppler shift frequency can then be extracted from the received signal by a process known as demodulation. One method of demodulation used in Doppler systems is shown in Figure 3.4. Here, the received signal is multiplied by the transmitted signal and the product is filtered to remove the high frequencies, thus providing the Doppler shift frequency. The received signal has a different frequency from the transmitted frequency, owing to the Doppler effect, and a lower amplitude, owing to attenuation of the signal by overlying tissue. As mentioned earlier, once the Doppler shift frequency has been extracted (by demodulation) and amplified, it can simply be output to a loudspeaker or investigated using a spectrum analyzer (Fig. 3.5). With experience, it is possible for the operator to recognize the different sounds produced by normal and diseased vessels.

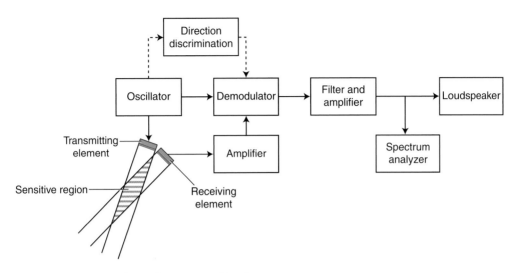

Figure 3.5   Elements of a simple continuous wave Doppler system.

The instruments described so far will not give information about the direction of flow relative to the transducer. This information is available in the returning signal, as objects moving toward the transducer will produce an increase in the detected frequency, while those moving away will produce a decrease in the detected frequency. Extracting directional information from the received Doppler signal requires more sophisticated electronics or software and this will not be explained in this textbook. When the flow directions have been separated, stereo loudspeakers can be used with one channel for forward flow and the other for reverse.

It is preferable to display both the forward and reverse Doppler signals simultaneously on the same spectrum. This is done by displaying the signals either side of a baseline, with flow toward the transducer displayed above the baseline and flow away from the transducer displayed below. Figure 3.6A shows the flow in the vertebral artery and vein displayed in different directions on the spectrum. Most Doppler systems allow the operator to invert this display, if desired, so that the flow away from the transducer can be displayed above the baseline, and it is important that the operator be aware that this has been done in order to correctly interpret any results. The fact that the display is inverted is usually indicated on the screen (Fig. 3.6B). The baseline can also be shifted up and down to make maximum use of the spectral display (Fig. 3.6C).

As well as obtaining Doppler shift frequencies from the flowing blood, the slow moving vessel walls act as large reflective surfaces, producing large-amplitude, low-frequency Doppler shift signals along with the low-amplitude high frequencies obtained from blood. These signals are known as wall thump, due to their sound, and are removed by high-pass filters. The high-pass filter will remove any signals with a frequency below the cutoff frequency of the filter, and this can be controlled by the operator. If this is set too low, the wall thump signal (Fig. 3.7A) will not be removed, whereas if it is set too high, important Doppler information will be removed, possibly altering the waveform shape (Fig. 3.7C) (e.g., by suggesting the absence of diastolic flow). The ideal filter setting (Fig. 3.7B) should remove unwanted signals such as wall thump without removing important blood flow information.

ANALYSIS OF THE DOPPLER SIGNAL

The Doppler signal can be investigated using spectral analysis, allowing waveforms to be displayed (as seen in Fig. 3.6) and blood velocity to be measured. The blood cells flowing through a vessel will be moving at different velocities within the vessel; for example, cells near the vessel wall will be moving more slowly than those in the center (see Ch. 5).

Figure 3.6 The use of an offset, or baseline, allows both forward and reverse flows to be displayed on the same spectrum (A), which can be inverted if required (B). The baseline can be altered to make maximum use of the spectral display (C). The values of the transmitted imaging and Doppler frequencies are often displayed on the screen.

The velocity of the blood cells will vary with time, owing to the pulsatile nature of arterial blood flow. This means that the Doppler shift signal obtained from flowing blood will contain a range of frequencies, due to the range of velocities present, and the frequency content will vary with time. It has already been explained in Chapter 2 (Figs 2.3 and 2.4) how a signal is made up of sine waves of different frequencies. Spectral analysis can be used to break down the Doppler signal into its component frequencies and to show how these component frequencies vary with time. Figure 3.8 shows how a spectrum is displayed, with time along the horizontal axis and the Doppler shift frequency along the vertical axis. The third axis, the brightness of the display, shows the back-scattered power of the signal at each frequency (i.e., the proportion of the blood cells moving at a particular velocity). Spectral analysis is carried out by computer using mathematical techniques such as the

A Wall thump

B

C

Figure 3.7   A: Wall thump gives a low-frequency, high-amplitude signal. B: A filter can be used to remove wall thump from the Doppler signal, but if the filter cut-off frequency is set too high (as in C), this can alter the appearance of the waveform.

fast Fourier transform (FFT). Figure 3.6C shows a typical spectral display produced by a Doppler system. In this case, each vertical line of data is produced every 5–10 ms (i.e., 100–200 lines of data per second).

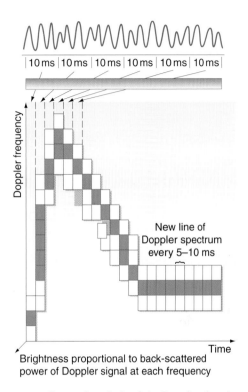

Figure 3.8   Spectral analysis of the Doppler signal enables the frequencies present within the signal to be displayed as consecutive spectra. This produces a display of the changes in blood velocity over time.

Continuous wave (CW) Doppler

Continuous wave (CW) Doppler continuously emits a single frequency while the receiving element continuously detects any echoes from the sensitive region of the beam (i.e., where transmitted and received beams overlap) (shaded region in Fig. 3.5). This region usually covers a depth of a few centimeters, and any flow within this area will be detected. This means that CW Doppler is unable to provide information about the depth from which the Doppler signal is returning. CW Doppler is therefore said to have poor range resolution. Veins often lie adjacent to arteries and so, in many cases, the CW Doppler will simultaneously detect arterial and venous flow.

Pulsed Doppler

The poor range resolution of CW Doppler can be overcome by using a pulse of ultrasound energy

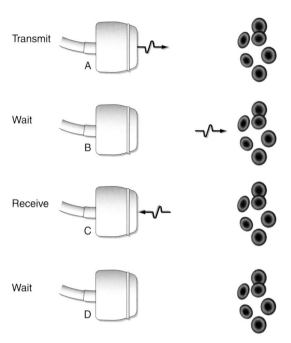

Figure 3.9   Pulsed Doppler ultrasound. The system transmits a pulse (A), waits for a specified time (B) and then only receives from a given depth (C); it waits again, with the receiver off (D), for all the echoes to return from greater depths before transmitting the next pulse.

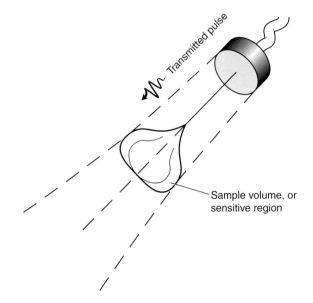

Figure 3.10   The sample volume, or sensitive region, of a single element pulsed Doppler system is shaped like a teardrop.

and only acquiring the returning signal at a known time after the pulse has been transmitted. Thus, by knowing the speed of sound in tissue, the depth from which the signal has returned can be calculated, in the same way as described for pulsed echo imaging (equation 2.3). As the piezoelectric element is only emitting ultrasound for a short period of time, it is possible to use the same element to receive the returning signal. Figure 3.9 shows how the pulse of ultrasound is transmitted and how the receiver then waits a given time before acquiring the signal over a short period of time. Although the system acquires no further signals, it has to wait for the echoes from greater depths to return before sending the next pulse. The time during which the received signal is acquired is known as the range gate, and this can be altered by the operator in order to determine the sample volume size. The sample volume is the region from which returning signals can be detected. Its size depends not only

on the size of the range gate but also on the shape of the transmitted pulse and the shape of the ultrasound beam; it is sometimes described as being teardrop-shaped (Fig. 3.10). The depth of the sample volume is determined by the time the electronic circuit waits before acquiring the signal, which also is controlled by the operator. The size of the sample volume has a significant effect on the Doppler spectrum produced. For example, a large sample volume is required if the operator wishes to record both the fast-moving blood in the center of the vessel and the slower moving blood near the walls. This is discussed further in Chapter 6.

In order to measure the frequencies present in the blood flow, thousands of pulses are sent along the beam path per second. The frequency at which these pulses are sent is known as the pulse repetition frequency (PRF) and is in the kHz range. The upper limit of the PRF is given by the constraint that the system has to wait for all the returning echoes from the last pulse before transmitting the next one. In fact, the pulsed Doppler method, unlike CW systems, does not actually measure the Doppler shift. However, the shape of the detected signal is similar to the Doppler shift that would be obtained from a CW system, so it can be described

Imaging frequency
band width
Doppler frequency
Sample volume size
Sample volume depth

Figure 3.11   The path of the Doppler ultrasound beam, sample volume size and position are displayed on the image.

A

B   45 min later

C   90 min later

D   135 min later

Figure 3.12   Aliasing. If the speed of a minute hand is observed once every 45 minutes, the hand will appear to be moving slowly anticlockwise.

by the Doppler equation and is typically referred to as the Doppler signal. The ultrasound pulses enable the changing velocity of the blood to be sampled, and the resulting signal can be analyzed to obtain a frequency spectrum using an FFT. The FFT requires either 64 or 128 consecutive pulses to produce one line of the spectrum, and Doppler systems are able to process these data fast enough to produce real-time Doppler spectra.

The path of the Doppler beam and the size and position of the sample volume are displayed on the pulse echo image. The values of the PRF, sample volume size and depth are usually displayed at the side of the image, as shown in Figure 3.11. Pulsed Doppler is able to provide good range resolution, but the disadvantage is that pulsed Doppler suffers from an artifact, known as aliasing, that puts an upper limit on the maximum frequency that can be detected.

Aliasing

Aliasing is the incorrect estimation of the frequency of a signal due to insufficient sampling of the signal. Imagine that you have a clock with only a minute hand and you wish to estimate the speed at which the hand is moving. If you look at the face every 45 min (Fig. 3.12), starting on the hour, first the hand would point at 12, then, 45 min later, it would point at 9, then at 6, at 3 and at 12 again. This would give the impression that the hand was travelling slowly anticlockwise. The speed of the hand would appear to be one complete revolution every 3 hours rather than as expected, once an hour. In order to correctly estimate the speed of the hand, the clock would have to be viewed at least twice in a complete cycle (i.e., at least twice an hour).

Figure 3.13 shows how the frequency of a simple sine wave, indicated by the solid line, can be underestimated when the signal is sampled less than twice in a complete cycle. If the dots (•) represent the points at which the signal is sampled, then the lowest frequency sine wave that would fit the sampled data is that shown by the dashed line. If, instead, the signal is sampled at least twice in a complete cycle, shown by the crosses (×), it is no longer possible to fit a lower frequency sine wave to the sampled data and the correct frequency is measured. Aliasing occurs when the sampling frequency is less than twice the frequency to be estimated, a limit known as the Nyquist frequency.

An example of aliasing of a Doppler signal can be seen in Figure 3.14A, where the frequency detected at peak systole is underestimated and displayed below the baseline of the spectrum. Aliasing can be overcome by increasing the sampling rate (i.e., increasing the PRF in this case from 2500 [Fig. 3.14A] to 3704 Hz [Fig. 3.14B]). There is, however, an upper limit to the PRF that can be

Figure 3.13   Aliasing. The frequency of a simple sine wave (solid line) can be underestimated (dashed line) when the signal is sampled less than twice in a complete cycle.

used, as the system has to wait for each pulse to return before the next pulse can be transmitted, in order to prevent confusion as to where a returning signal has originated. Therefore, there is also a limit to the maximum Doppler shift frequency that can be detected. This limits the maximum detectable Doppler frequency (f_{dmax}) and velocity (V_{max}) as follows:

$$f_{dmax} = \frac{PRF_{max}}{2} = \frac{2V_{max}f_t \cos\theta}{c} \quad (3.2)$$

This can be rewritten as

$$V_{max} = \frac{PRF_{max}c}{4f_t \cos\theta} \quad (3.3)$$

For a depth of interest, d, and speed of sound, c,

$$PRF_{max} = \frac{c}{2d} \quad (3.4)$$

The 2, in the equation above, arises from the fact that the pulse has to go to and return from the target. This gives

$$V_{max} = \frac{c^2}{8df_t \cos\theta} \quad (3.5)$$

The maximum velocity that can be detected without aliasing therefore depends on the depth of the vessel. When measuring very high blood flow

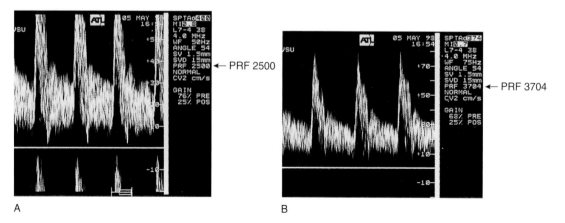

Figure 3.14   A: Aliasing leads to the high frequencies within the signal being underestimated and displayed below the baseline of the spectrum. B: Aliasing can be overcome by increasing the PRF.

velocities, especially at depth, some scanners will allow a 'high PRF' mode to be selected. This allows more than one pulse to be 'in flight' at a given time. The higher PRF allows higher velocities to be measured, but it also introduces range ambiguity (i.e., a loss of certainty as to the origin of the Doppler signal). In this mode, the scanner will typically show more than one sample volume displayed on the scan line. Using a lower transmitted frequency would produce a lower Doppler shift frequency. This lower frequency would not require as high a PRF to prevent aliasing. Therefore, reducing the transmit frequency would increase the maximum velocity that could be measured.

Limitations of CW versus pulsed Doppler

CW Doppler and pulsed Doppler have different limitations. There is no upper limit to the velocity of blood that can be detected by CW Doppler, but no information is available regarding the depth of the origin of the signal, and it is not always possible to detect arterial flow without the venous flow from a nearby vein also being detected. CW is most commonly used in simple hand-held systems to listen to blood flow, enabling ankle blood pressures to be measured (see Ch. 9) or for fetal heart detection. It can also be used in cardiology to allow high velocities to be measured through the heart valves. Pulsed Doppler provides information regarding the origin of the signal, enabling detailed studies of a specific vessel; however, this restricts the maximum velocity that can be detected. Pulsed Doppler is used in duplex systems for both spectral Doppler and color flow imaging.

DUPLEX ULTRASOUND

Duplex ultrasound systems, combining pulse echo imaging with Doppler ultrasound, have been commercially available for about 25 years. Combining the pulse echo imaging with Doppler ultrasound allows interrogation of a vessel in a known location and permits close investigation of the hemodynamics around areas of atheroma visualized on the image. Ideally, to produce a good image of a vessel wall, the vessel should be at right angles to the ultrasound beam. This is the case in the majority of peripheral vessels, as they mainly lie parallel to the skin. However, the Doppler equation shows that no Doppler signal will be obtained when the angle of insonation is at right angles to the direction of flow (as $\cos \theta = 0$). The greatest Doppler shift is detected when the beam is parallel to the direction of flow. Therefore, there is a conflict between the ideal angle of the beam used for imaging and that used for Doppler recordings. A compromise would involve the ability to steer or angle the Doppler beam independently of the imaging beam. Some early duplex systems did this by mounting a separate Doppler element, with an adjustable angle, next to the imaging element. Modern linear array and phased array transducers overcome this by producing a steered beam, as described in Chapter 2 (see Fig. 2.15). The transducer elements are most sensitive to the returning signals that are at right angles to the front face of the element. This means that, as the beam is steered, the sensitivity of the Doppler transducer will fall to some extent, and therefore the Doppler beam can only be steered by about 20° left and right of center. There is thus a compromise between the choice of Doppler angle and sensitivity.

Velocity measurements using duplex ultrasound

An important consequence of duplex ultrasound is that it allows the image of the vessel to be used to estimate the angle of insonation between the Doppler beam and the vessel. This enables the detected Doppler frequency to be converted into a velocity measurement using the Doppler equation (equation 3.1). Figure 3.11 demonstrates how the image of a vessel can be used to line up an angle correction cursor (which sits in the center of the sample volume display) with the vessel wall, so giving the angle of insonation. Very large errors in velocity measurement can be generated by incorrect alignment of the angle correction cursor. Although there are many potential sources of errors when using Doppler ultrasound to calculate blood flow velocity (see Ch. 6), it is a powerful technique for detecting and quantifying the degree of disease present in a vessel.

Reference

Fish P 1990 Physics and instrumentation of diagnostic
medical ultrasound. Wiley, Chichester

Further reading

Evans D H, McDicken W N 2000 Doppler ultrasound:
physics, instrumentation and signal processing.
Wiley, Chichester

Zagzebski J A 1996 Essentials of ultrasound physics.
Mosby, St Louis

Chapter 4

Creation of a color flow image

CHAPTER CONTENTS

Introduction 35
Collection of 2D Doppler information 35
Methods of estimating the velocity
    of blood 36
Elements of a color flow scanner 37
    Blood–tissue discrimination 38
    Color coding the Doppler information 38
Effect of angle of insonation on the color
    flow image 39
Aliasing in color flow imaging 41
Lower and upper limits to the velocity
    displayed 42
Frame rate 43
Resolution and sensitivity of color flow
    imaging 44
Power Doppler imaging 45
Enhanced flow imaging using contrast agents
    and harmonic imaging 46

INTRODUCTION

Ultrasound scanners also use the Doppler effect to form a color map of blood flow superimposed onto the anatomical map provided by pulse echo imaging. This map provides a means for rapid interrogation of a region of interest (ROI) and enables the operator to be selective in the points from which to obtain spectral Doppler information. The development of color flow imaging has greatly extended the capabilities of imaging small vessels and has also allowed for a reduction in investigation time, dramatically increasing the role of vascular ultrasound. The first real-time color flow images were produced in 1985 and were only possible due to the use of different mathematical methods to extract the mean velocity of flow relative to the beam (mean Doppler frequency). This made collection and analysis of the Doppler frequency information fast enough to enable the production of color flow maps capable of displaying pulsatile blood flow in real time.

COLLECTION OF 2D DOPPLER INFORMATION

The two-dimensional (2D) color flow map is created by detecting the back-scattered signals from hundreds of sample volumes along each scan line and using hundreds of scan lines to cover the ROI, as shown in Figure 4.1. The scanner divides the back-scattered signal into hundreds of samples along the scan line, each sample being at a different time delay after the transmitted pulse, and therefore returning

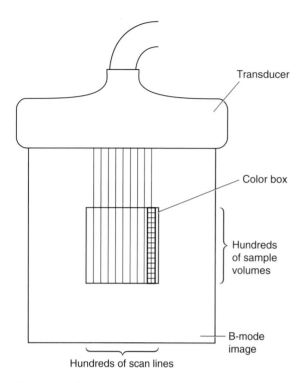

Figure 4.1   The color flow image is created by detecting the back-scattered ultrasound from hundreds of sample volumes along hundreds of different scan lines.

Figure 4.2   The color flow image displays the mean velocity of the flow relative to the ultrasound beam (equivalent to Doppler frequency) detected within each sample volume. This image of an artery, A, overlying a vein, V, demonstrates the difference in the velocity and direction of the blood flow in the two vessels. In this image, the color scale shows that flow in the artery is toward the transducer and is displayed as red, whereas flow in the vein is away from the transducer and is displayed as blue.

from a slightly different depth in the tissue. The depth from which a signal has returned can be calculated from this time delay, using the speed of sound in tissue, in the same way as is used in pulse echo imaging. Several pulses must be transmitted and received along the scan line for the movement of the blood to be detected. Once sufficient samples have been detected from each sample volume to allow estimation of the blood velocity relative to the beam, a second scan line adjacent to the first can be produced. Hundreds of scan lines may be used to produce the 2D color flow image. The estimated mean relative velocity (equivalent to the Doppler frequency) from each sample volume within the tissue can be displayed in color, as shown in Figure 4.2. In this image of an artery lying next to a vein, the Doppler shift frequencies produced by flow toward the transducer are displayed in red, and those produced by flow away from the transducer are shown in blue. The higher relative velocities are shown as yellow and turquoise, whereas the lower relative velocities are displayed as deep red and deep blue.

METHODS OF ESTIMATING THE VELOCITY OF BLOOD

Spectral Doppler ultrasound uses fast Fourier transform (FFT) to provide detailed information on the frequency content of the Doppler signal. However, the time needed to collect sufficient data to perform an FFT on the signals obtained from several scan lines would be so great that it would take several seconds to produce each color image. This would not be a suitable method for imaging pulsatile blood flow. The FFT would also produce more information than could be easily displayed on the image, as each color pixel can only represent one value of frequency at any point in the color image, unlike the range of frequencies that can be displayed on the spectral display. Real-time color flow imaging has been made possible by the use of alternative techniques to estimate the mean velocity of blood relative to the beam. It requires only a few pulses to estimate the mean relative velocity, making the process faster to perform. The method used relies on the facts that the ultrasound is back-scattered from groups of blood cells that remain in the same formation during the time taken to perform the velocity estimate and that the echo intensity pattern is different for different groups of cells. This allows a group of cells to be tracked as it moves through the sample volume. The velocity of

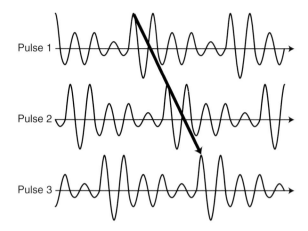

Figure 4.3 Signals from three consecutive pulses returning from a given group of cells as they move farther away from the transducer. Note the short delay introduced. (After Ferrara & DeAngelis 1997, with permission.)

the group of cells does not change significantly during the short time over which the blood flow velocity is being estimated. Figure 4.3 shows the shapes of three consecutive returning pulses as a group of blood cells passes through the sample volume. A short delay is introduced into the signal returning from a given group of cells as they move farther away from the transducer between pulses. An estimate of the velocity can be made by detecting this delay in the echo complex. This shift in the waveform can be understood in two ways. First, it can be considered as a time delay introduced between returning pulses as the group of cells moves. Second, it can be considered as a phase shift of the signal between two pulses scattered from the same sample volume. To understand the concept of a phase shift, consider an example using two clocks. If both the clocks are set to read the same time, both minute hands will be moving at the same speed, giving a frequency of one complete revolution of the clock face an hour. Both clocks will also be in phase with each other (i.e., the minute hand will appear at the '12' on both clocks at the same time), giving a phase shift of zero. If, however, one clock has the minute hand set 30 min behind the other, the minute hands will still complete one revolution of the clock face an hour, but the two clocks will now be out of phase and the clock hands will

appear at different places on the clock face. The time delay between the two clocks will be 30 min, or alternatively this delay could be measured as a phase shift, which in this case would be half a cycle of the clock face.

The delay between the returning ultrasound signals from the first and second pulses shown in Figure 4.3 can be measured in terms of a phase shift. We can see that the second signal is the same shape as the first but is delayed. This is analogous to the clock hands travelling at the same speed but with the second clock being half a cycle behind the first. A similar phase shift can be measured between signals 2 and 3. These phase shifts can be used to estimate the velocity of the blood. This method does not actually measure the Doppler shift frequency; however, the shape of the detected signal is similar to the Doppler shift that would be obtained from a continuous wave system and therefore can be described by the Doppler equation.

Modern color flow imaging scanners use the phase shift approach, employing a process known as autocorrelation detection to estimate the mean Doppler shift frequency. Autocorrelation compares two consecutive pulses returning from a given sample volume to produce an output that is dependent on the phase shift (i.e., dependent on the Doppler frequency). If the echoes are returning from stationary objects there will be no phase shift. The phase shifts between four or more pulses are used to estimate the frequency. The more pulses used, the more accurate is the result, as long as the time taken is not so great that the velocity of the blood cells has changed. This relatively small number of pulses required to estimate the mean relative velocity (Doppler shift frequency) enables several color images to be produced every second.

Another method, not currently used by ultrasound manufacturers, uses time-domain processing, which employs time delay rather than phase shift to estimate the velocity of blood. From the operator's perspective, both the frequency and time-domain processes produce similar color images.

ELEMENTS OF A COLOR FLOW SCANNER

Figure 4.4 shows the basic elements of a color flow scanner. Before any analysis of the returning

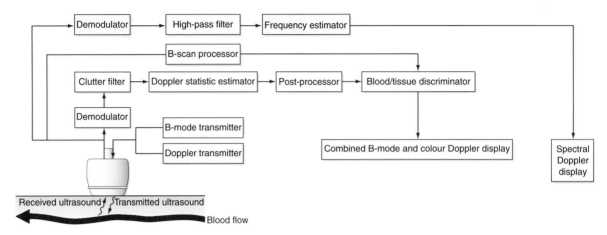

Figure 4.4   The basic elements of a color flow scanner.

echoes is carried out, the signal is filtered by the clutter filter to remove the high-amplitude signals returning from the surrounding stationary tissue and the slow moving vessel walls, while preserving the low-amplitude signals from the blood. The filtered signal is then analyzed to obtain an estimate of the mean relative velocity (Doppler shift frequency) in each sample volume, by the Doppler statistic estimator, as described earlier. Post-processing is then used to smooth the data in order to produce a less noisy color image. This can be done by combining the data obtained from consecutive images, known as frame-averaging. As each point on the image can only be assigned either a specific color or level of gray, a decision has to be made as to whether to display the pulse echo information or any flow information detected. This involves the process known as blood–tissue discrimination.

Blood–tissue discrimination

Generally, the returning pulse echo signals from the vessel lumen are very low in amplitude compared with those from the vessel walls and surrounding tissue. In addition, larger Doppler frequencies are detected from the rapidly moving blood in comparison to the low Doppler frequencies obtained from the slow moving vessel walls. No Doppler shift would be detected from stationary surrounding tissue. Ultrasound imaging systems are designed with an adjustable control called the 'color write enable' or 'color write priority' control. This control allows the operator to select the imaging signal

intensity above which the gray-scale image is displayed rather than the color information. If a Doppler signal is obtained from an area in which the gray-scale signal is higher than the level set by the operator, the scanner assumes that the Doppler signal results from moving tissue and therefore does not display it. Below this level of gray, providing there is an adequate Doppler shift frequency, it is assumed that any Doppler signal originates from blood, and color will overwrite the gray-scale in areas where a Doppler signal is detected. If, for instance, the operator wishes to demonstrate flow in a small vessel that does not have an anechoic (echo-free) lumen on the image, the threshold for displaying gray-scale information will need to be increased, thus giving priority to writing color information.

Most systems also have a flash filter. This is designed to remove color flashes, known as flash artifacts, that are generated by rapid movement between the transducer and tissue, such as when the sonographer moves the transducer during scanning.

Color coding the Doppler information

Having obtained a value of the mean Doppler frequency present in the multiple sample volumes, these data now have to be displayed on the image. This is done by color-coding the Doppler information. The color on the screen has three attributes: luminosity, hue and saturation. Luminosity is the degree of brightness or shade of the displayed color; hue is the wavelength (i.e., the actual color displayed, from violet through red), and saturation

Figure 4.5   A, B, C, D: Examples of different color scales, used to accentuate different parts of the range of velocities detected in various clinical situations. E: The inversion of the color scale shows that the image will now display flow toward the transducer as blue. The arrows on D and E show how the scanner displays the color write priority selected. The setting selected in D will display color in the presence of a brighter B-mode echo than the setting selected in E.

is the degree to which the color is mixed with white light (e.g., from red through light pink, producing up to 20 identifiable tints). These three attributes can be used to produce a variety of color scales, as shown in Figure 4.5, which can be displayed as a bar at the side of the image. The scale usually consists of a different color representing different flow directions, with red often used to show flow toward the transducer and blue depicting flow away from the transducer. Most scanners allow the operator to invert the color scale in order to display flow toward the transducer as blue and flow away as red. This is indicated by inverting the color scale displayed at the side of the image (Fig. 4.5E). It is essential for the operator to be aware of which colors represent which directions of flow within the image, otherwise serious diagnostic errors can occur. Ultrasound scanners provide a range of color scales, and certain scales are more appropriate in particular imaging situations. The various color scales may be selected to accentuate the different parts of the range of detected relative velocities seen in different clinical situations. For example, in an arterial scan, the color scale may accentuate the differences in the upper portion to highlight velocity changes in the higher range of velocities.

The velocity estimator can calculate not only the mean relative velocity but also the variance. The variance is a measure of the range of velocities present within the sample volume and may relate to the presence of a flow disturbance. The variance can be displayed along with the mean frequency by using a red and blue scale with increasing amounts of yellow or green introduced as the variance increases, although this form of display is not widely used. Another form of color display uses increasing luminosity of orange to display the increasing backscattered power detected. This is known as power Doppler and is discussed later in this chapter.

EFFECT OF ANGLE OF INSONATION ON THE COLOR FLOW IMAGE

As the colors used to display the flow depend on the Doppler frequencies detected, which in turn depend on the angle of insonation between the blood flow and the color Doppler beam, the appearance of the color image is very much dependent on the angle of insonation. Many of the peripheral vessels run parallel to the skin, perpendicular to the imaging beam. However, the color Doppler beam should ideally be less than 70° in order to obtain a Doppler signal. If the angle of insonation is near 90°, only a small Doppler shift will be detected; this will be removed by the high-pass filter, known as the clutter filter, and no signal will be displayed on the image.

When using a linear array transducer, it is possible to steer the beam, used to create the color image, from left or right as described in Chapter 2 (see Fig. 2.15). The direction of the color Doppler beam runs parallel to the sides of the color box displayed on the image. Figure 4.6 demonstrates the change in the color image seen when the color box is steered in three different directions relative to the flow. The beam can only be steered either left or right by a maximum of 20–25° because the sensitivity of the transducer decreases as the beam is steered. There is thus a compromise between optimizing the angle of insonation and maintaining the sensitivity. This is not usually apparent when imaging large vessels with good flow but can become a problem when imaging smaller diseased vessels with low flow, as the intensity of the Doppler signal may be very low and the vessel may have to be insonated at an angle above 70° to maintain transducer sensitivity. If demonstrating color filling of such a vessel proves difficult, it is worth changing the angle of insonation of the color beam to obtain the optimum compromise between the angle of insonation and sensitivity.

When imaging tortuous vessels, it is useful to obtain images with the color box steered in different directions to visualize the blood flow along the entire vessel. If the direction of the blood flow changes in relation to the Doppler beam, a different Doppler frequency will be detected even though the blood velocity is the same. The color image will demonstrate a change of color within the vessel as the path of the vessel alters direction. Figure 4.7 shows an image of an internal carotid artery as its path dips deep into the neck. The arrows on the image show how the blood flow changes direction relative to the color Doppler beam, causing a change in the Doppler frequency detected. This leads to a change in the color displayed, from red to orange and yellow then finally turquoise,

due to aliasing, even though the velocity of the blood within the vessel has remained unchanged.

Curvilinear and phased array transducers produce scan lines that fan out over the sector image. These probes do not usually have the facility to steer the Doppler beam along a path independently of the direction of the imaging scan lines. If a straight vessel is imaged with a curvilinear or phased array transducer, there will be a change in the angle of insonation along the vessel, unless the vessel is parallel to the Doppler beam. This will lead to a change in the Doppler frequencies detected and therefore will affect the color displayed on the image, as shown in Figure 4.8. On the left of the image, Doppler shift frequencies are detected, as there is a suitable angle of insonation and flow is

A   B   C

Figure 4.6 Effect of changing the angle of insonation (shown on the image), by steering the color box, on the image produced. A: A small angle gives a good image. B: A moderate angle displays flow but is not optimal. C: A large angle gives an unusable image.

Figure 4.7 An internal carotid artery as it dips deep in the neck. As the path of the artery changes relative to the Doppler beam (shown by the arrow), the relative velocity (Doppler frequency) detected will alter, leading to a change in the color displayed, despite the fact that the velocity of the blood flow has not changed.

Figure 4.8 As the scan lines of a curvilinear transducer diverge, the angle between the straight vessel and the beam will change. This will lead to a change in the detected velocity relative to the ultrasound beam (Doppler frequency), altering the color displayed. No flow is displayed in the center of the image, where the flow is at right angles to the beam.

toward the probe. In the very center, the angle of insonation is approximately 90°, so low or no Doppler frequency is detected or displayed. On the right side of the image, the angle of insonation is now such that the flow is away from the transducer, and it is therefore displayed in red.

When interpreting a color image, it is important to remember that it is the Doppler shift frequency (the velocity relative to the beam) that is being displayed, and it is essential to consider the angle of insonation used to produce each point of the image. To be certain of the velocities present, spectral Doppler can be used as this has the facility to provide angle correction for velocity estimates. Diagnosis should be made using a combination of color and spectral Doppler investigations.

ALIASING IN COLOR FLOW IMAGING

The range of frequencies displayed by the color scale is governed by the pulse repetition frequency (PRF) used to obtain the Doppler frequency shift. The maximum frequency that can be detected with color flow imaging is limited by the sampling frequency in the same way as described for spectral Doppler (see Ch. 3). Aliasing due to undersampling will limit the maximum frequency that can be displayed correctly, causing frequencies beyond this limit to be displayed as flow on the opposite side of the baseline. An example of aliasing occurring in a color image is shown in Figure 4.9A. The highest velocities present are in the center of the vessel, but because of aliasing, these are displayed as turquoise (i.e., as high velocities in the opposite direction)

instead of yellow (i.e., top of the color scale). If the PRF is increased, aliasing no longer occurs, and all the flow is displayed in the correct color (Fig. 4.9B). If the PRF is set too high, however, it may prevent low velocities, such as those near the vessel walls or during diastole, from being detected (Fig. 4.9C). One potential problem is differentiating aliasing from true flow reversal. True flow reversal, shown as a change in color within a vessel (i.e., from red to blue), can be seen where there is both forward and reverse flow present within a vessel due to a hemodynamic effect. Flow reversal is often seen in a normal carotid artery bulb, as described in Chapter 5. Apparent flow reversal can be due to an artifact and occurs when a vessel changes direction relative to the Doppler beam, although flow within the vessel has not changed direction.

Figure 4.10 shows an image of a slightly tortuous carotid artery, with flow away from the transducer on the right (shown in blue) and toward the

Figure 4.10 Image of a bend in a carotid artery showing flow toward and away from the transducer in different colors. The path of the flow is shown by the arrows. No flow is displayed in the center of the image, where the flow is at right angles to the beam.

A   B   C

Figure 4.9 Aliasing. A: This will lead to the assignment of the incorrect color to represent the velocity present within the vessel, shown here in blue. B: Increasing the PRF may overcome aliasing. C: If the PRF is set too high, it may prevent low velocities, present at the vessel walls, from being detected.

transducer on the left (shown in red). The arrows marked on the image show how the direction of flow changes relative to the ultrasound beam. In the center of the image, where the direction of flow is close to being at right angles to the ultrasound beam, low frequencies are detected; these are removed from the signal by the high-pass filter and therefore no color is displayed in this region.

It is possible to distinguish between aliasing and changes in the direction of flow relative to the transducer by the fact that the color transition seen in aliasing wraps around the farthest ends of the color scale. In contrast, the colors displayed when the flow changes direction are near the baseline and pass through black at the point where no or low Doppler shift frequencies have been detected. Figure 4.11 shows an image of a carotid artery that

Figure 4.11 Image demonstrating aliasing (A) and flow reversal (R) in an internal carotid artery. Aliasing can be recognized as a color change that wraps around from the top to the bottom of the color scale, or vice versa. A change in color due to a relative change in the direction of flow can be recognized as a change in color across the baseline, at the center of the color scale, passing through black (see color scale on right of image).

demonstrates both flow reversal and aliasing. The transitions in the colors displayed in both cases are shown on the color scales.

LOWER AND UPPER LIMITS TO THE VELOCITY DISPLAYED

The highest frequency that can be displayed without aliasing occurring is half the PRF, as with spectral Doppler. However, unlike spectral Doppler displays, aliasing does not necessarily make interpreting the image difficult and can sometimes be useful in highlighting sudden increases in velocity, as would be seen at a stenosis. The aliasing artifact can be overcome, up to a limit, by increasing the PRF, using a larger Doppler angle or using a lower ultrasound transmitting frequency.

When investigating low-velocity flow, such as that seen in the venous system, the lower limit of the velocity that can be detected is governed by the length of time spent interrogating the flow. Suppose you wanted to estimate the speed at which the hands of a clock are moving. You would have to watch the clock for a much longer time to estimate the speed of the hour hand than to estimate the speed of the minute hand. The same is true of color Doppler (i.e., the lower the velocity flow that is to be detected, the longer the time that has to be spent measuring it). The length of time over which pulses are sent along a scan line in order to estimate the frequency is known as the dwell time (Fig. 4.12). If a low PRF is selected, the time taken for the eight to ten pulses to be transmitted along the scan line will be longer, and consequently the dwell time will be greater than

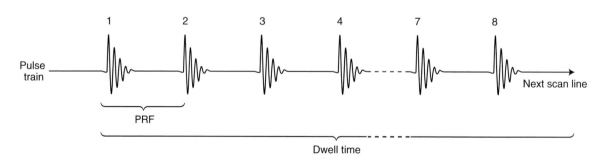

Figure 4.12 The dwell time is the time the beam spends interrogating the blood flow to produce one scan line. This depends on the number of pulses, the ensemble length, used to perform the frequency estimate and the pulse repetition frequency of the signal.

that produced by a higher PRF. It is therefore very important to select the appropriate PRF for the flow conditions to be imaged. If a low PRF is selected to image high-velocity flow, aliasing will occur, and if a high PRF is selected to image low-velocity flow, the flow may not be detected at all, as the dwell time will be too short (Fig. 4.9C). Ideally, a PRF should be selected that displays the highest velocities present with the colors near the top of the scale.

The cut-off frequency of the high-pass clutter filter will also affect the lowest frequencies that can be displayed. The high-pass filter will only allow frequencies greater than the cut-off frequency to be displayed, so that if this is set too high, the Doppler frequencies detected from the lower velocity blood flow will be removed. The level of the high-pass filter is usually displayed on the color scale (Fig. 4.13). Using the wrong filter setting has led to removal of the low velocities at the vessel walls or of low flow during diastole. The high-pass filter is linked to the PRF and therefore, as the PRF is increased, the high-pass filter is also automatically increased. However, some systems will allow the filter to be altered independently of the PRF, in which case the high-pass filter setting should be considered when the PRF is lower in order to image low-velocity flow.

FRAME RATE

The frame rate is the number of new images produced per second. For color flow imaging to be useful for visualizing pulsatile blood flow, a reasonably high frame rate is required. With pulse echo imaging alone, the frame rate can be greater than 50 images per second. However, the time required to produce a color flow image is much longer and therefore the frame rates are much lower. The frame rate is dependent on several factors when using color flow imaging (Fig. 4.14). The ROI refers to the color box, which can be placed anywhere within the image to examine blood flow. The size and position of the ROI have a significant effect on the frame rate. The width is especially important, as the wider the ROI, the more scan lines are required and therefore the longer it will take to collect the data for an image. The line density (the number of scan lines per centimeter across the image) also affects the time taken to produce the image as the pulses for each scan line have to return before the next line can be produced. The length of the color box is less important. This is because the scanner has to wait for all the returning echoes before sending the next pulse, even if the information is not used to produce the image, so as not to suffer from range ambiguity.

The depth of the ROI is, however, an important factor. To image at depth, lower frequency ultrasound is used, which will penetrate farther, allowing the ROI to be set at a greater depth. Therefore, the scanner will have to wait longer for the echoes to return from the greater depth and it will take longer to create each scan line, so reducing the frame rate.

A

B

Figure 4.13 Effect of using the filter. A: The filter is set too high, removing the low–velocity flow near the vessel walls (vertical arrows). B: The filter setting is reduced to display the low frequencies detected near the vessel walls. The filter setting may be displayed on the color scale (horizontal arrows).

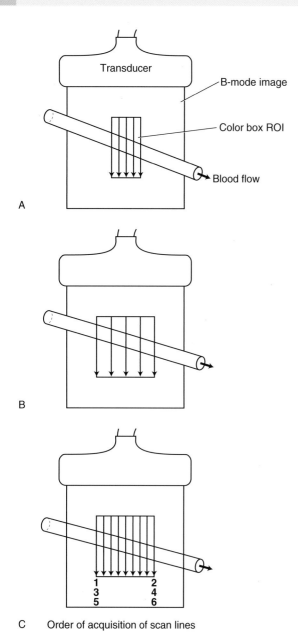

A

B

C   Order of acquisition of scan lines

Figure 4.14 The color image frame rate can be improved by (A) reducing the size of the color region of interest (ROI) or (B) reducing the density of the color scan lines. (C) The scanner may improve the frame rate by interleaving the acquisition of data from different parts of the ROI. (After Ferrara & DeAngelis 1997, with permission.)

Interleaving the acquisition from different scan lines that are a distance apart can enable more than one pulse to be transmitted at a time, allowing an improvement in the frequency estimate without a decrease in the frame rate. Figure 4.14C shows how the data from scan line 2 can be acquired while data from scan line 1 are being obtained, as scan line 1 will not detect pulses transmitted along scan line 2. The same is true for scan lines 3 and 4, and so forth. Extra lines of data can be created by averaging two adjacent lines to produce a scan line between them. As no new information is acquired to perform this, no change in the frame rate occurs.

The number of pulses used to produce each scan line of the color image is known as the ensemble length. Typically, an ensemble length of between 2 and 16 pulses is used to estimate the Doppler frequency. However, the more pulses that are used, the more accurate the estimate will be, and in situations in which the returning Doppler signal is poor, a high number of pulses is required. There is, therefore, a compromise between the accuracy of the frequency estimate and frame rate. The time taken for these 2 to 16 pulses to be transmitted and to return, the dwell time, obviously depends on the rate at which the pulses are transmitted (i.e., the PRF). When a low PRF is used, it will take longer for the pulse ensemble to be transmitted, leading to a lower frame rate.

These various limitations require a compromise to be made between the area over which the color Doppler information is acquired, the accuracy of the Doppler frequency estimate and the time it takes to acquire it. The selection of PRF, position of the ROI and frequency of the transducer are governed by the region of the body being imaged and the type of blood flow in that region. However, it is possible to optimize the frame rate by using as narrow an ROI as possible for the examination. The quality of the color image may be improved by averaging consecutive images, to reduce the noise, and displaying the image for a longer period of time. This control is sometimes known as the persistence.

RESOLUTION AND SENSITIVITY OF COLOR FLOW IMAGING

The spatial resolution of the color image can be considered in three planes, as described for B-mode imaging (see Fig. 2.21). However, as blood flow imaging is dynamic, the temporal resolution (i.e., the ability to display changes that occur during a short period of time) is also an important factor. The axial resolution of the color image is governed by the length of the individual sample volumes along each scan line. The lateral resolution of the color image depends on the width of the beam and the density of the scan lines across the field of view. The ability of the color image to follow the changes in flow over time accurately depends on the system having an adequate frame rate. Imaging arterial flow effectively usually requires a higher frame rate than does demonstrating venous flow, as changes in arterial flow occur much more rapidly.

The sensitivity of an ultrasound system to flow is another indication of the quality of the system and depends on many factors. First, the ultrasound frequency and output power must be appropriately selected to allow adequate penetration. Second, the time spent detecting the flow must be long enough to distinguish blood flow from stationary tissue. The filters used to remove wall thump and other tissue movement must be set so as not to remove signals from blood flow. The resolution and sensitivity of modern color flow systems have rapidly improved over the last decade, improving the range and quality of vascular examinations.

POWER DOPPLER IMAGING

So far, this chapter has described how the Doppler shift frequency can be displayed as a color map superimposed onto the gray-scale image. However, instead of displaying the detected frequency shift, it is possible to display the back-scattered power of the Doppler signal. The color scale used shows increased luminosity with increased back-scattered power. This allows the scanner to display the presence of moving blood, but it does not indicate the relative velocity or direction of flow, as shown in Figure 4.15. This method of display has some advantages in that the power Doppler display is not dependent on the angle of insonation, and it has improved sensitivity compared with conventional Doppler frequency displays. The diagram in Figure 4.16A shows how the beam used to produce the scan lines actually produces a range of angles of insonation within a vessel due to the range of elements used to form the beam. When the center of the beam is at an angle of 90° to the vessel, parts of the beam will actually produce an angle of

Figure 4.15 Power Doppler image of a diseased internal carotid artery, showing a narrow flow channel.

insonation of less than 90°, and the blood flow will be toward part of the beam and away from other parts of the beam. Therefore, the range of frequencies detected will be as shown in Figure 4.16B, with the blood appearing to be travelling both toward the beam (producing a positive Doppler shift) and away from the beam (producing a negative Doppler shift). The mean of this range of Doppler frequency shifts is zero, and therefore no flow would be displayed with a color Doppler frequency map. If, however, the total power (i.e., the area under the curves in Fig. 4.16B) is displayed, this will not be too dissimilar to a signal obtained at a smaller angle of insonation. The display of back-scattered power is therefore practically independent of the angle. As the frequency is not displayed, power Doppler does not suffer from aliasing. The back-scattered power will, however, be affected by the attenuation of the tissue through which the ultrasound has travelled and will be lower for deep-lying vessels than for superficial vessels.

At the vessel walls, where the sample volume may be only partially filled by the vessel, the detected back-scattered power will be lower, and the power Doppler will be displayed by darker pixels than at the center of the vessel. Color Doppler imaging displays the mean frequency detected

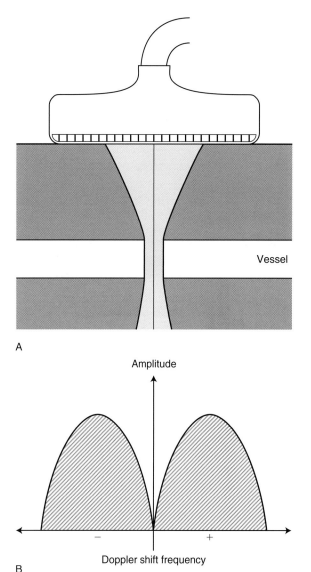

Figure 4.16 A: The beam used to detect the flow actually produces a range of angles of insonation. B: When the beam is at right angles to the blood flow, this will result in both negative and positive Doppler shift frequencies within the signal.

the Doppler signal. If the color gain is increased to visualize the background noise, the operator will see the noise as a speckled pattern of all colors within the color box. This is because the noise generated within the scanner is a low-amplitude signal containing all frequencies. As the noise occurs in all frequencies, this noise is impossible to remove using the high-pass filter. As power Doppler displays power rather than frequency, it is less susceptible to this low-amplitude noise since it is displayed as a darker color or not displayed at all.

The main disadvantage with power Doppler is that in order to improve sensitivity, a high degree of frame-averaging is used, which means that the operator has to keep the transducer still to obtain a good image. Therefore, this modality is less suitable for rapidly scanning along vessels. The lack of angle dependence makes power Doppler useful in imaging tortuous vessels. Power Doppler also provides improved edge definition (e.g., around plaque). Some ultrasound systems provide a color flow display that combines the power Doppler display with directional information. In this mode, the power of the signal is displayed as red for flow detected travelling toward the transducer, and the power of the signal detected from blood moving away from the transducer is displayed as blue. No velocity information is displayed in this mode.

ENHANCED FLOW IMAGING USING CONTRAST AGENTS AND HARMONIC IMAGING

A limiting factor in ultrasound imaging of flow is that the power of the ultrasound back-scattered from blood is much lower than that reflected from the surrounding tissue. Increasing the output power of the scanner will not overcome this problem as it would increase the signal from the surrounding tissue as well as from the blood. The concept behind the use of contrast agents in ultrasound is to introduce a substance into the blood that provides a higher back-scattered power than is available from blood alone. Contrast agents used clinically at present consist of microparticles to which gas microbubbles adhere. It is these microbubbles that provide the increase in back-scattered power. Contrast agents are divided into two types: right heart and left heart agents. Right heart agents are

within a sample volume and therefore does not depend on whether the sample volume is totally or partially filled with the blood flow. Power Doppler is therefore able to provide better definition of the boundaries of the blood flow than color Doppler.

The improved sensitivity of the power Doppler is due to the relationship between the noise and destroyed as they pass through the lungs and, therefore, when injected intravenously, are only suitable for imaging the right side of the heart. Left heart, or transpulmonary, agents can pass through the lungs and can therefore be used to enhance the back-scattered signal from peripheral arteries. These agents effectively enhance the Doppler signal for approximately 5–10 min, so are only really suitable for investigations that do not take longer than this to perform.

Bubbles insonated with ultrasound will oscillate and will back-scatter ultrasound both at the frequency at which they were insonated and at higher frequencies. These higher frequencies are harmonics of the original frequency (i.e., they are multiples of the fundamental frequency) (see Ch. 2). If, for example, a broad-band transducer is used to insonate the contrast agent at a frequency of 3 MHz, the scanner will be able to detect a back-scattered signal from the microbubbles at a frequency of 6 MHz. The surrounding tissue, however, does not oscillate to the same extent and will therefore not produce as big a back-scattered signal at the higher harmonic frequency. The Doppler shift imposed on the harmonic frequency can be extracted and displayed on a color image or as a Doppler spectrum. This technique, known as harmonic imaging, used in conjunction with contrast agents, may improve the sensitivity of Doppler ultrasound. One of the negative aspects of the use of contrast agents is that the ultrasound examination becomes an invasive procedure.

Reference

Ferrara K, DeAngelis G 1997 Color flow mapping. Ultrasound in Medicine and Biology 23(3):321–345

Further reading

Evans D H, McDicken W N 2000 Doppler ultrasound: physics, instrumentation and signal processing. Wiley, Chichester

Hoskins P R, Thrush A, Martin K, Whittingham T (eds) 2003 Diagnostic ultrasound: physics and equipment. Greenwich Medical Media, London

Zagzebski J A 1996 Essentials of ultrasound physics. Mosby, St Louis

Chapter 5

Blood flow and its appearance on color flow imaging

CHAPTER CONTENTS

Introduction 49

Structure of vessel walls 49

Why does blood flow? 50

Resistance to flow 51

Velocity changes within stenoses 52

Flow profiles in normal arteries 53
  Pulsatile flow 54
  Flow at bifurcations and branches 56
  Flow around curves in a vessel 57

Flow through stenoses 58
  Transition from laminar to turbulent
    flow 59

Venous flow 60
  Changes in flow due to the cardiac cycle 60
  Effects of respiration on venous flow 60
  Changes in venous blood pressure due to
    posture and the calf muscle pump 61
  Abnormal venous flow 62

INTRODUCTION

Arterial blood flow is complex and consists of pulsatile flow of an inhomogeneous fluid through viscoelastic arteries that branch, curve and taper. However, a useful understanding of hemodynamics can be gained by first considering simple models, such as steady flow in a rigid tube. Factors affecting venous flow will also be considered. This will allow us to interpret spectral Doppler and color Doppler images of blood flow more easily. However, when interpreting color flow images it is important to remember that the color represents the mean Doppler frequency obtained from the sample volumes and that this will depend on the angle between the ultrasound beam and blood flow. The pulse repetition frequency (PRF) and filter setting used and the length of time over which the image is created may also affect the appearance of the image. Artifactual effects also have to be considered carefully before drawing conclusions about the blood flow.

STRUCTURE OF VESSEL WALLS

The arterial and venous systems are often thought of as a series of tubes that transport blood to and from organs and tissues. In reality, blood vessels are highly complex structures that respond to nervous stimulation and interact with chemicals in the blood stream to regulate the flow of blood throughout the body. Changes in cardiac output and the tone of the smooth muscle cells in the arterial walls are crucial factors that affect blood flow. The structure of a blood vessel wall varies considerably depending on its position within the vascular system.

Arteries and veins are composed of three layers of tissue, with veins having thinner walls than arteries. The outer layer is called the adventitia and is predominantly composed of connective tissue with collagen and elastin. The middle layer, the media, is the thickest layer and is composed of smooth muscle fibers and elastic tissue. The intima is the inner layer and consists of a thin layer of epithelium overlying an elastic membrane. The capillaries, by contrast, consist of a single layer of endothelium, which allows for the exchange of molecules through the capillary wall. It is possible to image the structure of larger vessel walls using ultrasound and to identify the early stages of arterial disease, such as intimal thickening.

The arterial tree consists of elastic arteries, muscular arteries and arterioles. The aorta and subclavian arteries are examples of elastic or conducting arteries and contain elastic fibers and a large amount of collagen fibers to limit the degree of stretch. Elastic arteries function as a pressure reservoir, as the elastic tissue in the vessel wall is able to absorb a proportion of the large amount of energy generated by the heart during systole. This maintains the end diastolic pressure and decreases the load on the left side of the heart. Muscular or distributing arteries, such as the radial artery, contain a large proportion of smooth muscle cells in the media. These arteries are innervated by nerves and can dilate or constrict. The muscular arteries are responsible for regional distribution of blood flow. Arterioles are the smallest arteries, and their media is composed almost entirely of smooth muscle cells. Arterioles have an important role in controlling blood pressure and flow, and they can constrict or dilate after sympathetic nerve or chemical stimulation. The arterioles distribute blood to specific capillary beds and can dilate or constrict selectively around the body depending on the requirements of organs or tissues.

WHY DOES BLOOD FLOW?

Energy created by the contraction of the heart forces blood around the body. Blood flow in the arteries depends on two factors: (1) the energy available to drive the blood flow, and (2) the resistance to flow presented by the vascular system.

A scientist named Daniel Bernoulli (1700–1782) showed that the total fluid energy, which gives rise to the flow, is made up of three parts:

- Pressure energy (p)—this is the pressure in the fluid, which, in the case of blood flow, varies due to the contraction of the heart and the distension of the aorta.
- Kinetic energy (KE)—this is due to the fact that the fluid is a moving mass. KE is dependent on the density (ρ) and velocity (V) of the fluid

$$KE = \frac{1}{2}\rho V^2 \qquad (5.1)$$

- Gravitational potential energy—this is the ability of a volume of blood to do work due to the effect of gravity (g) on the column of fluid with density (ρ) because of its height (h) above a reference point, typically the heart. Gravitational potential energy ($\rho g h$) is equivalent to hydrostatic pressure but has an opposite sign (i.e. $-\rho g h$). For example, when a person is standing, there is a column of blood—the height of the heart above the feet—resting on the blood in the vessels in the foot (Fig. 5.1A) causing a higher pressure, due to the hydrostatic pressure, than that seen when the person is lying down (Fig. 5.1B). As the heart is taken as the reference point, and the feet are below the heart, the hydrostatic pressure is positive. If the arm is raised so that it is above the heart, the hydrostatic pressure is negative, causing the veins to collapse and the pressure in the arteries in the arm to be lower than the pressure at the level of the heart.

The total fluid energy is given by:

Total fluid energy = pressure energy
+ kinetic energy
+ gravitational energy

$$E_{tot} = p + (-\rho g h) + \frac{1}{2}\rho V^2 \qquad (5.2)$$

Figure 5.2 gives a graphical display of how the total energy, kinetic energy and pressure alter with continuous flow through an idealized narrowing. Usually the kinetic energy component of the total energy is small compared with the pressure energy. When fluid flows through a tube with a narrowing, the fluid travels faster as it passes through the narrowed section. As the velocity of the fluid increases in a narrowed portion of the vessel, the kinetic energy increases and the potential energy (i.e., the

Figure 5.1 Schematic diagram showing typical pressures in arteries and veins with the subject standing (A) and lying (B). The component due to hydrostatic pressure when the subject is vertical is shown alongside A.

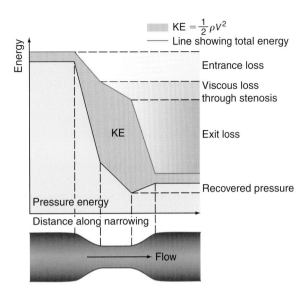

Figure 5.2 Diagram showing how energy losses can occur across a narrowing. (After Oates 2001, with permission.)

pressure) falls. The pressure within the narrowing is therefore lower than the pressure in the portion of the vessel before the narrowing. As the fluid passes beyond the narrowing, the velocity drops again and the kinetic energy is converted back to potential energy (the pressure), which increases. Energy is lost as the fluid passes through the narrowing (Fig. 5.2), with the extent of the entrance and exit losses depending on the geometry and degree of the narrowing (Oates 2001). In normal arteries, very little energy is lost as the blood flows away from the heart toward the limbs and organs, and the mean pressure in the small distal vessels is only slightly lower than in the aorta. However, in the presence of significant arterial disease, energy may be lost from the blood as it passes through tight narrowings or small collateral vessels around occlusions, leading to a drop in the pressure greater than that which would be expected in a normal artery; this can lead to reduced blood flow and tissue perfusion distally. Because the entrance and exit losses account for a large proportion of the pressure loss, it is likely that two adjacent stenoses will have a more significant effect than one long one (Oates 2001).

RESISTANCE TO FLOW

In 1840, a physician named Poiseuille established a relationship between flow, the pressure gradient along a tube and the dimensions of a tube. The relationship can simply be understood as:

$$\text{Pressure drop} = \text{flow} \times \text{resistance} \quad (5.3)$$

where the resistance to flow is given by:

$$R = \frac{\text{viscosity} \times \text{length} \times 8}{\pi \times r^4} \quad (5.4)$$

where r is the radius.

Viscosity causes friction between the moving layers of the fluid. Treacle, for example, is a highly viscous fluid, whereas water has a low viscosity and therefore offers less resistance to flow when travelling through a small tube. Poiseuille's law shows that the resistance to flow is highly dependent on changes in the radius (r^4). In the normal circulation, the greatest proportion of the resistance is thought to occur at the arteriole level. Tissue perfusion is controlled by changes in the diameter of the arterioles. The presence of arterial disease in the arteries, such as stenoses or occlusions, can significantly alter the resistance to flow, with the reduction in vessel diameter having a major effect on the change in resistance seen. In severe disease, the arterioles distal to the disease may become maximally dilated in order to reduce the peripheral resistance, thus increasing blood flow in an attempt to maintain tissue perfusion. Poiseuille described nonpulsatile flow in a rigid tube, so his equation does not completely represent arterial blood flow; however, it gives us some understanding of the relationship between pressure drop, resistance and flow.

VELOCITY CHANGES WITHIN STENOSES

We have already seen that fluid travels faster through a narrowed section of tube. The theory to determine these changes in velocity is described below. The volume flow through the tube is given by:

Flow = velocity of the fluid × cross-sectional area

$$Q = V \times A \qquad (5.5)$$

where V is the mean velocity across the whole of the vessel, averaged over time, and A is the cross-sectional area of the tube. If the tube has no outlets or branches through which fluid can be lost, the flow along the tube remains constant. Therefore, the velocity at any point along the tube depends on the cross-sectional area of the tube. Figure 5.3 shows a tube of changing cross-sectional area (A_1, A_2); now, as the flow (Q) along the tube is constant:

$$Q = V_1 \times A_1 = V_2 \times A_2 \qquad (5.6)$$

This equation can be rearranged to show that the change in the velocities is related to the change in the cross-sectional area, as follows:

$$\frac{V_2}{V_1} = \frac{A_1}{A_2} \qquad (5.7)$$

As the cross-sectional area depends on the radius r of the tube ($A = \pi r^2$), we have:

$$\frac{V_2}{V_1} = \frac{A_1}{A_2} = \frac{r_1^2}{r_2^2} \qquad (5.8)$$

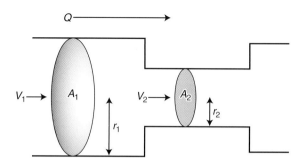

Figure 5.3   Change in cross-sectional area. As the flow is constant through the tube, the velocity of the fluid increases from V_1 to V_2 as the cross-sectional area decreases from A_1 to A_2.

This relationship actually describes steady flow in a rigid tube, but it does give us an indication as to how the velocity will change across a stenosis in an artery.

Figure 5.4 shows how the flow and velocity within an idealized stenosis vary with the degree of diameter reduction caused by the stenosis, based on the predictions from a simplified theoretical model. On the right-hand side of the graph, where the diameter reduction is less than 70–80%, the flow remains relatively unchanged as the diameter of the vessel is reduced. This is because the proportion of the resistance to flow due to the stenosis is small compared with the overall resistance of the vascular bed that the vessel is supplying. However, as the diameter reduces farther, the resistance offered by the stenosis becomes a significant proportion of the total resistance, and the stenosis begins to limit the flow. This is known as a hemodynamically significant stenosis. At this point, the flow decreases quickly as the diameter is reduced.

The graph also predicts the behavior of the velocity as the vessel diameter is reduced and shows that the velocity increases with diameter reduction. Noticeable changes in velocity begin to occur at much smaller diameter reductions than would produce a flow reduction. Therefore, measurement of velocity changes is a more sensitive method of detecting small-vessel lumen reductions than measurement of flow. Measurements of velocity made using Doppler ultrasound are also more accurate than measurement of flow, as will be discussed later (see Ch. 6). Therefore, it is often the change in velocity of blood within a diseased artery that is used

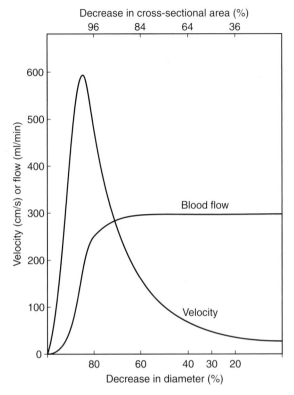

Figure 5.4   Changes in flow and velocity as the degree of stenosis alters, predicted by a simple theoretical model of a smooth, symmetrical stenosis. (After Spencer & Reid 1979 Quantitation of carotid stenosis with continuous-wave (C-W) Doppler ultrasound. Stroke 10(3):326–330, with permission.)

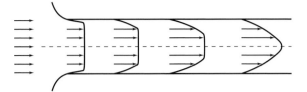

Figure 5.5   The change in velocity profile with distance along a vessel from a blunt to a parabolic. (After Caro et al 1978, with permission.)

FLOW PROFILES IN NORMAL ARTERIES

There are three types of flow observed in arteries:

- laminar
- disturbed
- turbulent.

The term laminar flow refers to the fact that the blood cells move in layers, one layer sliding over another, with the different layers being able to move at different velocities. In laminar flow, the blood cells remain in their layers. Turbulent flow occurs when laminar flow breaks down, which is unusual in normal healthy arteries but can be seen in the presence of high-velocity flow caused by stenoses, as discussed later in this chapter.

Figure 5.5 is a schematic diagram showing how the flow profile is expected to change as fluid enters a vessel. When flow enters a vessel from a reservoir (in the case of blood flow, this is the heart), all the fluid is moving at the same velocity, producing a flat velocity profile. This means that the velocity of the fluid close to the vessel wall is similar to that at the center of the vessel. As the fluid flows along the vessel, viscous drag exerted by the walls causes the fluid at the vessel wall to remain motionless, producing a gradient between the velocity in the center of the vessel and that at the walls. As the total flow has to remain constant (as there are no branches in our imaginary tube), the velocity at the center of the vessel will increase to compensate for the low velocity at the vessel wall. This leads to a change in the velocity profile from the initial blunt flow profile to a parabolic flow profile. This is often known as an entrance effect. The distance required for the flow profile to develop from the blunt to the parabolic profile depends on vessel diameter and velocity, but it is

to quantify the degree of narrowing. Eventually, there comes a point at which the resistance to flow produced by the narrowing is so great that the flow drops to such an extent that the velocity begins to decrease, as shown on the left side of the graph. This is seen as 'trickle flow' within the vessel. It is especially important to be able to identify trickle flow within a stenosis as the peak velocities seen may be similar to those seen in healthy vessels, but the color image and waveform shapes will not appear normal.

As blood flow is pulsatile and arteries are non-rigid vessels, it is difficult to predict theoretically the velocity increase that would be seen for a particular diameter reduction. Instead, velocity criteria used to quantify the degree of narrowing are produced by comparing Doppler velocity measurements with arteriogram results, as arteriography is considered to be the 'gold standard' for the diagnosis of arterial disease.

Figure 5.6 Color flow image showing high velocities (shown as yellow) in the center of a normal superficial femoral artery, with lower velocities (shown as red) nearer the vessel wall.

usually several times the vessel diameter. With blood flow, the velocity profiles are complicated by the pulsatile nature of the flow.

A color flow image obtained from the superficial femoral artery, during systole, is shown in Figure 5.6. This image shows high velocities in the center of the mid-superficial femoral artery and lower velocities near the artery wall.

Pulsatile flow

The flow profiles considered in Figure 5.5 describe steady flow, but clearly arterial flow is pulsatile. So how will this affect the velocity profile across the vessel? The mean velocity profile of the pulsatile flow will develop as described for steady-state flow but will have a pulsatile component superimposed upon it. The flow direction and velocity are governed by the pressure gradient along the vessel. The pressure pulse generated by the heart is transmitted down the arterial tree and is altered by pressure waves reflected from the distal vascular bed. Figure 5.7A shows the pressure waveforms, typical of those seen in the femoral arteries, from two different points along the vessel, 'a' and 'b'. The pressure difference between these two points is given by a − b, as shown in Figure 5.7B, such that a negative pressure gradient is produced at periods during the cardiac cycle. This leads to periods of reverse flow as seen in a typical Doppler waveform obtained from a normal superficial femoral artery (Fig. 5.8). If we consider a slowly oscillating pressure gradient applied to the flow, this will slow down, stop and then reverse the direction of flow. If this oscillation is gradual, the parabolic velocity profile will be maintained, but if the pressure gradient is

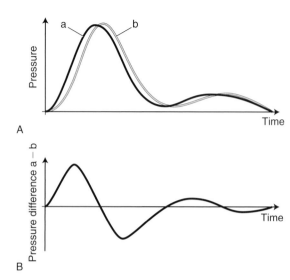

A

B

Figure 5.7 A: Idealized pressure waveforms obtained from two sites (a and b) along the femoral artery. B: The direction of blood flow between 'a' and 'b' will be governed by the pressure difference, given by 'a − b'. (After Nichols & O'Rourke 1990, with permission.)

Figure 5.8 Velocity waveform in a normal superficial femoral artery. The arrows represent points in the cardiac cycle where both forward and reverse flows are seen simultaneously.

Figure 5.9 Color flow image showing forward and reverse flow simultaneously in a normal superficial femoral artery. The red represents forward flow near the vessel wall while the blue represents reverse flow in the center of the vessel.

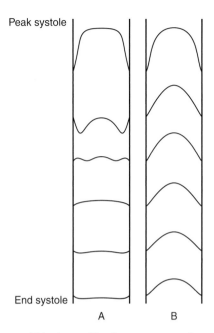

Figure 5.10 Velocity profiles from a common femoral artery (A) and a common carotid artery (B), calculated from the mean velocity waveforms. (After Evans & McDickens et al 1999, with permission.)

cycled more frequently, the velocity profile will become increasingly complex.

As the laminae of flowing blood near the vessel wall tend to have a lower velocity (due to the effect of viscosity), and hence lower momentum, they will reverse more easily when the pressure gradient along the vessel reverses. This can lead to a situation in which flow near the vessel wall is in a different direction to flow at the center of the vessel. Figure 5.9 shows a color image obtained from a normal superficial femoral artery during diastole. The image shows forward flow near the vessel wall, while flow in the center of the vessel is reversed. This would occur at the point in the cardiac cycle marked by the long arrow in Figure 5.8. The short arrow shows another point at which both forward and reverse flow may occur simultaneously. Figure 5.10 shows velocity profiles, as they vary over the cardiac cycle, for the common femoral artery (Fig. 5.10A) and the common carotid artery (Fig. 5.10B) that have been calculated from mean velocity waveforms. They show that reversal of flow is seen in the common femoral artery, but that, although the flow is pulsatile, reverse flow is not seen in the normal common carotid artery. Reversal of flow will only be seen if the reverse pulsatile flow component is greater than the steady flow component upon which it is superimposed. This greatly depends on the distal vascular bed. Total reversal of flow is rarely seen in normal renal or internal carotid arteries, both of which supply highly vascular beds with low resistance. However, there are hemodynamic effects at bifurcations and branches that may cause areas of localized flow reversal. There is a different appearance between waveform shapes obtained from vessels supplying a low-resistance vascular bed (i.e., organs such as the brain and kidney) and those obtained from peripheral vessels in the arms and legs, which supply high-resistance vascular beds.

Changes in peripheral resistance will change the flow pattern. For example, the waveform in the dorsalis pedis artery in the foot changes from bi-directional flow at rest (Fig. 5.11A) to hyperemic monophasic flow (i.e., flow that is always in the same direction; Fig. 5.11B) following exercise. Hyperemic flow can also be induced by temporary occlusion of the calf arteries using a blood pressure cuff. The lack of blood flow during the arterial occlusion with the cuff, or the increase in demand during exercise, causes the distal vessels to dilate in order to reduce peripheral resistance and maximize blood flow, and this is reflected in the change in shape of the waveform seen directly after cuff release. The hyperemic flow soon returns to bi-directional flow once adequate perfusion has occurred. This change in shape can also be seen when hyperemic flow is induced by infection. Monophasic flow is also seen in the lower limb, distal to severe stenoses or occlusions (Fig. 5.11C). This waveform shape is

Figure 5.11 Doppler spectra obtained from a normal dorsalis pedis artery in the foot showing bi-directional flow at rest (A) and monophasic hyperemic flow following exercise (B). Low volume monophasic flow seen in the foot distal to an occlusion (C).

Figure 5.12 A: Color flow image showing reverse flow in the origin of a normal internal carotid artery. B: Spectral Doppler waveform obtained from the area of flow separation shown by the arrow in A.

systolic rise time may be longer. The systolic rise time is the time between the beginning of systole and peak systole.

Flow at bifurcations and branches

The arterial tree divides many times, and each branch will affect the velocity profiles seen. The hemodynamics of the carotid bifurcation has been extensively investigated using multigate pulsed Doppler systems, and more recently using color Doppler systems, and these investigations show that localized reversed flow is seen at the carotid bifurcation in normal subjects. Figure 5.12A shows reversal of flow, due to flow separation, at the origin of a healthy internal carotid artery. The schematic diagram in Figure 5.13 indicates how the asymmetric flow profile in a normal proximal internal carotid artery develops, with the high-velocity flow occurring toward the flow divider and the reverse flow occurring near the wall away from the origin of the external carotid artery. The effect is primarily due to a combination of the pulsatile flow, the relative dimensions of the vessels, the angle of the bifurcation and the curvature of the vessel walls, making it difficult to predict these profiles. Figure 5.12B is a spectral Doppler signal obtained from the area of flow separation shown by an arrow in Figure 5.12A, illustrating reverse flow during

also due to distal vasodilatation, in an attempt to maximize flow distal to the diseased vessel, but this can usually be distinguished from hyperemic flow as the velocity of the flow is low and the

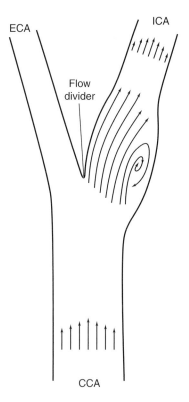

Figure 5.13   Schematic diagram of the velocity patterns commonly observed in the normal carotid bifurcation. The velocity profile is flat and symmetric in the CCA and flat but slightly asymmetric in the ICA. In the carotid bulb the velocities are highest near the flow divider. Flow separation with flow reversal is observed on the opposite side to the flow divider. (From Reneman et al 1985 Flow velocity patterns in and distensibility of the carotid artery bulb in subjects of various ages. Circulation 71(3): 500–509, with permission.)

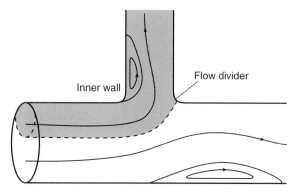

Figure 5.14   Flow in a right-angle junction. The dashed line shows the surface that divides fluid flowing into the side branch from that continuing down the parent vessel. (After Caro et al 1978, with permission.)

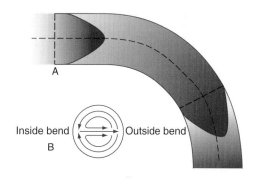

Figure 5.15   A: Distortion of parabolic flow caused by tube curvature. B: Secondary flow, in the form of two helical vortices. (After Caro et al 1978, with permission.)

systole in that part of the vessel. This normal finding could potentially be misleading if the whole bifurcation is not observed and, typically, spectral Doppler recordings are made beyond the bifurcation unless the presence of disease indicates otherwise (see Ch. 8).

Flow reversal can also occur when a daughter vessel branches at right angles from the parent vessel. Figure 5.14 is a schematic diagram of the results obtained with dye in steadily flowing water in a tube with a right-angled branch and shows how the flow is divided between the main vessel and its branch. The flow is seen to separate from the inner

wall of the junction and a region of reverse flow develops, primarily due to the sharp bend.

Flow around curves in a vessel

Curvature of vessels can also have an effect on the velocity profile. When a fluid flows along a curved tube, it experiences a centrifugal force, as well as the viscous forces at the vessel wall, and the combination of these forces results in secondary flow, in the form of two helical vortices (Oates 2003). In the case of parabolic flow, the fluid in the center of the vessel has the highest velocity and will thus experience the greatest force. These vortices will cause the high-velocity flow to move toward the

A

B

C

Figure 5.16   A: Color flow image from a tortuous internal carotid artery, with flow going from right to left, shows the highest velocities beyond the bend (left), represented in orange due to aliasing, skewed toward the outside of the bend. Spectral Doppler recordings showing that the peak velocity recorded on the outside of the bend (B) measures 70 cm/s compared to the peak velocity on the inside of the bend (C), which measures 55 cm/s.

outside wall of the vessel, as seen in Figure 5.15. Figure 5.16 shows a color flow image obtained from a tortuous internal carotid artery, with flow going from right to left. The image shows the highest velocities beyond the bend (left), represented in orange due to aliasing, skewed toward the outside of the bend. This is confirmed by spectral Doppler recordings showing that the peak velocity recorded on the outside of the bend (Fig. 5.16B) measures 70 cm/s compared to the peak velocity on the inside of the bend (Fig. 5.16C), which measures 55 cm/s. If the flow profile is blunt, when it enters a bend in the vessel (as seen in the ascending aorta), the profile becomes skewed in the opposite direction (i.e., toward the inner wall of the curve). Secondary helical flow also occurs at bifurcations, as the daughter vessels bend away from the path of the parent vessel, leading to skewed velocity profiles in the daughter vessels (Fig. 5.13).

FLOW THROUGH STENOSES

Flow separation leading to flow reversal can also be seen in diseased arteries. At an arterial stenosis, the velocity of the blood has to increase because the same volume of blood needs to pass through a smaller cross-sectional area. If the vessel lumen rapidly returns to its normal diameter following the narrowing, flow separation can occur. Whereas the velocity increases as the blood passes through the constriction, the pressure within the stenosis falls, but the pressure rises again just distal to the stenosis as the lumen expands, having the effect of retarding the flow. As the flow near the vessel wall has a lower velocity, and therefore lower inertia, it will reverse, while the higher velocity flow in the center of the vessel is reduced but not reversed. A schematic diagram of this effect is shown in Figure 5.17. The color image in Figure 5.18 demonstrates the increase in velocity as the blood flows through a stenosis, with flow reversal occurring along the distal wall beyond the stenosis as the vessel lumen returns to its normal diameter.

The geometry of stenoses is very variable, and these narrowings are often not symmetrical, sometimes producing eccentric jets, so it is impossible to predict the typical velocity profiles. As the degree of narrowing increases, the velocity within the vessel will increase, making the breakdown of laminar flow to turbulent flow more likely. Turbulent flow can withstand more acute geometric changes than laminar flow, so flow separation is less likely to be seen beyond a stenosis that has produced turbulent flow.

Figure 5.17   Schematic diagram of flow through a constriction followed by a rapid expansion downstream, showing the regions of flow reversal. The velocity increases as the blood flows through a stenosis (from right to left) followed by an area of flow reversal beyond the narrowing. (After Caro et al 1978, with permission.)

Figure 5.18   The increase in velocity as the blood flows from right to left through a stenosis (arrow) produces the color change from red to turquoise (due to aliasing). Beyond the stenosis, flow reversal occurs along the posterior wall, represented by the deep blue, as the vessel lumen returns to its normal diameter.

Transition from laminar to turbulent flow

Turbulent flow occurs when laminar flow breaks down and the particles in the fluid move randomly in all directions with variable speeds. The transition from laminar flow to disturbed and then to turbulent flow is shown in Figure 5.19. Turbulent flow is more likely to occur at high velocities (V), and the critical velocity at which flow becomes turbulent depends on the viscosity (μ) and the density (ρ) of the fluid and the diameter of the vessel (d). Reynolds described this relationship, which defines a value called the Reynolds number (Re):

$$Re = \frac{dV\rho}{\mu} \qquad (5.9)$$

Once the Reynolds number has exceeded the critical value of approximately 2000, turbulent flow will occur. Table 5.1 gives typical values of the Reynolds number in various arteries in the body and shows that in normal vessels the velocity of blood is such that turbulent flow does not occur, with the

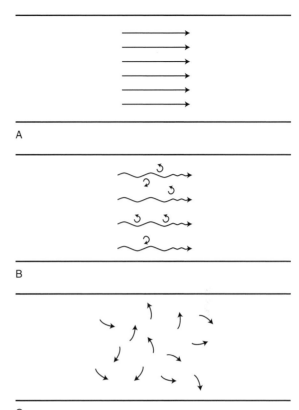

Figure 5.19   A: Laminar flow. B: Disturbed flow. C: Turbulent flow. (After Taylor et al 1995, with permission.)

Table 5.1   Typical values of the Reynolds number in various arteries in the body (after Evans & McDicken 1999, with permission)

Artery	Reynolds number
Ascending aorta	1500
Abdominal aorta	640
Common carotid	217*
Superficial femoral	200
Posterior tibial	35*

*Estimated values.

exception of the proximal aortic flow during heavy exercise, for which cardiac output is increased. The presence of an increase in the blood velocity, due to arterial disease, can cause turbulent flow. Figure 5.20 is a Doppler waveform demonstrating turbulent

Figure 5.20 Doppler waveform demonstrating turbulent flow.

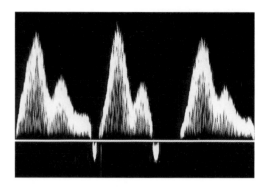

Figure 5.21 Doppler waveform showing the effect of changes in the pressure in the right atrium on blood flow in the jugular vein.

flow. In the presence of turbulence, not all the blood is travelling in the same direction, resulting in the angle of insonation being smaller for some parts of the blood flow. This results in turbulent spikes seen on the Doppler spectrum. It is possible for turbulent flow to occur only during the systolic phase of the cardiac cycle, when the systolic flow exceeds the critical velocity and the diastolic flow does not.

The presence of turbulent flow causes energy to be lost, leading to an increased pressure drop across the stenosis. It is thought that bruits in the tissue near a stenosis (see Fig. 11.18A) may be due to perivascular tissue vibration caused by turbulence, and this may also lead to post-stenotic dilatation of the vessel. Vortices or irregular movement of a large portion of the fluid are more correctly referred to as disturbed flow rather than turbulent flow.

VENOUS FLOW

The venous system acts as a low-resistance pathway for blood to be returned to the heart. Veins are collapsible, thin-walled vessels capable of distending to a larger cross-sectional area than their corresponding arteries, so acting as a blood volume storage system which is important in the regulation of cardiac output. In addition, they also have a thermoregulation role in which blood is diverted to the superficial veins to reduce body temperature. The venous system can be divided into the central system (within the thorax and abdomen), the deep peripheral system and the superficial peripheral veins.

An important structural feature of the vein is the presence of very thin, but strong, bicuspid valves which prevent retrograde flow away from the heart. The vena cava and common iliac veins (see Fig. 12.3)

are valveless. Valves are found in the external iliac or common femoral veins in a proportion of the population. Generally the more distal the vein, the greater the number of valves.

Venous flow back to the heart is influenced by respiration, the cardiac cycle and changes in posture.

Changes in flow due to the cardiac cycle

The central veins include the thoracic and abdominal veins, which drain to the right side of the heart via the inferior and superior venae cavae. The flow pattern and pressure in the central venous system are affected by changes in the volume of the right atrium, which occur during the cardiac cycle. Reverse flow occurs in the thoracic veins when the right atrium contracts, as there is no valve in the vena cava. This flow reversal can also be seen in the proximal veins of the arm and neck (Fig. 5.21) due to their proximity to the chest. During ventricular contraction, the atrium expands, increasing venous flow into the right atrium, and then flow gradually falls during diastole, only increasing briefly as the tricuspid valve opens. Flow patterns in the lower limb veins and peripheral arm veins are not significantly affected by the cardiac cycle due to vein compliance (which allows damping of the pressure changes), the presence of valves and changes in intra-abdominal pressure during respiration.

Effects of respiration on venous flow

Respiration has an important effect on venous pressure and flow because of changes in the volume of

Figure 5.22 Doppler waveform demonstrating the effect of respiration on the blood flow in the common femoral vein. The large arrow indicates the cessation of flow during inspiration and the small arrows show small changes in flow due to the cardiac cycle, which may not always be seen in the common femoral vein.

the thorax brought about by movement of the diaphragm and ribs. Inspiration during calm breathing expands the thorax, leading to an increase in the volume of the veins in the chest, which in turn causes a reduction in the pressure in the intra-thoracic veins. This creates a pressure gradient between the veins in the upper limb and head and those in the thorax, producing an increase in flow into the chest. Flow is decreased during expiration as the volume of the thorax decreases, leading to an increase in central pressure.

The reverse situation is seen in the abdomen as the diaphragm descends during inspiration, increasing intra-abdominal pressure. This leads to a decrease in the pressure gradient between the peripheral veins and the abdominal veins, thus reducing flow. During expiration the diaphragm rises, producing a reduction in intra-abdominal pressure, and the pressure gradient between the abdominal veins and peripheral veins increases, causing increased blood flow back to the heart. The effects of respiration are observed as phasic changes in flow in proximal deep peripheral veins (Fig. 5.22). Breathing maneuvers are often used to augment flow when investigating venous disorders (see Ch. 12).

Changes in venous blood pressure due to posture and the calf muscle pump

Large pressure changes occur in the venous system, due to the effects of hydrostatic pressure generated by posture (Fig. 5.1). If an individual is lying supine,

for example, there is a relatively small pressure difference between the venous pressures at the ankle and right atrium. However, when an individual is standing, there is a column of blood between the right atrium and the veins at the ankle. If the hydrostatic pressure is assumed to be zero in the right atrium, the hydrostatic pressure at the ankle will be equal to the distance between the two, which is obviously dependent on the person's height, but is usually between 80 and 100 mmHg. Therefore, in a standing position, there is a significant pressure gradient to overcome in order for blood to be returned to the heart; this is achieved by the calf muscle pump mechanism assisted by the presence of the venous valves.

The muscle compartments in the calf contain the deep veins and venous sinuses, which act as blood reservoirs. Regular small contractions occur in the deep muscles of the calf, causing compression of the veins, thereby propelling blood flow out of the leg, with the venous valves preventing the blood refluxing back down. This also generates a pressure gradient between the superficial and deep veins in the calf, and blood drains through the perforating veins and major junctions from the superficial to the deep venous system. The valves in the perforators prevent blood flowing from the deep to the superficial veins. During more active exercise, such as walking or running, the calf muscle pump mechanism is able to produce a significant pressure reduction in the deep and superficial venous systems to approximately 30 mmHg. The pressure change that occurs during exercise is called the ambulatory venous pressure. At rest, because the hydrostatic pressure is the same on both the arterial and venous sides, the pressure drop across the capillary bed is the same whether the person is standing or lying down. However, after exercise the pressure on the venous side of the capillary bed will drop, but the pressure on the arterial side will remain the same, creating a pressure drop across the capillary bed and aiding the return of blood to the heart. Once the muscle contraction stops, the venous pressure in the lower leg will begin to rise due to filling of the venous system from the arterial system via the capillaries.

It is possible to measure the ambulatory venous pressure by inserting a small cannula into a dorsal foot vein, which is then connected to a pressure transducer and recorder. The pressure in the vein is first recorded with the patient standing. The patient is asked to perform 10 tiptoe maneuvers and then to stand still. The pressure recording demonstrates the pressure reduction during the exercise, and the venous refilling time can also be calculated. With normal veins, the refilling of the venous system occurs gradually by capillary inflow and takes 18 s or more to return to pre-exercise pressures (Fig. 5.23A). If there is significant failure of the venous valves in either the superficial or the deep venous system, reflux will occur, leading to a shorter refilling time and a higher post-exercise pressure (Fig. 5.23B). Reflux in the deep or superficial venous systems, or in both, can lead to chronic venous hypertension in the lower leg and may result in the development of venous ulcers. Failure of the calf muscle pump due to poor flexion of the ankle and poor contraction of the calf muscle can lead to a reduction in the volume of blood ejected from the calf. This results in an inability to lower venous pressure adequately and can cause chronic venous hypertension. Patients at greatest risk due to poor calf muscle pump mechanism include those with limited ankle flexion due to chronic injury, osteoarthritis or rheumatoid arthritis.

Figure 5.23 Typical ambulatory venous pressures recordings. A: Normal venous refilling. B: Incompetent veins leading to a shorter refilling time.

Abnormal venous flow

Venous disease can dramatically alter the flow patterns seen in the veins. Valve incompetence allows retrograde flow in the veins, which can easily be demonstrated with color flow imaging and spectral Doppler (see Figs 12.15 and 12.16). Venous outflow obstruction results in the loss of the spontaneous phasic flow generated by respiration seen in normal veins. Congestive heart failure may lead to increased pulsatility of the flow in the femoral and iliac veins (see Fig. 13.17). Ultrasound now plays an important role in the diagnosis of venous disease, which is discussed further in Chapters 12 and 13.

References

Caro C G, Pedley T J, Schroter R C, Seed W A 1978 The mechanics of the circulation. Oxford University Press, Oxford

Evans D H, McDicken W N 1999 Doppler ultrasound: physics, instrumentation, and signal processing. Wiley, Chichester

Nichols W N, O'Rourke M F 1990 McDonald's blood flow in arteries. Edward Arnold, London

Oates C P 2001 Cardiovascular haemodynamics and Doppler waveforms explained. Greenwich Medical Media, London

Reneman R S, van Merode T, Hick P, Hoeks A P G 1985 Flow velocity patterns in and distensibility of the carotid artery bulb in subjects of various ages. Circulation 71(3):500–509

Spencer M P, Reid J M 1979 Quantitation of carotid stenosis with continuous-wave (C-W) Doppler ultrasound. Stroke 10(3):326–330

Taylor K J W, Burns P N, Wells P N T 1995 Clinical applications of Doppler ultrasound. Raven Press, New York

Chapter 6

Factors that influence the Doppler spectrum

CHAPTER CONTENTS

Introduction 63
Factors that influence the Doppler spectrum 63
    Blood flow profile 63
    Nonuniform insonation of the vessel 64
    Sample volume size 64
    Pulse repetition frequency, high-pass filter
      and gain 65
    Intrinsic spectral broadening 65
Velocity measurements 66
    Converting Doppler shift frequencies to velocity
      measurements 66
    Errors in maximum velocity measurements
      relating to the angle of insonation 67
    Errors relating to the direction of flow relative to
      the vessel walls 68
    Errors relating to the out-of-imaging plane angle
      of insonation 68
    Creation of a range of insonation angles by the
      Doppler ultrasound beam aperture 68
    Optimizing the angle of insonation 69
    Other potential sources of error in maximum
      velocity measurements 70
Measurement of volume flow 70
    Sources of error in vessel diameter
      measurement 70
Waveform analysis 72
    Pulsatility index 72
    Pourcelot's resistance index 72
    Spectral broadening 72
    Pulse wave velocity 72
    Subjective interpretation 73

INTRODUCTION

The shape of the Doppler spectrum can provide much useful information about the presence of disease and enables the sonographer to make measurements to quantify the degree of vessel narrowing. However, the shape of the spectrum will also depend on other factors, such as the velocity profile of the blood flow being interrogated and how evenly the ultrasound beam insonates the vessel. Factors that relate to the equipment rather than the blood flow can also affect the shape of the waveform. It is important to understand how these factors influence the waveform shape in order to be able to interpret the Doppler waveform. The sonographer should also be aware of potential errors involved in any measurements made.

FACTORS THAT INFLUENCE THE DOPPLER SPECTRUM

Blood flow profile

The Doppler spectrum displays the frequency content of the signal along the vertical axis, with the relative brightness of the display representing the proportion of back-scattered power at each frequency, and the time along the horizontal axis. The velocity profiles seen within arteries can be quite complex and will vary over time, as discussed in Chapter 5. The frequency content displayed in the Doppler spectrum will depend on the velocities of the cells present within the blood. If we assume that the vessel is uniformly insonated by the Doppler beam, all the different velocities of blood present

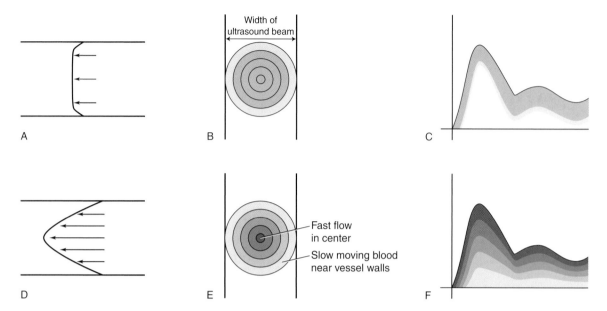

Figure 6.1 A, D: Velocity profiles for blunt flow and parabolic flow, respectively. B, E: If a wide ultrasound beam is used to insonate the vessel, all the velocities present will be detected. C, F: Idealised Doppler spectra that would be obtained from complete insonation of blunt flow and parabolic flow, respectively.

within the vessel will be detected and displayed on the spectrum. If blood is travelling with a blunt flow profile, most of the blood cells will be moving with the same velocity, and the spectrum will show only a small range of frequencies (Fig. 6.1A–C). If, however, the blood is travelling with a parabolic flow profile, then the blood in the center of the vessel will be travelling faster than that near the vessel walls and therefore the Doppler spectrum will display a wide range of frequencies (Fig. 6.1D–F).

The spread of frequencies present within the spectrum at a given point in time is known as the degree of spectral broadening. Figure 6.1 shows the way in which the degree of spectral broadening depends on the velocity profile of the flow being interrogated, with greater spectral broadening seen in Figure 6.1F than in Figure 6.1C. The presence of turbulent flow (e.g., as a result of a stenosis) will increase spectral broadening, as the blood cells will be travelling with different velocities in random directions (see Fig. 5.20). Therefore, increased spectral broadening may indicate the presence of disease. However, the degree of spectral broadening can also be influenced by Doppler instrumentation, and this is known as intrinsic spectral broadening (discussed later in this chapter).

Nonuniform insonation of the vessel

The examples of idealized spectra given in Figure 6.1 assume that the beam evenly insonates the whole cross-section of the blood vessel in order to detect the correct proportions of all the blood velocities present. This is, however, an unrealistic situation as the Doppler beam can be quite narrow (of the order of 1 to 2 mm wide) and therefore may insonate only part of the artery or vein. If the beam passes through the center of the vessel (Fig. 6.2A), only part of the flow near the vessel walls (i.e., near the anterior and posterior walls) will be detected. The blood flow along the lateral walls will not be detected as it is not insonated by the Doppler beam. Therefore, in the presence of parabolic flow, the low-velocity flow near the walls will only be partially detected and the Doppler spectrum will no longer truly represent the low-velocity flow present within the vessel.

Sample volume size

The size and position of the sample volume, which can be controlled by the operator, will also affect the proportion of the vessel insonated. A small sample volume placed in the center of a large vessel

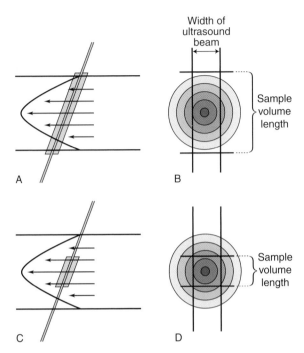

Figure 6.2   Incomplete insonation of the vessel will occur when a narrow beam is used. A, B: Large sample volume length. C, D: Small sample volume length.

Figure 6.3   Doppler spectrum demonstrating the appearance of a mirror image below the baseline when the scanner's Doppler gain control is set too high.

may not detect any of the flow near the vessel wall at all (Figs 6.2C and D). However, a larger sample volume, which could cover the whole depth of the vessel (Figs 6.2A and B), would detect the flow near the anterior and posterior walls but not the lateral walls. The size of the sample volume (i.e., the sensitive region of the beam) will therefore affect the range of Doppler frequencies detected and should be taken into account when interpreting the degree of spectral broadening. A narrow Doppler beam with a small sample volume placed in the center of the vessel may detect only the fast-moving blood and therefore, in normal circumstances, would not demonstrate much spectral broadening. However, in the presence of disease, increased spectral broadening may be seen due to the presence of turbulent flow.

Pulse repetition frequency, high-pass filter and gain

The high frequencies present in the Doppler signal will be incorrectly displayed on the Doppler spectrum if aliasing has occurred as a result of a low pulse repetition frequency (PRF) (see Fig. 3.14A). This results in misleading waveform shapes and errors in velocity measurement. The effect of aliasing is easily visualized, as the Doppler waveform appears to 'wrap around' from the top of the spectrum to the bottom. Aliasing can be corrected by increasing the PRF.

The shape of the Doppler spectrum can also be altered if the high-pass filter is set too high, removing important information from the spectrum, such as the presence of low-velocity diastolic flow (see Fig. 3.7C). The gain used to amplify the Doppler signal may also alter the appearance of the spectrum. If the gain is set too low, flow may not be detected. Increasing the gain can increase the appearance of spectral broadening. An inappropriately high gain can lead to the overloading of the instrument, causing poor direction discrimination, and this may result in a mirror image of the spectrum appearing in the reverse direction on the display (Fig. 6.3).

Intrinsic spectral broadening

Intrinsic spectral broadening (ISB) is broadening of the Doppler spectrum that is an artifact, related to the scanner rather than the blood flow interrogated. Linear array transducers use several elements

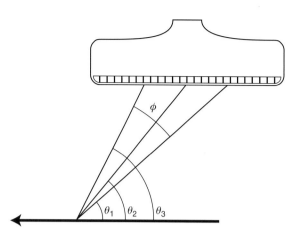

Figure 6.4 A schematic diagram showing the range of angles of insonation produced by a linear array transducer when making blood velocity measurements. θ_1 and θ_3 represent the smallest and largest angles of insonation generated by the array, respectively, and θ_2 represents the angle produced by the midpoint of the active elements. ϕ is the angle produced by the aperture of the active elements generating the Doppler beam. The arrow represents the direction of the blood flow. (From Thrush & Evans 1995, with permission.)

A

B

Figure 6.5 A: The moving string test object mounted in a water tank at 45° to the ultrasound transducer. B: A typical spectrum obtained from the moving string, showing the spread of frequencies detected. (From Thrush & Evans 1995, with permission.)

to form the beam (see Ch. 2). Figure 6.4 shows how the ultrasound beam from a linear array transducer can produce a range of angles of insonation, with the Doppler signals being detected at many angles. As the Doppler shift frequency detected is proportional to the cosine of the angle of insonation, θ, this will lead to a range of frequencies being detected even in the presence of a single target. A test object constructed of a string driven at a constant speed by a motor can be used to investigate this effect (Fig. 6.5A). The spectrum obtained from the moving string shows that a large range of Doppler shift frequencies have been detected despite the fact that the target is a single object moving at a constant velocity (Fig. 6.5B). This is due to the range of angles of insonation produced from different elements within the active portion of the probe and is the effect known as ISB. The degree of ISB depends on the range of angles over which back-scattered ultrasound is received by the transducer (ϕ in Fig. 6.4)—i.e., it depends on the aperture of the transducer—and on the angle of insonation of the beam (θ).

VELOCITY MEASUREMENTS

Converting Doppler shift frequencies to velocity measurements

The combination of imaging and spectral Doppler ultrasound allows an estimate of the angle of insonation (θ) between the Doppler ultrasound beam and the blood flow. The angle of insonation is measured by lining up the angle correction cursor with the estimated direction of flow.

The Doppler equation (equation 3.1) can be used to estimate the velocity of the blood (V) from the measured Doppler shift frequency (f_d), as the transmitted frequency of the Doppler beam (f_t) is known and the speed of sound in tissue (c) is assumed to be constant (1540 m/s). As the velocity of the blood usually varies across the vessel, a range of velocities will be recorded at any given point in time. The velocity of blood also varies with time, due to the pumping action of the heart. This means that the velocity of the blood is not actually a single value. A choice has to be made as to which value to use to represent the velocity of the blood. The value most commonly used in vascular ultrasound is maximum peak systolic velocity. This is the maximum velocity recorded within the spectrum at the point in time that represents peak systolic flow, as shown on the sonogram in Figure 6.6A. This velocity represents the fastest moving blood in the vessel. The maximum velocity can similarly be measured at end diastole. These measurements do not take into account the slower moving blood near the vessel walls.

An alternative is to measure mean velocity at any point in time. This can be calculated by the scanner by finding the average of all the velocities recorded at an instant in time, as shown as a black line superimposed on the Doppler spectrum in Figure 6.6B. As with maximum velocity, the mean velocity will obviously change during the cardiac cycle. If the mean velocity for each line of the sonogram is averaged over a complete cardiac cycle, this will give the value known as the time-averaged velocity (TAV). This can be used to estimate volume flow (discussed later in this chapter).

Many diagnostic criteria are based on velocity ratios rather than on absolute velocity measurements. For example, stenoses may be categorized by the velocity ratio of the maximum peak systolic velocity within the stenosis, V_{sten}, divided by the maximum peak systolic velocity in the normal proximal vessel, V_{prox}:

$$\text{Velocity ratio} = \frac{V_{sten}}{V_{prox}} \quad (6.1)$$

Figure 6.6 A: Doppler spectrum showing the measurement of maximum peak systolic velocity, S, and maximum end diastolic velocity, D. B: The mean velocity can be calculated from the Doppler spectrum, displayed by the black line. A large sample volume will allow the blood velocity at the anterior and posterior walls, as well as in the center of the vessel, to be estimated but may not detect the flow along the lateral wall. The time-averaged mean velocity, TAM, can be found by averaging the mean velocity over one or more complete cardiac cycles. Volume flow can be calculated by multiplying the TAM measurement by the cross-sectional area of the vessel (displayed bottom left).

Errors in maximum velocity measurements relating to the angle of insonation

An estimate of the angle of insonation is required to convert the detected Doppler shift frequency into a velocity measurement. Any inaccuracy in placing the angle correction cursor parallel to the direction of flow will lead to an error in the estimated angle of insonation. This in turn will lead

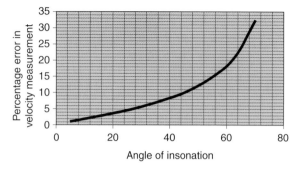

Figure 6.7 Graph showing the relationship between the percentage error in the velocity measurements as the angle of insonation increases, for a 5° error in the placement of the angle correction cursor. (After Evans D H & McDicken W N 2000 Doppler ultrasound: physics, instrumentation, and signal processing. © John Wiley & Sons Limited, with permission.)

to an error in the velocity measurement. The velocity calculation depends on the $\cos \theta$ term, so the error created will be greater for larger angles of insonation. Figure 6.7 shows the relationship between the percentage error in the velocity measurement as the angle of insonation increases where there is a 5° error in the placement of the angle correction cursor. For example, Figure 6.7 shows that this 5° error in cursor placement causes an error in velocity measurement of 23% when the angle of insonation is 65°. In order to minimize this error, angles of insonation of greater than 60% should not be used. However, estimating the angle of insonation is not always straightforward, especially in the presence of disease. Some of the limitations are listed below.

Errors relating to the direction of flow relative to the vessel walls

The direction of the blood flow may not be parallel to the vessel wall, especially in the presence of a stenosis, vortices or helical flow. Therefore, in these cases lining the angle correction cursor parallel to the walls may lead to large errors. If there is a clear image of the flow channel through a narrowing it may be possible to line up the angle cursor with the flow channel. However, the maximum velocity may be just beyond the stenosis, and the direction of flow may be less obvious at that point. The color image may be used to identify the site of

maximum velocity, although this can be misleading as the color image displays mean frequency, which is related to the blood motion in the direction of the beam, rather than the actual blood velocity. What appears to be the maximum velocity on the image may instead be the site at which the angle between the Doppler beam and the direction of the blood flow is smallest. It is important to consider this when estimating the site of maximum velocity and the direction of flow from the color image. The blood velocity may need to be measured at a few points through and beyond a stenosis to ensure the highest velocity has been obtained.

Errors relating to the out–of–imaging plane angle of insonation

It is important to remember that the interception of the ultrasound beam with the blood flow occurs in a three-dimensional space and not just in the two-dimensional plane shown on the image. An underestimate of the true velocity will be obtained if the out-of-imaging plane angle of insonation is not close to 0°. Therefore, the transducer should be aligned with a reasonable length of the vessel, as seen on the image, to ensure a minimal error.

Creation of a range of insonation angles by the Doppler ultrasound beam aperture

The large aperture used by linear array transducers not only results in ISB but also leads to another problem. For velocity to be calculated from the Doppler shift frequency, the $\cos \theta$ term is required, but clearly only a single value for the angle can be used. Substituting the two extreme angles shown in Figure 6.4 (θ_1 and θ_3) into the Doppler equation would obviously give different values for the velocity. A decision has to be made as to which angle is most suitable for use in converting the detected Doppler frequency into velocity. Typically, ultrasound scanners use the angle between the center of the active elements and the direction of flow (i.e., angle θ_2). This would be an appropriate angle to select for estimation of the mean velocity, but it leads to an overestimation of the calculated maximum velocity. In fact, in order to obtain a correct value for the peak velocity from the frequency spectrum, the smallest angle of insonation present

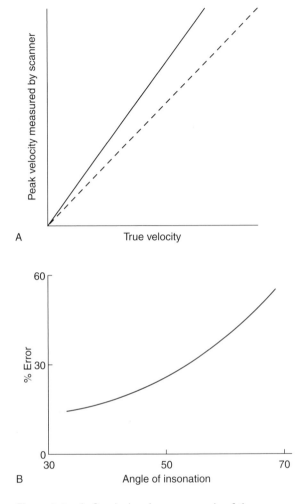

Figure 6.8 A: Graph showing an example of the overestimation of peak velocity measured at a given angle of insonation by a typical linear array transducer due to intrinsic spectral broadening (solid line). Dashed line shows correct value of velocity. B: Graph showing an example of how the error in peak velocity measurements may increase with an increase in the angle of insonation.

unless the ISB produced by a given scanner is taken into account when developing velocity criteria for the quantification of disease. Early duplex scanners, before the development of linear array transducers, used single-element Doppler probes that produce low ISB. The velocity measurements made using these older ultrasound scanners were not prone to ISB errors, and therefore the velocity criteria produced using them may differ from those produced using linear array transducers. The error produced due to spectral broadening can vary with changes in the active aperture that accompany changes in the sample volume depth. The error also varies among manufacturers. It is therefore recommended that departments compare their ultrasound results with those obtained from angiography or other imaging techniques.

Diagnosis of vascular disease often depends on velocity ratio measurements, and these are not affected by the errors produced by ISB as long as both measurements used to calculate the ratio are made with a similar angle of insonation. If the velocity ratios are calculated using two velocity measurements made with significantly different angles of insonation, significant errors may be introduced.

Optimizing the angle of insonation

Ideally, the angle of insonation for estimating velocity measurement should be zero to minimize errors; however, as peripheral vessels often lie parallel to the skin, this is not possible. No single choice of angle of insonation is completely reliable, especially when comparisons between velocity measurements are being made. The possibilities are discussed below:

Velocity ratio measurements

Ideally the angle of insonation used to make the velocity measurement proximal to and at the stenosis should be similar. This will result in the two velocities having similar errors that will cancel out when calculating the ratio.

Absolute velocity measurements

There are two schools of thought about selecting the angle of insonation when making absolute

(i.e., θ_1) should be used; however, this is not under the sonographer's control. Figure 6.8 gives an example of the possible errors in peak velocity measurements on a typical ultrasound scanner caused by ISB. The graphs show that the larger the angle of insonation, the greater the potential source of error in velocity measurement. It is therefore important not to use a Doppler angle greater than 60°. These overestimates in peak velocity measurements could lead to an overestimate in the degree of narrowing velocity measurements:

- Always set the angle of insonation to 60°

This ensures that any error in alignment of the angle correction cursor only leads to a moderate error in the velocity estimate (Fig. 6.7) and that the errors caused by ISB are kept similar between measurements. However, it can be difficult to insonate all vessels at a fixed 60° angle.

- Always select as small an angle of insonation as possible

This ensures that any error in the alignment of the angle correction cursor produces as small an error in velocity estimation as possible. The error due to ISB will also be minimized. However, this error will be different for measurements made at different angles of insonation. This makes comparisons between measurements made at different angles less meaningful.

Doppler criteria developed over the years may not have been produced with a full understanding of all these possible sources of error. Different models of ultrasound system may produce different results for the same blood flow. However, despite these sources of error, velocity measurements have been successfully used to quantify vascular disease for the past two decades. A greater understanding of the sources of error in velocity measurement may lead to improvements in accuracy.

Other potential sources of error in maximum velocity measurements

Figure 3.7 has already shown how high-pass filters can be used to remove unwanted signals. The high-pass filter setting will not affect the peak systolic velocity measurements, but the shape of the peak velocity envelope (the outline of the spectrum) may be affected if the filter is set so high that it removes the diastolic flow. This would lead to an incorrect finding that the end diastolic velocity is zero. Figure 3.14 shows how aliasing will lead to an underestimation in the mean velocity and the maximum velocity due to the incorrect estimation of the high frequencies present within the signal. Noise may be introduced into the Doppler signal, especially if the signal is recorded at depth, requiring

significant amplification. The maximum Doppler frequency may be difficult to define in the presence of high levels of noise.

MEASUREMENT OF VOLUME FLOW

Volume flow is a potentially useful physiological parameter (see Fig. 5.4) that can be measured using ultrasound, although it involves several possible sources of error (Evans & McDicken 2000). An estimation of the volume flow of blood can be made if the cross-sectional area of the vessel and the velocity of the blood through the vessel are known. Ultrasound scanners usually have the facility to perform volume flow measurements by enabling the sonographer to measure diameter or cross-sectional area from the image and then to measure the TAV from the Doppler spectrum, calculating the flow as follows:

$$\text{Flow} = \text{cross-sectional area} \times \text{TAV} \qquad (6.2)$$

The most straightforward method of obtaining the vessel cross-sectional area is to measure the vessel diameter (d) and calculate the area as follows:

$$A = \frac{\pi d^2}{4} \qquad (6.3)$$

Some scanners also allow the sonographer to outline the circumference of the vessel, imaged in transverse section, using a cursor. This method tends to be less reliable as it requires a steady hand and a good image of the lateral walls of the vessel. The cross-sectional area can then be multiplied by the TAV to give the flow, as shown in Figure 6.6B.

Sources of error in vessel diameter measurement

Errors in either the velocity measurement or the diameter measurement will introduce errors into the estimation of volume flow. As flow is proportional to the cross-sectional area of the vessel, which in turn depends on the square of the radius, any error in the diameter will produce a fractional error in the flow measurement that is double the fractional error in the radius. The possible sources of error in vessel diameter measurement are discussed below.

Image resolution

The ability to image an object is dependent on the resolution of the scanner, as described in Chapter 2. The resolution along the axis of the beam is better than that across the image (i.e., the lateral resolution). The axial resolution is of the order of the wavelength of the ultrasound. For example, the wavelength of a 3 MHz transducer is 0.5 mm, whereas the wavelength of a 10 MHz transducer is 0.15 mm, the latter therefore providing more accurate distance measurements. Lateral measurements are much less accurate, as a result of the poorer image resolution and reduced image quality due to the beam being parallel to the vessel wall. The vessel diameter is especially difficult to measure in the presence of disease.

Calliper velocity calibration

Accurate diameter measurements rely on correct calliper velocity calibration. Most scanners assume the mean velocity in tissue to be 1540 m/s; however, the velocity of sound in blood is actually 1580 m/s. This results in a systematic underestimate of the order of 2.6% in diameter measurement, leading to a 5% error in cross-sectional area.

Variable vessel diameter

The arterial diameter is not, in fact, constant but varies during the cardiac cycle due to the changing pressure within the vessel. This means that a single measurement of the diameter may not be representative of the mean diameter. It has been shown that vessel wall pulsatility may result in up to a 10% change in vessel diameter between systole and diastole. This cyclical variation in diameter will lead to errors in volume flow estimation, but it may be reduced by taking several diameter measurements and finding a mean value. Ideally, an instantaneous diameter measurement should be multiplied by the instantaneous mean velocity to obtain a more accurate volume flow measurement, but this technique is not currently available on commercial ultrasound scanners.

Noncircularity of the vessel lumen

The calculation of cross-sectional area from the diameter measurement assumes that the vessel lumen is circular, which may not be the case, especially in the presence of disease.

Errors in measuring TAV

Incomplete insonation of the vessel will lead to an underestimation of the proportion of slower moving blood at the vessel wall, which in turn will lead to errors in the mean velocity measurements. For example, if a Doppler recording is obtained from a vessel with parabolic flow using a narrow beam (as shown in Fig. 6.2A and B), the high-velocity flow in the center of the vessel will be adequately sampled, but a large proportion of the slower moving blood at the vessel wall will not be detected. When the mean velocity is calculated from the spectra, this will be an overestimate of the true mean velocity due to the undersampling of the flow at the lateral edges of the vessel. This is true even if the sample volume is set to cover the near and far walls of the vessel as the out-of-imaging plane flow will not be sampled. Incomplete insonation of the vessel can lead to errors of up to 30% in the TAV (Evans & McDicken 2000).

Alternatively, the mean TAV can be estimated from the maximum TAV if the flow is measured at an adequate distance from geometric changes (e.g., bifurcations or stenosis) and the shape of the flow profile in the vessel is known. If there is a blunt flow, the maximum velocity will be equal to the mean velocity across the vessel. However, if the velocity is parabolic then the maximum velocity will be twice the value of the mean. One advantage of the maximum velocity measurement is that it is not affected by the width of the beam, provided the beam passes through the center of the vessel.

If the wall thump filter is set too high, the low-frequency signals from the slower moving flow will be removed, and this would lead to an overestimate in the mean velocity. Aliasing would lead to underestimation of the mean velocity due to the incorrect estimation of the high frequencies present within the signal. The presence of high-amplitude noise will bias the estimate of the mean velocity,

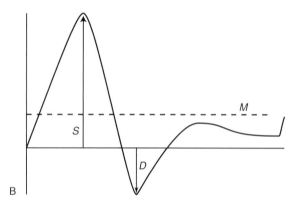

Figure 6.9 Pulsatility index (A & B) and resistance index (A) can be calculated from the peak systolic, S, minimum diastolic, D, end diastolic, E, and the mean velocity (or frequency), M, shown here on two different waveforms.

as the Doppler system is unable to differentiate between the noise and the Doppler signals.

WAVEFORM ANALYSIS

As well as the blood velocity and flow changing with the presence of significant disease, the shape of the waveform will also be altered (as discussed in Ch. 5). The waveform may indicate whether the disease is proximal or distal to the site at which the Doppler signal is obtained. Over the years, several researchers have attempted to quantify these changes in waveform shape by defining various indices, and many modern scanners incorporate facilities to calculate such quantities, some of which are listed below.

Pulsatility index

The pulsatility index (PI) is probably the most commonly used of all the indices. It can be used to

quantify the degree of pulse wave damping at different measurement sites. It is defined as the maximum height of the waveform, S, minus the minimum diastolic, D (which may be negative), divided by the mean height, M, as shown in Figure 6.9A and B:

$$PI = \frac{S - D}{M} \qquad (6.4)$$

Damped flow beyond significant disease will have a lower PI value than a normal pulsatile waveform.

Pourcelot's resistance index

The resistance index (RI) was first used on common carotid waveforms as an indicator of the peripheral resistance and has also been used to study neonatal cerebral hemodynamics. It is defined as follows (Fig. 6.8A):

$$RI = \frac{S - E}{S} \qquad (6.5)$$

where E is end diastolic velocity. The value of RI can be calculated by the scanner and displayed on the screen.

Spectral broadening

There have been several definitions of spectral broadening (SB) described over the years in an attempt to quantify the spread of frequencies present within a spectrum. One such definition is as follows:

$$SB = \frac{f_{max} - f_{min}}{f_{max}} \qquad (6.6)$$

Increased SB indicates the presence of arterial disease but can, to some extent, also be introduced by the scanner itself, as in ISB (described above).

Pulse wave velocity

The pressure pulse and the associated velocity wave travel along the vessel at a different speed from the flowing blood. The speed at which the pulse is transmitted along the vessel depends on the elasticity of the vessel wall. For example, the pulse will travel much faster down the stiff-walled artery of a

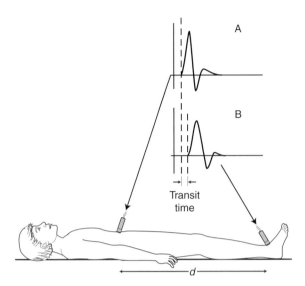

Figure 6.10   The pulse wave velocity can be calculated using two transducers at a distance '*d*' apart along the vessel and measuring the transit time of the pulse.

diabetic patient than down the normal artery of a younger person. The pulse wave velocity of a pulse can be measured using two Doppler transducers to detect the transit time of the pulse along a known length of vessel. The transit time is given by the delay in the beginning of the pulse detected distally compared with that detected by the proximally positioned transducer (Fig. 6.10). The pulse wave velocity is given by the distance along the vessel between the two transducers divided by the transit time. Measurement of the pulse wave velocity has been used by researchers to study vessel wall elasticity changes (e.g., with age or diabetes).

Subjective interpretation

Subjective interpretation of the Doppler spectrum can give many clues as to the level and extent of any disease. For example, changes in the pulsatility of the waveform shape can help to identify disease. The systolic rise time of the waveform is influenced by changes in the cardiac impulse and circulation proximal to the measurement site, whereas the decay of the velocity tends to relate to the distal circulation. Even if these various indices are not quantified, understanding the concept behind them can help when interpreting waveform shapes.

References

Evans D H, McDicken W N 2000 Doppler ultrasound: physics, instrumentation, and signal processing. Wiley, Chichester

Thrush A J, Evans D H 1995 Intrinsic spectral broadening: a potential cause of misdiagnosis of carotid artery disease. Journal of Vascular Investigation 1(4):187–192

Chapter 7

Optimizing the scan

CHAPTER CONTENTS

Introduction   75
The patient   76
Starting the scan   76
B-mode controls   76
Imaging artifacts   76
Color Doppler controls   78
  Color pulse repetition frequency   78
  Color box angle and size   79
Color imaging artifacts   80
Spectral Doppler optimization   81
Repetitive strain injury and occupational
  hazards   82
Safety of diagnostic ultrasound   82
  Ultrasound intensity   82
  Mechanical and thermal indices   82
  User's responsibility   83
  Infection control   83

INTRODUCTION

The preceding chapters have covered some of the basic scientific principles behind ultrasound, the Doppler effect and hemodynamics. The sonographer should now have a clearer understanding of how a B-mode image is created and how color flow imaging can be used to rapidly interrogate blood flow in vessels, allowing the blood flow in selected areas to be assessed with spectral Doppler. This has made duplex scanning a powerful technique for the investigation of patients with vascular diseases, and many vascular surgeons are making clinical decisions on the basis of duplex scanning alone. It is therefore vitally important that the operator understands the use of the scanner controls and the limitations of the technique. Some manufacturers have introduced auto-optimization controls, but there are still many situations in which the controls will need to be adjusted manually. Manufacturers often use different names or terms for the same scanner control or function, such as power imaging and color angiography, both of which relate to power Doppler imaging. It is important to consult the operator's manual or ask the manufacturer if the function of any control is not clear.

Contemporary duplex scanners have a range of examination-specific presets that optimize the system for a particular examination. However, in many instances the scanner controls need adjusting, or optimizing, to demonstrate pathology. In addition, a number of imaging and Doppler artifacts may be confused or misinterpreted as significant disease, leading to serious diagnostic errors. The aim of this chapter is to introduce the sonographer to the practical aspects of scanning, covering the basic use of scanner controls and reiterating some of the principles discussed in the preceding chapters. Imaging artifacts will also be discussed to assist the sonographer in the interpretation of images. It is likewise essential that the sonographer has a good understanding of the principles relating to ultrasound safety in order to minimize any exposure risks to the patient.

THE PATIENT

It is an ironic fact that a sonographer may use a state of the art duplex scanner but fail to obtain any useful diagnostic information because of an inadequate approach to the examination and the patient. For example, an introduction and simple explanation of the test may put patients more at ease and willing to cooperate, especially if they are nervous or in some discomfort. Local protocols that are rigid and do not allow any flexibility can also lead to problems. For example, a protocol that requires that patients always be completely flat with the head fully extended during carotid scans may lead to severe discomfort for patients with breathing difficulties, dizziness, angina or spondylosis of the neck. It is possible they will not be able to tolerate the examination at all. An alternative would be to perform the scan with the patient sitting up on a low chair. It is still possible to obtain good images from this scanning position. Most problems can be solved with a little careful thought and the occasional inventive approach.

STARTING THE SCAN

The scan should be carried out in a dimly lit room to optimize visualization of the black and white image. The transducer selected should be of the highest frequency that allows adequate penetration to the area to be examined. Most duplex systems use a broad-band transducer, and some allow the sonographer to alter the imaging, color and spectral Doppler transmit frequencies to optimize the image or enable better penetration. When scanning, it is important to adopt a logical approach. Using a systematic technique cuts down on examination time and ensures that pathology is less likely to be missed. The scan is best started by examining the region of

interest with B-mode imaging alone, to identify relevant structures. In general, a cross-sectional survey should be performed before a longitudinal scan as this helps to relate structures to each other. Avoid switching on the color flow or spectral Doppler straight away, unless they are essential for identifying vessels, as the imaging frame rate will be reduced and the display may be confusing if anatomy has not been clearly identified.

B-MODE CONTROLS

Always set the focal zones at the depth of interest on the scan image. B-mode frame rates of modern scanners are generally high even when multiple focus zones have been selected, but reducing the number of focal zones will increase the frame rate even further. If the region of interest in the B-mode image is very small, or very deep, consider using the zoom control to magnify the area. This will improve the frame rate. Scanners usually allow the operator to adjust the size and position of the area to be magnified. Most systems have a write zoom facility that will improve image resolution. Many vascular sonographers prefer B-mode images with a reasonable degree of contrast using a lower dynamic range. Duplex systems have examination-specific presets that are optimized to produce the best images of vascular structures. It is also worthwhile experimenting with different pre- and post-processing controls in order to understand the function of these controls. Try this when imaging a carotid plaque and note the difference in the appearance of the image. Optimize the total gain and depth gain compensation sliders so that the returning echoes are of relatively uniform intensity throughout the image. In general, the gain should be set so that the lumen of any large nondiseased vessel appears clear or black but any further increase in gain would introduce noise or speckle. Harmonic imaging can be especially useful in the abdomen and may produce clearer and less noisy images. The use of compound imaging, if available, may also improve the overall image.

IMAGING ARTIFACTS

An imaging artifact is a feature on the image that does not relate exactly to a structure within the

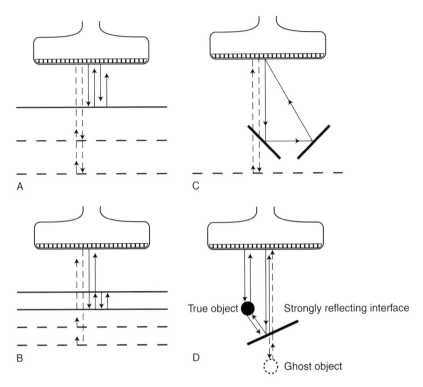

True object ● │ Strongly reflecting interface

B D

Ghost object

Figure 7.1 Imaging artefacts can be produced by multiple reflections from strongly reflecting surfaces. The solid line shows the true path of the ultrasound beam. The dashed lines show the path of the beam assumed by the ultrasound scanner and the assumed interfaces displayed on the ultrasound images. A: Multiple reflections between the transducer and a strongly reflecting boundary. B: Multiple reflections between two parallel, strongly reflecting surfaces. C: Multiple reflections not returning along the same path. D: Mirror image produced in the presence of a strongly reflecting surface.

tissue being investigated. This can be due to a feature being misplaced on the image, a feature appearing that is not present within the tissue or an existing structure that is absent from the image. The creation of an image relies on the assumption that the ultrasound beam travels in a straight path between the transducer and the structures within the tissue and returns along the same path once reflected. It is also assumed that the attenuation of tissue is constant. Any process that alters this situation can lead to the misplacement or absence of information. This can be caused by the following:

- Multiple reflections can lead to reverberation artifacts, seen as several equidistant echoes that reduce in brightness with depth. This is due to multiple reflections, along the same path, between the transducer and a strongly reflecting boundary (Fig. 7.1A) or between two parallel, strongly reflecting surfaces (Fig. 7.1B). If the multiple reflections do not return along the same path, the structure may be misplaced on the image (Fig. 7.1C).
- A mirror image of a structure can be produced in the presence of a strongly reflecting surface.

Figure 7.1D shows how the true position of a structure is displayed, with a second ghost image also displayed. The ghost image has been detected by an ultrasound beam that has undergone multiple reflection from the strongly reflecting surface.

- Refraction can lead to bending of the path of the ultrasound when the beam passes through an interface between two media in which the speed of sound is significantly different (see Fig. 2.7).
- Range ambiguity can occur if an echo from the previously transmitted pulse is received back from a distant boundary after the current ultrasound pulse has been transmitted. The scanner will assume that the echo is from the current pulse and place it nearer to the top of the image rather than at its true depth.
- Grating lobes are areas of lower intensity ultrasound outside the main beam and are produced as a function of the multi-element structure of array transducers. These grating lobes can lead to strongly reflecting surfaces outside the main beam being displayed in the image.

Figure 7.2   An image showing how an artefact (arrow) can give the impression of a dissection or tear, of the carotid artery wall.

Figure 7.3   Differences in attenuation can be observed in this image of a synthetic bypass graft. The graft has spaced external supporting rings that are causing increased attenuation in the tissue lying below the rings (arrows).

The image in Figure 7.2 shows how an artifact can give the appearance of a dissection, or tear, of the carotid artery wall. If an artifact is suspected, the vessel should be imaged in different planes or from different angles. The artifact may then appear in a different position relative to the vessel or may not appear at all, confirming that it is not a true structure that has been visualized. It is usually easier to identify artifacts in real-time imaging than on a frozen image. If there is a significant difference in the attenuation seen by different scan lines, the tissue at depth may appear as different levels of gray, despite having similar backscatter properties (Fig. 7.3). For example, the tissue beneath a low-attenuation, anechoic region, such as a cyst, may appear brighter than adjacent areas. Highly attenuating tissue, however, such as calcified plaque, can cause loss of ultrasound information beneath the region, leading to a shadow (see Fig. 9.12).

COLOR DOPPLER CONTROLS
Color pulse repetition frequency

The pulse repetition frequency (PRF) should be adjusted to optimize the image of the blood flow in the vessel under examination. Many duplex systems display the value of the PRF in Hz. However, some systems only indicate the PRF as a mean velocity on the color bar, in cm/s, or specify the sampling rate as high-, medium- or low-velocity flow. The examination preset selects a nominal PRF to start a specific examination. The PRF is generally set moderately high for sampling normal arterial flow, typically a PRF of 3000–4000 Hz, so that the peak systolic phase of the cardiac cycle appears in the upper portion of the color scale without aliasing, as demonstrated in Figure 4.9B. If the PRF is set too low, aliasing will be demonstrated in a normal vessel during the peak systolic phase, making it more difficult to identify areas of true flow disturbance. If the PRF is set too high, the peak systolic phase of the cardiac cycle will appear in the lower region of the color scale, flow changes will be less well differentiated on the image and minor flow disturbances could be overlooked. Low-velocity flow in diastole may also go undetected.

In situations in which there is significant pathology, the flow velocities may be much lower than normal. For example, the flow velocities in a calf artery distal to a long superficial femoral and popliteal artery occlusion may be very low. Using a default PRF setting of 3000 Hz may not adequately demonstrate the low-velocity flow in the patent calf artery because the sampling rate is too high (Fig. 7.4). The PRF should be lowered to demonstrate the low-velocity flow, showing the systolic phase in the upper part of the color scale (Fig. 7.4C). An alternative technique to altering the PRF to optimize the flow display is to change the position of

A   B   C

Figure 7.4   A: Poor color filling is seen in the posterior tibial artery distal to a long arterial occlusion because the PRF is set too high at 2500 Hz, and the color controls have not been optimized. B: The Doppler waveform confirms low-velocity damped flow with a peak systolic velocity of 10 cm/s. C: In order to improve the color flow display, the PRF has been lowered to 1000 Hz, the color write priority increased and the color sensitivity control increased. Note that only 79% color gain is needed in image C, compared to 85% in image A.

the color baseline to either extend or decrease the range of velocities displayed in one direction. By optimizing the PRF for the flow velocities present in a vessel, it is possible to investigate longer segments of an artery using color flow imaging, reducing the amount of time spent taking spectral Doppler measurements, provided that the color display remains unchanged. Color aliasing is an artifact rather than the representation of a true change in flow direction. If a vessel changes direction it can result in a change in insonation angle (and thus to detected frequency), leading to a change in color. In this situation, angle-corrected spectral Doppler should be used to record the flow velocities in the vessel, to confirm the absence of a stenosis, as the peak systolic velocity should remain the same despite the change in vessel direction.

The flow velocities recorded in the venous system are lower than those recorded in the arterial system and therefore the PRF will have to be lowered. A PRF setting of 1000 Hz is a typical starting value for many venous examinations. Most ultrasound systems link the high-pass filter to the PRF, and in most examinations there may be little need to make any adjustments to the filter setting. However, in situations in which there may be very low-velocity flow, such as that found in a suboccluded internal carotid artery, the filter should be lowered as far as possible to avoid missing the flow. Conversely, the color filter can be increased to cut out the low-frequency noise, such as that produced by bowel movement seen when scanning

the iliac arteries. In practice, many experienced sonographers can cope with additional color noise in the image.

Color box angle and size

When using linear array transducers it is possible to steer the color box to the left or right by 20° to 25° depending on the system. It is therefore possible to optimize the color box angle to the flow direction in order to obtain the highest Doppler shift frequencies. Inexperienced sonographers often find this one of the most confusing aspects of duplex scanning when learning color Doppler techniques, and it may be a case of trial and error to get used to optimizing the color image. Areas of poor filling in the image may be caused by a poor angle of insonation, preventing the signal from being detected. It may be necessary to image a vessel with the color box steered in more than one direction in order to demonstrate flow in all parts of the vessel (Fig. 7.5). For curvilinear array transducers, it is necessary to optimize the transducer position and the position of the color box in the sector display to obtain suitable Doppler angles. An example is shown in Figure 9.8B.

It is important to keep the color box size reasonably small and to keep the area of interest within it by adjusting the color box or transducer position. Increasing the color box width means that more time is spent producing the color flow image, and consequently the imaging frame rate will decrease.

Figure 7.5   Images of a carotid artery showing how a vessel may need to be imaged with the color box steered in more than one direction to demonstrate flow in the whole vessel.

This is less of a problem in modern duplex systems. As the time taken to produce an image lengthens, especially when imaging with a large color box or at depth, a time delay may be introduced between the signals detected from different sides of the image. This can result in the color image displaying flow detected at different parts of the cardiac cycle. For example, both end diastolic and peak systolic flow in a vessel may be displayed on different sides of the image. Many systems have a control for increasing the color sensitivity, which increases the number of pulses sent down each scan line. This can improve the color image but decreases the overall frame rate. In certain situations, pulsatile low-volume flow in a vessel may be seen as a brief flash of color on the image, and it may be difficult to follow the vessel. Increasing the color persistence will display the color in the vessel for a longer period of time and can make the vessel easier to follow. The color write priority control can be adjusted to write color on an image where a high B-mode gain is necessary (see below).

COLOR IMAGING ARTIFACTS

Color flow imaging artifacts can lead to failure to display flow when, in fact, it is present, as shown in Figure 7.5. A bright black and white imaging artifact (as seen in Fig. 7.2) may be displayed in preference to the color flow information, and this may give the appearance of a structure within the vessel lumen, around which the flow is displayed. If the color write priority is set too low in the presence of a noisy black and white image, flow detected may not be displayed due to the lack of a clear vessel lumen. Giving priority to the color flow imaging means that the B-mode image can be reasonably bright without losing color information on the screen.

A strongly reflective surface can lead to the loss of ultrasound signals beyond the interface. For example, calcification within the vessel wall or the presence of bowel gas can produce shadowing on both the black and white image and color flow image and will prevent spectral Doppler recordings (see Fig. 8.26).

Artifacts can also be introduced into the color image whereby color is displayed when blood flow is not present. This can occur when the color gain is set too high, giving the appearance of the color 'bleeding' out of the vessel (Fig. 7.6). Alternatively, anechoic areas can be filled with speckled color due to noise, if the gain is set high or if there is low-velocity tissue motion present (e.g., due to respiration). Tissue bruits (e.g., near a stenosis) may result in color appearing outside the vessel wall (see Fig. 11.18A).

Multiple reflection can produce color image artifacts. Figure 7.7 shows a mirror image of the subclavian artery produced by multiple reflections from the pleura overlying the lung. This mirror image artifact can be seen where a vessel overlies a strongly reflecting surface, such as the tissue–air interface present at the pleura. The tibial vessels or

Figure 7.6   The color flow image may give the impression of flow 'bleeding out' of the vessel if the color gain is set too high (arrow shows position of posterior artery wall).

Figure 7.7   Color image of the subclavian artery (S) with a mirror image (M) below the pleura (P).

bypass grafts may also suffer from this artifact when lying above bone. The path of the reflected ultrasound that has undergone multiple reflections is different from that of the ultrasound back-scattered directly from the blood to the transducer. Therefore, the Doppler shift frequency detected

and displayed for the mirror image may not be the same as for the vessel itself. The artifactual Doppler signal displayed on the color image can also be detected with spectral Doppler, if the sample volume is placed over the mirror image.

The color image may not give a true representation of the relative blood velocities within the vessel. Changes in the angle of insonation, owing to changes in vessel direction, can lead to color imaging artifacts, giving the false impression of changes in blood velocity (see Fig. 4.7). Aliasing artifacts will also change the appearance of the color image (see Figs 4.9A and 4.11).

SPECTRAL DOPPLER OPTIMIZATION

The spectral Doppler PRF should be set to avoid aliasing and the high-pass filter should be set to remove wall thump but not useful Doppler signals. The spectral Doppler PRF may be referred to as 'scale' or 'flow rate' on some systems. The selection of the size of the sample volume is an important consideration. If detailed investigation of flow within a stenosis is to be performed, a small sample volume is required. The sample volume should be placed in the center of the vessel or at the point of maximum velocity indicated by the color image. However, if the presence of flow within a vein is to be detected, a large sample volume may be more appropriate. The issue of spectral Doppler angle correction remains a contentious subject. Some units insist that all measurements be taken with the cursor lined up with the direction of flow at a fixed angle of 60° whereas other departments use the smallest angle of insonation possible (see Ch. 6). In practice, the decision on which technique to use may be dictated by local protocols. The position of the angle correction cursor should be carefully lined up with the vessel wall, or the direction of blood flow, to minimize angle-related errors. There are three possible reasons why a Doppler signal may be displayed both above and below the baseline, and the sonographer should be able to identify these:

- aliasing (see Fig. 3.14A)
- mirroring due to the gain being set too high (see Fig. 6.3)
- flow reversal during the cardiac cycle (see Fig. 5.8).

REPETITIVE STRAIN INJURY AND OCCUPATIONAL HAZARDS

Sonographers are at high risk of developing occupational injuries due to prolonged periods of bad posture during ultrasound examinations. Back problems and repetitive strain injuries of the wrist and shoulder are increasingly common. To minimize the risk it is essential that vascular ultrasound units be equipped with variable height examination tables that have adjustable upper and lower sections. Ideally, it should be possible to tilt the table, especially for venous examinations. The operator's chair should have a variable height adjustment, adjustable back rest and swivel capability. Sonographers should vary the workload and types of scans performed during the day and take regular breaks. The ability to scan with either hand also reduces strain on one side. The probe should not be gripped too hard, and excessive pressure should not be used to make contact between the patient and the probe. Most vascular examinations can be performed with relatively light probe contact. If the sonographer develops problems, these should be treated at an early stage as long-term chronic problems may be difficult to resolve. Care should be taken when moving apparatus around the hospital, as it is easy to strain muscles, trap hands between the scanner and door frames or run over toes.

SAFETY OF DIAGNOSTIC ULTRASOUND

During the scan, the patient is exposed to ultrasound energy, and it is therefore important that the sonographer be aware of the possible risks and how to minimize them. Over the years there has been a steady increase in the output power generated by ultrasound systems. The potential risks have been regularly assessed by various safety committees, including that of the World Federation of Ultrasound in Medicine and Biology (WFUMB 1998). Information on safety issues can be found on the website of the European Federation of Societies for Ultrasound in Medicine and Biology (EFSUMB 2002). The British Medical Ultrasound Society has also produced a statement on the safe use and potential hazards of diagnostic ultrasound equipment (BMUS Safety Group 2002).

Table 7.1 The upper limits of exposure required by the United States Food and Drug Administration

Application	Derated I_{spta} (mW cm^2)	Derated I_{sppa} (W cm^2)	MI	TI
All except ophthalmology	720	190	1.9	(6.0)*
Ophthalmology	50	NS	0.23	1.0

*The upper limit of 6.0 is advisory. At least one of the quantities MI and I_{sppa} must be less than the specified limit. NS: not specified.

It is believed that the two main potential risks of tissue damage due to ultrasound exposure are tissue heating and cavitation. Cavitation refers to the formation, growth, oscillation and violent collapse of small, gas-filled cavities within the ultrasound beam. Inertial cavitation—that is, large variation in size and possible violent collapse of bubbles—occurs above a threshold of negative acoustic pressure (Duck & Shaw 2003).

Ultrasound intensity

The intensity is the energy crossing a unit area (usually 1 cm^2) in unit time. The spatial peak temporal average intensity, I_{spta}, is the peak within the beam averaged over time. Another value of intensity that is used is the spatial peak pulse average intensity, I_{sppa}, which is the spatial peak intensity averaged over the duration of the pulse. These have been used by the Food and Drug Administration (FDA) in the United States to define the upper limit of exposure produced by ultrasound systems for diagnostic use (Table 7.1). Manufacturers often supply data on the maximum I_{spta} and I_{sppa} in the operator's manual.

Mechanical and thermal indices

The output power produced by a system will vary with the modality used and the control settings. So that the ultrasound user can be aware of the potential risks of any given scanner set-up, two new, potentially more meaningful indices have been developed. These are the thermal index (TI) and the mechanical index (MI). These indices are displayed on the screen of modern scanners in real time and will demonstrate any changes in the potential risk as the scanner modalities or controls are altered.

The TI has been developed to indicate the potential risk of producing thermal effects during the scan. It is the ratio of acoustic power emitted at the time to the power required to heat the tissue by $1°C$. A TI of 1 would therefore indicate the potential to heat the tissue in the beam by $1°C$. A TI of 2 indicates a potential rise of $2°C$, and so forth. An ultrasound exposure that does not produce a temperature rise of greater than $1.5°C$ above normal body temperature of $37°C$ is not thought to pose any risk of producing thermal damage. The power required to heat the tissue will depend greatly on what tissue is lying in the path of the ultrasound beam and is especially affected by the presence of bone, as bone is a strongly absorbing medium. For this reason, three models for the TI have been developed:

- soft tissue (TIS)
- tissue with bone present at the focus (TIB)
- the cranial thermal index (TIC), used in transcranial Doppler.

The appropriate TI should be displayed depending on the scanner examination set-up selected. The development of these indices suffers from some limitations, as it is not straightforward to estimate the heat lost from the various regions of the body that are scanned.

The mechanical index (MI) indicates the likelihood of the onset of inertial cavitation. It is related to the peak negative pressure of the ultrasound pulses being used at the time. For an MI <0.7, the physical conditions probably cannot exist for bubble growth and collapse to occur (Duck & Shaw 2003). However, if this threshold is exceeded, it does not mean that bioeffects due to cavitation will occur. The higher the value of MI above this threshold, the greater the potential risk. There is currently no evidence that diagnostic ultrasound causes cavitation in the soft tissue, except in the presence of gas, such as in the lung and intestines, and in the presence of contrast agents.

Another potential thermal hazard that the sonographer should be aware of is heating of the transducer itself, which may occur if the transducer has been damaged. Malfunction of the scanner may potentially lead to a higher than expected output power.

User's responsibility

Diagnostic ultrasound has been used for many years with no reported evidence of harmful effects. However, it is prudent to keep patient exposure to the minimum required to obtain an optimal diagnostic result. This can be done by keeping the time of the examination of a particular area to a minimum, especially when using color and spectral Doppler ultrasound, as these modes are more likely to cause heating. Controls such as the gain should be optimized before increasing the output power. Changes in the TI and MI with changes in scanner set-up should be monitored. It is important to keep up-to-date with current guidelines on the safe use of diagnostic ultrasound (BMUS Safety Group 2000, EFSUMB).

Probably the biggest risk of ultrasound is misdiagnosis, and it is therefore important to obtain an adequate scan. The sonographer should be aware of new technologies and new developments in scanning techniques. If the sonographer is in any doubt of the result at the end of the scan, the limitations of the scan should be reported.

Infection control

Cross-infection of patients by the ultrasound transducer is a possible risk, therefore the transducer should be cleaned between each examination. The front face of transducers can be made of delicate material and the use of strong cleaning fluids is often not recommended. Consult the operating manual or manufacturer for advice on suitable cleaning procedures. The best method to overcome this problem, when there is a known risk, is to use a disposable probe cover. If the scan is to be performed near an open wound, a sterile probe cover and sterile gel should be used. Alternatively, a sterile transparent plastic dressing may be used to cover the wound, ensuring no air bubbles are trapped under the dressing that would prevent imaging. Disposable gloves should always be worn if scanning infected or discharging regions.

References

Duck F A, Shaw A 2003 Safety of diagnostic ultrasound. In: Hoskins P R, Thrush A, Martin K, Whittingham T A (eds) Diagnostic ultrasound: physics and instrumentation. Greenwich Medical Media, London, pp 179–203

BMUS Safety Group 2000 British Medical Ultrasound Society Statement on the safe use, and potential hazards of diagnostic ultrasound www.bmus.org

EFSUMB 2002 Clinical safety statement for diagnostic ultrasound (2002) www.efsumb.org/safstat.htm

WFUMB 1998 Conclusions and recommendations on the thermal and non-thermal mechanisms for biological effects. Ultrasound in Medicine and Biology 24(Suppl 1):xv–xvi

Further reading

ter Harr G, Duck F A (eds) 2000 The safe use of ultrasound in medical diagnosis. BMUS/BIR, London

European Committee for Medical Ultrasound Safety (ECMUS) Tutorials on behalf of the European Federation for Societies of Ultrasound in Medicine and Biology (EFSUMB) www.efsumb.org/ecmus.htm

Chapter 8

Ultrasound assessment of the extracranial cerebral circulation

CHAPTER CONTENTS

Introduction 85
Anatomy 86
  Collateral pathways and anatomical
    variants 86
Possible symptoms of carotid and vertebral artery
  disease 88
Scanning 88
  Objectives and preparation 88
  Technique 89
B-mode imaging 93
  Normal appearance 93
  Abnormal appearance 93
Color imaging 95
  Normal appearance 95
  Abnormal appearance 95
Spectral Doppler waveforms 96
  Normal appearance 96
  Abnormal appearance 96
Grading the disease 97
  Imaging 98
  Spectral Doppler 100
Combining B-mode, color imaging and
  spectral Doppler information 102
Normal and abnormal appearances of vertebral
  artery flow 103
Problems encountered in imaging carotid artery
  flow 103
  Calcified atheroma 103
  Vessel tortuosity 104
Postoperative and post-angioplasty carotid artery
  appearance on ultrasound 105
Nonatheromatous carotid artery diseases 105
Transcranial Doppler ultrasound 106
Reporting 107

INTRODUCTION

Ultrasound can be used to evaluate the extracranial cerebral circulation in order to investigate patients who may be at risk of suffering a stroke or who have already suffered a stroke. Stroke is the third most common cause of death in the United Kingdom, with the stroke rate being approximately 2 in 1000 of the population per year. Approximately 80% of strokes are ischemic (i.e., thrombotic or embolic or both) as opposed to hemorrhagic. Up to 80% of ischemic strokes occur in the carotid territory, the area of the brain supplied by the carotid arteries. Recent trials have shown that patients with significant carotid artery disease and relevant symptoms may benefit from surgery in order to prevent a stroke. The majority of carotid artery disease develops at the carotid bifurcation, and in the presence of a significant stenosis, carotid endarterectomy can be performed. In this procedure, the diseased inner wall of the artery, the plaque, is removed, thus eliminating a potential source of emboli or flow-limiting stenosis. Carotid ultrasound examinations can be used to screen patients for carotid artery disease before further investigation with angiography. Alternatively, many centers now use ultrasound examination to select patients directly for surgery, without preoperative angiography, as angiography is known to carry its own risks of transient and permanent neurological deficit. Developments in magnetic resonance angiography (MRA) may make this a safer alternative to x-ray angiography for confirming ultrasound findings prior to surgery or for further investigations, when ultrasound has provided only limited results.

ANATOMY

The brain is supplied by four vessels—the right and left internal carotid and vertebral arteries—and receives 15% of the cardiac output. The term extra-cranial cerebral arteries refers to all the arteries that carry blood from the heart up to the base of the skull. The left and right sides of the extracranial circulation are not symmetrical (Fig. 8.1). On the left side, the common carotid (CCA) and subclavian arteries arise directly from the aortic arch, whereas on the right side the brachiocephalic artery, also known as the innominate artery, arises from the aorta and divides into the subclavian artery and CCA. The CCA, which has no branches, divides into the internal and external carotid arteries, but the level of the carotid bifurcation in the neck is highly variable. In approximately 90% of cases, the internal carotid artery (ICA) lies posterolateral or lateral to the external carotid artery (ECA) and, unlike the ECA, has no branches below the skull. The proximal branches of the ECA are the superior thyroid, lingual, facial and maxillary arteries. The carotid artery widens, at the level of the bifurcation, to form the carotid bulb. In some cases, the carotid bulb may only involve the proximal ICA, and not the distal CCA, and the degree of widening of the carotid bulb is quite variable. Within the skull, the distal segment of the ICA follows a curved path, known as the carotid siphon. The most important branch of the ICA is the ophthalmic artery, which supplies the eye. The terminal branches of the ophthalmic artery, the supratrochlear and supraorbital

arteries, unite with the terminal branches of the ECA. The ICA finally divides into the middle cerebral artery (MCA) and the anterior cerebral artery (ACA).

The posterior circulation of the brain is mainly supplied by the left and right vertebral arteries, via the basilar artery. The vertebral artery is the first branch of the subclavian artery, arising from the highest point of the subclavian arch. At the sixth cervical vertebra, the vertebral artery runs posteriorly to travel upward through the transverse foramen of the cervical vertebrae. It is common for one vertebral artery to be larger than the other, with the left often being larger than the right. The two vertebral arteries join, at the base of the skull, to form the basilar artery, which then divides to form the posterior cerebral arteries. Figure 8.2A shows how the circle of Willis, situated at the base of the brain, joins the cerebral branches of the ICAs and basilar artery via the anterior and posterior communicating arteries. Blood flow to the brain is regulated by changes in cerebrovascular resistance, with carbon dioxide playing a major role in vasodilation.

Collateral pathways and anatomical variants

In the presence of severe vascular disease, the cerebral circulation has many possible collateral (alternative) pathways, both extracranially and intracranially. Not all of these can be assessed using ultrasound; however, two pathways that can be assessed are the following:

- *The ophthalmic artery.* The ECAs do not normally supply blood to the brain, but in the presence of severe ICA disease, branches of the ECA can act as important collateral pathways. One important collateral pathway is via the terminal branches of the ECA, communicating with the terminal branches of the ophthalmic artery. This collateral pathway can be observed using continuous wave (CW) Doppler to detect reversal of flow in the supraorbital artery, a terminal branch of the ophthalmic artery, as retrograde flow travels from the ECA branches toward the brain.

- *The circle of Willis.* In the normal circulation, there is little blood flow through the communicating arteries in the circle of Willis, but in the presence

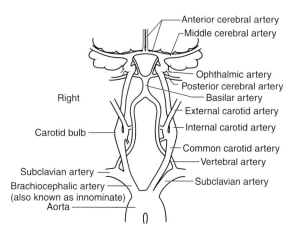

Figure 8.1 Diagram of cerebrovascular anatomy.

of severe vascular disease they perform an important role in flow distribution. For example, in the presence of a left ICA occlusion, it is possible for the right ICA to supply blood flow to the left MCA via the right ACA, the anterior communicating artery and the left ACA, with flow reversal occurring in the left ACA (Fig. 8.2B).

The vertebral arteries may also supply flow to the MCA via the posterior communicating arteries of the circle of Willis. If the circle is well developed, it is possible for a single extracranial artery to provide adequate cerebral blood flow. However, in about 75% of the population, parts of the circle may be hypoplastic (very small) or absent, making the circle incomplete and therefore preventing the development of good collateral flow (von Reutern &

von Büdingen 1993), but this may only become apparent in the presence of severe disease. Adequate collateral pathways have a better chance to develop in the presence of slowly developing disease.

An unusual collateral pathway can occur when the CCA is occluded and flow in the proximal ECA reverses, being supplied by retrograde flow in an ECA branch, to supply a patent ICA. Severe narrowing or occlusion of the proximal subclavian or brachiocephalic artery can result in a collateral pathway that 'steals' blood from the brain to supply the arm. In this case, blood will be seen to flow retrogradely down the ipsilateral vertebral artery to supply the distal subclavian artery beyond the diseased segment (Fig. 8.3). This is known as subclavian steal syndrome.

There are few variations in the extracranial circulation. In rare cases, the left CCA and subclavian artery may share a common origin or a single trunk. Other anomalies are the left vertebral artery arising directly from the aortic arch and, even more unusually, the right vertebral origin arising from the aortic arch.

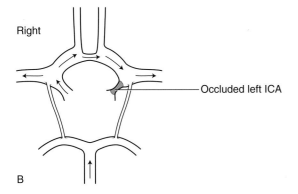

Figure 8.2 Diagram of the circle of Willis. A: Arrows indicate normal flow direction. B: Arrows indicate cross-over flow from the right ICA to the left MCA in the presence of a left ICA occlusion.

Figure 8.3 Arrows indicate the direction of collateral flow in subclavian steal syndrome, via reverse flow in the vertebral artery to supply the arm, in the presence of a severe stenosis or occlusion of the proximal subclavian artery.

POSSIBLE SYMPTOMS OF CAROTID AND VERTEBRAL ARTERY DISEASE

Patients with carotid artery stenosis may suffer from transient ischemic attack (TIA) or amaurosis fugax, a form of visual disturbance. Symptoms of TIA may only last a few minutes and the patient will make a full recovery within 24 hours, whereas patients suffering from a stroke will have symptoms lasting more than 24 hours and may not make a full recovery. Symptoms include single or multiple episodes of loss of power or sensation in an arm or leg (monoparesis), in both (hemiparesis), or in one side of the face; slurring or loss of speech (dysphasia); or visuospatial neglect (Box 8.1). As the right side of the brain controls the left-hand side of the body and the converse, the symptoms will relate to the contralateral carotid artery. The speech is usually controlled by the dominant side of the brain (i.e., a right-handed patient's speech will typically be controlled by the left side of the brain). Patients suffering from episodes of amaurosis fugax often complain of 'a curtain drawing across one eye' lasting for a few minutes, which is due to emboli within the retinal circulation. In this situation, the symptoms in the eye will relate to the ipsilateral carotid artery. Typical vertebrobasilar symptoms are shown in Box 8.1. Vague symptoms, such as dizziness and blackout, are not usually associated with carotid artery disease. Subclavian steal syndrome does not usually cause significant symptoms. Patients with symptoms of TIA are thought to have a risk of stroke of the order of 7–8% per year for the first 2–3 years following a TIA. Patients suffering from crescendo TIA (i.e., very frequent TIA) may require urgent surgery and should be scanned, as a matter of priority, to assess the severity of any carotid disease.

Symptoms similar to TIA can also be caused by other neurological problems, such as epilepsy, intracranial tumor, multiple sclerosis or migraine. Asymptomatic carotid disease is usually discovered clinically by the presence of a carotid bruit, heard as a murmur when listening to the neck with a stethoscope. However, the presence of a carotid bruit may not be due to an ICA stenosis, but could instead relate to an ECA or aortic stenosis or to no stenosis at all. A large proportion of patients with a >70% stenosis will not have a carotid bruit, and therefore its presence or absence is not accurate enough to predict the presence of disease.

Only about 15% of patients suffer symptoms of TIA prior to a stroke. Fifty per cent of ischemic strokes are due to thromboembolism of the ICA or MCA or both, whereas 25% are due to small vessel disease and 15% are due to emboli originating from the heart. Only 1–2% of all strokes are hemodynamic strokes (i.e., due to flow-limiting stenoses) (Naylor et al 1998).

Trauma to the neck can lead to dissection of the carotid artery wall, possibly causing the vessel to occlude. This condition may be suspected in patients suffering a stoke following a neck injury. Ultrasound examination may also be requested in the presence of a pulsatile swelling in the neck to identify the presence of a carotid aneurysm or carotid body tumor, both of which are quite rare.

Box 8.1 Typical carotid territory and vertebrobasilar symptoms (after Naylor et al 1998, with permission)

Typical carotid territory symptoms
- Hemimotor/hemisensory signs
- Monocular visual loss (amaurosis fugax)
- Higher cortical dysfunction (dysphasia— incomplete language function, visuospatial neglect, etc.)

Typical vertebrobasilar symptoms
- Bilateral blindness
- Problems with gait and stance
- Hemi- or bilateral motor/sensory signs
- Dysarthria
- Homonymous hemianopia (loss of visual field in both eyes)
- Diplopia, vertigo and nystagmus (provided it is not the only symptom)

SCANNING

Objectives and preparation

The purpose of the carotid scan is to identify the extent of any atheroma within the CCA and extracranial ICA and ECA and to determine the degree of narrowing of the vessels. The examination should also demonstrate the presence and direction of flow in the vertebral arteries. No specific preparation is required, but the patient must be capable of lying or sitting still during the examination. The optimal position for scanning the carotid arteries is with the sonographer sitting behind the patient's head. This allows easy access to the neck and enables the operator to rest the arm on the examination table while performing the scan (Fig. 8.4). Alternatively the sonographer can sit by the side of the patient while resting the arm on the patient's upper chest. The patient should lie supine on the couch with the head resting on a pillow. The neck should be extended and the head turned in the opposite direction to the side being examined. If the patient has difficulty in breathing or has back problems it may be necessary to sit the patient in a more upright position. If the patient is in a wheelchair (e.g., following a disabling stroke), it may be easier to do the scan in the wheelchair with the head resting on a pillow for support, preventing unnecessary movement of the patient.

The examination can be performed with a medium- to high-frequency (e.g., broad-band 4–7 or 5–12 MHz) flat linear array transducer. The higher the frequency, the better the resolution of the vessel wall structure; however, in some cases the carotid bifurcation lies deep in the neck, requiring a lower frequency transducer for visualization. Blood flow velocities detected in the majority of normal and diseased carotid arteries are reasonably high, so the scanner should be configured to visualize

high-velocity pulsatile flow. Most ultrasound systems have examination presets available that are suitable for the majority of carotid examinations, but it may be necessary to alter these to enable the detection of low-velocity flow when differentiating carotid artery occlusion from a subtotal occlusion. A small spectral Doppler sample volume is usually used to interrogate the carotid arteries, as it allows for more selective investigation of areas of velocity increase or flow disturbance.

Technique

The carotid arteries are best visualized through the sternocleidomastoid muscle, which provides a good ultrasonic window, and this is done using a lateral rather than an anterior approach. The procedure is as follows:

1. Using B-mode imaging only, the CCA should be visualized in transverse section (Fig. 8.5A), starting at the base of the neck. On the right side, it is usually possible to visualize the distal brachiocephalic artery and the origin of the CCA and subclavian arteries. On the left side, the origin of the CCA cannot be visualized as it lies too deep in the chest. The CCA should be scanned along its length, in transverse section, up to the bifurcation, and along the ICA and ECA (Fig. 8.5B) as high up the neck as can be seen. This allows the sonographer to ascertain the level and orientation of the carotid bifurcation and also gives the first indications of the presence and location of any arterial disease. The jugular vein lies over the CCA (Fig. 8.5A) and is usually easily compressed. However, it is important not to apply too much transducer pressure when scanning the carotid arteries as there is a possibility of dislodging an embolus from the vessel wall.

2. The CCA is now visualized in longitudinal section using B-mode imaging, starting at the base of the neck. A longitudinal image of the CCA can be easily obtained by imaging the CCA in transverse section and then, keeping the CCA in the center of the image, rotating the probe so the CCA first appears as an ellipse and finally can be seen in longitudinal section. Prior knowledge of the orientation of the ICA and ECA

Figure 8.4 The optimal position for scanning the carotid arteries.

A   B

Figure 8.5 Transverse B-mode images. A: CCA and jugular vein. B: The ICA and ECA just above the carotid bifurcation.

Figure 8.6 Longitudinal scan planes used to visualize the carotid arteries. A: Posterior. B: Lateral. C: Anterior.

Figure 8.7 Longitudinal B-mode image of the carotid bifurcation with the ICA and ECA seen in the same plane. The arrows mark where the intima-media layer can be seen.

gained from transverse imaging is helpful for locating the correct longitudinal imaging plane to view the bifurcation. It is necessary to use a range of longitudinal scan planes to visualize the carotid arteries, especially at the bifurcation (Fig. 8.6). Typically, the ICA lies posterolateral or lateral to the ECA and is usually the larger of the two vessels. In a small percentage of cases, the bifurcation will appear as a tuning fork arrangement (Fig. 8.7), but in the majority of cases the ECA and ICA will not be seen in the

same plane and will have to be imaged individually. This is achieved by keeping the lower portion of the probe face over the CCA and slowly rotating the upper portion through a small angle to image first the ICA and then the ECA, or vice versa. Only small probe movements are required when imaging the ICA and ECA, as the vessels usually lie close together.

3. Having located the three vessels and observed any evidence of disease in the B-mode image, color flow imaging can be used to investigate

Figure 8.8 B-mode image of the ECA showing the superior thyroid branch (arrow).

A

B

C

Figure 8.9 Typical normal Doppler spectra obtained from the CCA (A), the ICA (B) and the ECA (C). The effect of temporal tapping on ECA diastolic flow is marked with arrows.

the flow from the proximal CCA up into the ICA and ECA. Identification of ECA branches (either on B-mode or color imaging) serves as a further indication as to which vessel is the ECA, as the ICA has no branches below the jaw (Fig. 8.8). Color flow imaging can provide evidence of disease, such as velocity changes due to stenosis, areas of filling defects due to the presence of atheroma and the absence of flow due to occlusion. Diagnosis should not be made based on the color flow imaging alone, but it greatly aids the sonographer in selecting areas that require close investigation with the spectral Doppler.

4. The spectral Doppler is now used to observe the inflow to the carotid arteries by placing the sample volume in the proximal CCA at the base of the neck. The shape of the waveform may reveal the presence of proximal or distal disease, such as an ICA occlusion. In the absence of significant distal or proximal disease, the left and right CCA waveforms should appear symmetrical.

5. The examination so far has provided many clues as to which of the two vessels beyond the bifurcation is the ICA, such as the relative size and position of the two vessels and the presence of ECA branches. Spectral Doppler can now be used to confirm the identification of the ICA and ECA, as the ICA waveform shape is less pulsatile and has higher diastolic flow than the ECA (Fig. 8.9). Differentiation of the vessels may be further helped by tapping the temporal artery, an ECA branch (which runs in front of

the upper part of the ear), as this will cause changes in the ECA flow during diastole (Fig. 8.9C) but will have little effect on the ICA. It is imperative that the ICA and ECA should be correctly identified, as it is the presence of

Figure 8.10 A: A color image of an occluded ICA showing flow in the CCA with retrograde flow seen in the stump of the ICA occlusion and an absence of flow in the ICA beyond. B: Doppler spectrum obtained from a CCA proximal to an ICA occlusion showing low-volume, high-resistance flow.

Figure 8.11 Color image showing a narrow channel of low-velocity flow detected in a subtotal occlusion of the ICA. A low PRF (arrow) is required to detect the low-velocity flow.

disease in the carotid bifurcation and ICA, not the ECA, that is the possible cause of carotid artery symptoms. If significant disease is present in the ICA, the upper limit of the disease in relation to the level of the jaw should be assessed. If no clear vessel can be seen beyond the stenosis, angiography may be required to confirm the endpoint of the disease.

6. Using spectral Doppler, peak systolic and end diastolic velocity measurements should be made in the CCA, ICA and ECA and at the site of the maximum velocity increase within any stenoses to allow the degree of narrowing to be graded. Untypical waveform shapes should also be noted.

7. If no flow is detected in the ICA (Fig. 8.10) or CCA using the high-flow scanner settings, it is necessary to rule out the presence of low-volume flow due to a critical stenosis or subtotal occlusion (Fig. 8.11) before reporting the vessel to be occluded. This is achieved by optimizing the scanner controls to detect low-velocity flow (i.e., by lowering the PRF and high-pass filter setting). If low-velocity flow is detected, the cause should be identified. For example, low-velocity flow may be detected in the CCA because of an ICA occlusion (Fig. 8.10B), or it may be detected in the ICA due to a very severe stenosis of the ICA origin.

8. To conclude the first side of the examination, the vertebral artery should be located using B-mode or color imaging. The patient's head should be turned slightly to one side. First image the mid-CCA in longitudinal section and then slowly angle the transducer into a more anteroposterior plane. The vertebral processes, seen as bright echoes, should slowly be seen to stand out. Only short sections of the vertebral artery and vein can be seen at this level as they run through the transverse foramen of the vertebrae. The walls of the vertebral artery and vein can often be seen on the B-mode image, but color flow imaging can also help visualize the vessels (Fig. 8.12). Spectral Doppler is then used to confirm the direction and quality of flow in the vertebral artery.

9. Having completed the first side of the examination, the patient is asked to turn the head in the opposite direction, and the other side is examined in the same way. It is important to remember that the carotid and vertebral arteries on both sides are linked via several possible collateral pathways and that the presence of severe disease in one extracranial vessel may affect flow in another extracranial vessel if it is supplying a collateral pathway.

Figure 8.12   Color flow image of the vertebral artery (A) and vein (V) seen between the vertebral processes of the spine (marked by the arrows).

B-MODE IMAGING

Normal appearance

The normal vessel walls will often appear as a double-layer structure when imaged in longitudinal section (Fig. 8.7), especially if a high-frequency transducer is used. This represents the intima-media layer and adventitia (Ch. 5) and is most clearly seen on the posterior wall in the CCA, when the vessel lies at right angles to the ultrasound beam. The normal thickness of the intima-media layer is of the order of 0.5 mm (Pignoli et al 1986). A normal vessel lumen should appear anechoic, but it is possible for the sonographer to remove echoes from within the lumen by reducing the time gain compensation (Ch. 2), so careful use of the imaging controls is important. Reverberation artifacts can also give the appearance of structures within the lumen. Occasionally, it is difficult to obtain adequate B-mode images of the bifurcation. In this case, color flow imaging may help locate the vessels and enable spectral Doppler measurements to be made.

Abnormal appearance

The ultrasound appearance of the early stages of carotid artery disease is a thickening of the intima-media layer. As the disease progresses, more substantial areas of atheroma can be visualized, and this is most likely to occur at the carotid bifurcation. However, in a small proportion of patients, significant disease may be seen in the CCA and may even involve the CCA origin. It is important to remember the way ultrasound interacts with tissue and the effects of scanner setup, such as gain control and compression curve selection (Ch. 2), before drawing conclusions about the appearance of plaque surface or composition. A high-frequency transducer should be used when investigating plaque composition. There have been many studies carried out comparing the ultrasound appearance of atheromatous plaque with histological investigation of specimens removed during carotid endarterectomy (Fig. 8.13) in an attempt to predict which plaques are more likely to be the source of emboli. Several of these studies show an association between the symptoms and the presence of intraplaque hemorrhage (i.e., bleeding into the plaque) (Merrit & Bluth 1992). If the surface of a plaque containing intraplaque hemorrhage or lipid pools ruptures, the contents of the plaque are discharged into the vessel lumen, causing distal embolization and leading to symptoms such as TIA or stroke. A multicenter European study (European Carotid Plaque Study Group 1995) showed that the echogenicity on the B-mode image was inversely related to the content of soft tissue (including hemorrhage or lipid) and directly related to the presence of calcification. In this study, they described the plaque by using a scale of 1 to 3, with 1 representing 'strong' echoes and 3 representing low echogenicity or anechoic areas. The plaques were also described as being homogeneous or heterogeneous. Irregularity of the plaque surface was not found to relate well to the presence of ulceration.

An international consensus meeting (de Bray et al 1997) used a similar method of describing plaque features: echogenicity (from anechoic to hyperechoic), surface (from smooth to cavitated) and texture (from homogeneous to heterogeneous). It was suggested that echogenicity can be standardized against blood (anechoic), mastoid muscle (isoechogenic) or bone (hyperechogenic cervical vertebrae). Lumen surface was classified as regular, irregular (0.4–2 mm) and ulcerated (>2 mm depth and 2 mm in length with well-defined back

Figure 8.13   Atheroma removed from the carotid bifurcation during carotid endarterectomy.

Figure 8.14   An image of a heterogeneous plaque with a crater (arrow) suggesting an ulcer.

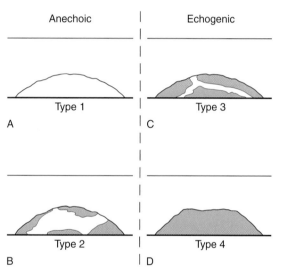

Figure 8.15   Plaque categorization based on ultrasound imaging described by Bock & Lusby. (From Bock & Lusby 1992, with permission.)

wall at its base, with flow vortices seen on color imaging). Figure 8.14 shows a heterogeneous plaque with a crater, filled with blood flow, suggesting an ulcer.

A slightly different method of categorizing the plaque, imaged in longitudinal views, was reported by Bock & Lusby (1992) whereby the plaque was graded from 1 to 4, as shown in Figure 8.15. Type 1 appears as an anechoic area seen to have a thin cap (Fig. 8.16A). Anechoic areas were shown to relate to either lipid or intraplaque hemorrhage. Echogenic plaques were categorized as type 4 and were considered to be more benign. Figure 8.16D demonstrates a more echogenic plaque. Types 2 and 3 were heterogeneous plaques (Fig. 8.16B and C), with type 3 appearing more echogenic than type 2. Plaque types 1 and 2 were seen significantly more frequently in symptomatic patients, whereas types 3 and 4 were more commonly found in asymptomatic patients.

These and many other studies over recent years suggest that the most useful quality of the B-mode appearance of a plaque is the proportion of anechoic areas or areas of low echogenicity within the plaque. Clearly the appearance of a plaque is dependent on the scanner controls being set to give an optimal image. Studies have shown a correlation of histological appearance with an increased risk of ischemic cerebrovascular events (Mathiesen et al 2001); however, the benefits of surgery over medical treatment in the management of asymptomatic patients based on plaque appearance have not been proven. Several research centers

Figure 8.16 A: Anechoic plaque (arrow) with a thin cap, type 1. B: Type 2 plaque. C: Type 3 plaque. Types 2 and 3 are heterogeneous, with type 3 appearing more echogenic than type 2. D: Homogeneous echogenic plaque, type 4.

have attempted to use image analysis methods to objectively quantify features in images of plaques, which may in time improve plaque characterization.

Large areas of atheroma will often be seen in the origin of an occluded ICA and, if the occlusion is long-standing, the occluded ICA may appear much smaller as its lumen contracts over time (Fig. 8.18).

COLOR IMAGING

Normal appearance

Flow in normal carotid arteries is pulsatile, with forward flow present throughout the cardiac cycle. With the appropriate PRF selected, color should continually fill the vessel lumen up to the walls. The flow may appear more pulsatile in the ECA than in the ICA and CCA. At the bifurcation, changes in the vessel geometry often lead to areas of flow reversal within the bifurcation, on the opposite side of the

vessel to the ECA origin, giving the normal appearance seen in Chapter 5 (see Fig. 5.12A).

Abnormal appearance

The lack of color filling to the vessel wall may indicate the presence of atheroma. However, it is important to ensure that filling defects are not due to a poor Doppler angle, inappropriately high PRF or high-pass filter setting or to the presence of an image artifact preventing the color from being displayed. The presence of a filling defect at the vessel wall, where atheroma is not apparent on the B-mode image, may indicate an area of anechoic atheroma.

Increased velocity within a stenosis usually causes a change in the color displayed on the image, often associated with aliasing (Fig. 8.17A) and sometimes with flow recirculation (see Fig. 5.18). The color flow image can help to locate the area of

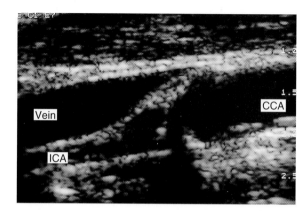

Figure 8.18 A long-standing ICA occlusion.

Figure 8.17 A: Color image showing a narrowed proximal ICA. B: Doppler recording obtained from within the narrowing, demonstrating a significant velocity increase (peak systolic velocity 500 cm/s, end diastolic velocity 300 cm/s) with increased spectral broadening, suggesting a significant stenosis (>80% diameter reduction).

greatest narrowing within a diseased segment of a vessel, which should then be investigated with the spectral Doppler (Fig. 8.17B). High-velocity jets may be seen within and just beyond a stenosis and the path of the flow may no longer be parallel to the vessel wall. In this case, the color image allows more accurate angle correction for velocity measurements. The complete absence of color Doppler filling within a vessel could indicate that the vessel is occluded, but this should be confirmed by optimizing the color controls for detection of low-velocity flow to rule out the presence of a very tight stenosis somewhere along the vessel. The apparent lack of color filling within the CCA or ICA during diastole may indicate high-resistance flow due to an occlusion or tight stenosis distally. Spectral Doppler should be used to confirm the absence of diastolic flow, and both color and spectral Doppler should be used to investigate the distal vessels carefully.

SPECTRAL DOPPLER WAVEFORMS

Normal appearance

Spectral Doppler recordings obtained from the ECA show a high-resistance flow pattern with a pulsatile waveform shape and low diastolic flow (Fig. 8.9C) compared with the low-resistance waveform shape seen in the ICA (Fig. 8.9B). The normal CCA waveform (Fig. 8.9A) has a shape somewhere between that of the ICA and the ECA. The peak systolic velocities seen in the carotid arteries depend on the relative size of the vessel but are typically less than 110 cm/s in the normal ICA. The flow profiles in the normal bifurcation seen in color flow imaging (see Fig. 5.12) will affect the spectral Doppler waveform shapes detected in the ICA origin, which may appear disturbed or demonstrate areas of reverse flow. Distal to the bifurcation, the waveform shapes should no longer appear disturbed.

Abnormal appearance

The presence of a narrowing within the carotid arteries will lead to an increase in the velocity of the blood across the stenosis, and this can be measured using spectral Doppler. Significant changes in the velocity within and just beyond a stenosis will be detected once the vessel is narrowed by a >50% reduction in diameter. The increase in velocity is related to the degree of narrowing (see Ch. 5). These velocity changes can be used to grade the degree of narrowing. The Doppler waveforms obtained within or just beyond a significant stenosis

Figure 8.19 High-resistance waveform detected in a non-diseased ICA origin proximal to an MCA occlusion.

Figure 8.21 Doppler recording demonstrating turbulent flow beyond a significant stenosis.

Figure 8.20 CCA waveform showing reverse diastolic flow in the presence of aortic valve regurgitation.

(Fig. 8.21). These untypical waveform shapes can give the sonographer useful clues as to the presence of significant disease. The total absence of flow within a vessel, as demonstrated by color flow imaging, can be confirmed using spectral Doppler. However, it is sometimes possible to pick up low-velocity signals, due to wall thump, at a point just within the occluded vessel. The presence of small veins in the area of the bifurcation can also produce misleading Doppler signals, as venous flow in the neck can appear pulsatile.

GRADING THE DISEASE

The results from two large multicenter trials have been published, the North American Symptomatic Carotid Endarterectomy Trial Collaborators (NASCET) (1991, 1998) and the European Carotid Surgery Trialists' Collaborative Group (ECST) (1998). These trials compared the benefits of carotid surgery, which carries some risk of mortality and morbidity, with the best medical treatment for patients with symptomatic carotid artery disease. The carotid disease was quantified using angiography. However, the method used to report the degree of narrowing from an angiogram differed between the European and North American trials. In the ECST trial, the degree of stenosis was measured by comparing the residual lumen diameter with the estimated diameter of the carotid bulb, whereas the NASCET trial compared the residual lumen diameter with the diameter of the normal

will also demonstrate an increase in spectral broadening (Fig. 8.17B).

Unusually low velocities can indicate the presence of disease proximal or distal to the site at which the Doppler recording is made. High-resistance waveforms, with an absence of flow during diastole, obtained from the CCA may indicate a severe ICA stenosis or occlusion (Fig. 8.10B). Figure 8.19 shows another example of a high-resistance waveform, obtained from a disease-free origin of the ICA proximal to an MCA occlusion. A reversal of flow during the whole of diastole in the carotid arteries (Fig. 8.20) may relate to a heart problem, such as aortic valve regurgitation (Malaterre et al 2001). In this case this abnormal appearance will be seen in both the left and right carotid arteries and not be associated with only one side.

The waveform detected distal to a very severe, flow-limiting stenosis will often demonstrate turbulent flow with an increased systolic rise time distal ICA, as shown in Figure 8.22. Using these two different methods can lead to significant differences in grading the disease. For example, the narrowing in Figure 8.22 would be reported as a 70% diameter reduction by the European method but as only a 50% reduction by the North American method. Figure 8.22 also gives the approximate equivalent degree of stenosis, measured (from the same stenoses) using the different methods employed by the NASCET and ECST trials. It has been proposed that a better method of measurement may be to compare the residual lumen with the diameter of the distal CCA.

The difference in methods used to grade the degree of narrowing has made the comparison of the results from the two trials complicated. The ECST study showed that surgery reduced the risk of stroke in patients with [ECST]70–99% stenosis. However the NASCET reported similar results for patients with [NASCET]70–99%, which is equivalent to a [ECST]80–99% stenosis. Taking the results of both trials together Rothwell (2000) concluded that carotid endarterectomy reduces the overall risk of stroke in patients with a recently symptomatic [ECST]70–99% stenosis ([NASCET]50–99%). Rothwell states that using these criteria, it would be necessary to operate on 8 to 10 patients to prevent one stroke over the next 3 years. Another trial studying patients with significant (60–99%) asymptomatic stenosis, the Asymptomatic Carotid Atherosclerosis Study (ACAS) (1995), showed limited benefit of surgery in this group. Future developments in patient selection may enable the group of patients at high risk of stroke to be more closely targeted. The fact that the symptoms are likely to relate to embolic rather than hemodynamic phenomena means that there is still some clinical debate as to whether plaque type and volume, along with the degree of vessel narrowing, are critical factors in the cause of stroke.

Angioplasty and stenting can also be used to treat carotid artery stenosis, as an alternative to endarterectomy, but the risks involved still make this a controversial method requiring randomized controlled trials comparing the two methods of treatment (Rothwell 2000). Stents are expandable mesh tubes that can be used to keep a diseased vessel patent. Although stent placement does not involve a general anesthetic, unlike carotid endarterectomy, there is a potential risk of stroke during the procedure.

Imaging

Angiographic grading of carotid artery disease, as with other arterial disease, is described in terms of diameter reduction. Therefore, ultrasound grading of stenoses is also typically described in terms of diameter reduction, although the use of area reduction would seem more appropriate, especially in the presence of eccentric disease. Table 8.1 gives the percentage area reduction associated with a given percentage diameter reduction, assuming a symmetrical lumen reduction; however, these values are not correct in the presence of eccentric disease. B-mode imaging is the most appropriate method to evaluate the degree of narrowing, if the degree of lumen diameter reduction is less than 50%. However, if disease is eccentric, it is possible to overestimate the degree of narrowing if the atheroma lies on the anterior or posterior wall when imaged longitudinally. It is equally possible to underestimate the degree of narrowing on a

NASCET	ECST
30	65
40	70
50	75
60	80
70	85
80	91
90	97

Approximate equivalent degree of ICA stenosis according to NASCET and ECST measurement methods

$$NASCET \quad \frac{A - B}{A}$$

$$ECST \quad \frac{C - B}{C}$$

Figure 8.22 The NASCET and ECST trials used different methods of reporting the degree of narrowing seen on carotid angiograms. (After Donnan et al 1998, with permission.)

longitudinal image if the plaque is situated on the lateral walls (Fig. 8.23). Therefore, the diseased vessel should be visualized in transverse section first, in order to select the optimal longitudinal imaging plane, although this is obviously limited by the range of longitudinal scan planes available.

The percentage diameter reduction can be estimated from diameter measurements as follows:

$$\% \text{ diameter reduction} = \left(1 - \left[\frac{\text{diameter of patent lumen}}{\text{total diameter of vessel}}\right]\right) \times 100$$

Color flow imaging can help in identifying any lumen reduction. It is possible to obtain a color flow image in longitudinal and transverse section and this may help in estimating the degree of

Table 8.1 Relationship between diameter reduction and cross-sectional area reduction assuming a concentric stenosis

Diameter reduction (%)	Cross-sectional area reduction (%)
30	50
50	75
70	90

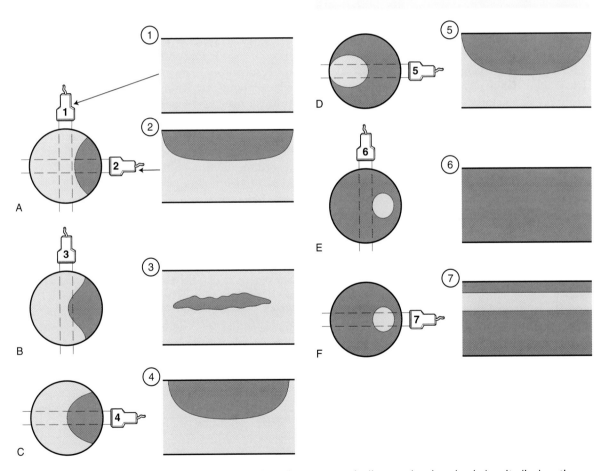

Figure 8.23 It is possible to overestimate and underestimate eccentric disease when imaging in longitudinal section. The schematic diagrams show examples of disease imaged in transverse and longitudinal section from the numbered transducer positions. A: An area of atheroma may not be seen in one longitudinal plane (1) and may appear more significant in another (2). B: Atheroma on the lateral walls may protrude into the centre of the vessel and give the appearance of atheroma floating in the vessel. C, D: These longitudinal images give a similar appearance despite very different degrees of narrowing. The longitudinal image may give the appearance of the vessel being occluded (E) or stenosed (F) depending on the imaging plane used.

narrowing, but there are potential pitfalls. Spurious flow voids can be created due to a poor angle of insonation or inappropriate PRF or filter settings, which may lead to an overestimate of the degree of narrowing. If the color gain is set too high, it is possible for the color to appear to 'bleed' out of the vessel lumen, and this can lead to an underestimate of the degree of narrowing (Fig. 7.6).

Spectral Doppler

As the quantity of atheroma in the vessel increases, it becomes more difficult to estimate the degree of narrowing from the image, especially in the presence of calcified or anechoic atheroma. However, velocity criteria are used to grade the degree of stenosis once the vessel becomes narrowed by a >50% reduction in diameter. Over the years, several criteria have been produced for grading carotid artery disease, many of which have been published, and this has revealed many discrepancies.

The various criteria have been produced by comparing Doppler measurements with those of angiography, which has its own limitations, as the gold standard.

Most criteria for grading carotid stenoses are based on the peak systolic velocity (PSV) and end diastolic velocity (EDV) in the ICA, and the ratio of the PSV in the ICA to that in the CCA. Unlike the grading of stenosis in other parts of the arterial system, where there is often a proximal segment of normal vessel which can be used to calculate a velocity ratio, the geometry of the carotid bulb makes the situation less straightforward. The ratio of the PSV in the ICA to that in the CCA will partly depend on the relative dimensions of the CCA and ICA, and this is further complicated by the variable geometry of the carotid bulb. Many criteria use absolute velocities in grading the narrowing. Using a combination of absolute velocity measurements and velocity ratios potentially reduces the pitfalls of using velocity criteria alone. For example, an increase in PSV can arise due to hypertension, age-related changes in vessel wall compliance or increased flow to supply a collateral pathway. However, an increase would be seen in both the CCA and ICA, and the absence of a significant velocity increase would reassure the sonographer

that there was no significant evidence of a stenosis. Conversely, an abnormal velocity ratio in the presence of low velocities, possibly due to low cardiac output, may help to identify a stenosis.

Table 8.2 gives some examples of criteria for grading carotid stenosis that have been developed by investigators at different centers over the years. These centers have divided the degree of narrowing into different bands. Following the ECST and NASCET trials, it is especially useful to distinguish between stenoses of <70% and ≥70% in order to select the group of patients who would benefit from surgery, given the appropriate symptoms. Bluth et al (1988) produced their criteria using an early duplex scanner with a stand-off Doppler element, as opposed to a linear array transducer. These older systems were less prone to intrinsic spectral broadening and therefore produced different results from many modern linear array systems, which tend to overestimate peak velocities. Intrinsic spectral broadening (see Ch. 6) may lead to errors in velocity measurements that are dependent on the angle of insonation. Some centers choose to overcome angle-dependent variations in velocity recordings by using a fixed angle of 60°.

Most of the sets of criteria listed in Table 8.2 have been correlated against angiography using the NASCET method of reporting angiographic findings. Therefore a ≥70% stenosis as defined by these criteria would relate to a >80% diameter reduction as measured by the ECST method. Staikov et al (2002) compared ultrasound criteria for detecting stenosis using both the NASCET and ECST methods of measuring angiograms and showed that the velocity criteria produced for a ≥70% stenosis by the NASCET method are similar to the criteria produced for a ≥80% stenosis using the ECST method. The criteria suggested by Sidhu & Allan (1997) are based on results reported by Moneta et al (1993, 1995). Table 8.2 includes criteria published following the Carotid Artery Stenosis Consensus conference (Grant et al 2003). The consensus makes many recommendations, including the use of plaque estimate (% diameter reduction) with B-mode and color Doppler ultrasound, along with ICA PSV criteria as primary parameters. ICA/CCA PSV ratio and ICA EDV are recommended as additional parameters. Nicolaides et al (1996) have described another velocity ratio,

Table 8.2 Summary of a selection of reported Doppler ultrasound criteria for diagnosing stenosis

Author	Percentage stenosis diameter reduction	ICA PSV (cm/s)	ICA EDV (cm/s)	ICA PSV to CCA PSV ratio
Bluth et al (1988)	40–59	<130	40*	<1.8
	60–79	>130	>40*	<1.8
	80–99	>250	>100*	>3.7
Robinson et al (1988) (NASCET)	<50	<150	<50	<2
	>50	>150	>50	>2
	>70	>225	>75	>3
Hunik et al (1993) (NASCET)	70–99	≥230		
Fraught et al (1994) (NASCET)	50–69	<130	≤100	
	70–99	>130	>100	
Sidhu & Allan (1997)	50–59	>130	<40	<3.2
	60–69	>130	40–110	3.2–4
	70–79	>230	110–140	>4
	80–95	>230	>140	>4
	96–99	'String flow'		
	100	'No flow'		
Filis et al (2002) (NASCET)	<50	<150	<50	<1.8
	50–59	150–200	50–70	<2.2
	60–69	200–250	70–90	2.2–2.8
	70–79	250–330	90–130	2.8–3.8
	80–89	330–400	130–180	3.8–5
	90–99	>400	>180	>5
	Occlusion	'No flow detected at ICA by PW/CDI using sensitive scale settings. Unilateral blunted CCA flow'		
Staikov et al (2002)	70–99 (NASCET)	≥220	≥80	
	70–99 (ECST & CC[†])	≥190	≥65	
	80–99 (ECST)	≥215	≥90	
Grant et al (2003) (NASCET)	<50	<125	<40	<2.0
	50–69	125–230	40–100	2.0–4.0
	≥70 but less than near occlusion	>230	>100	>4.0
	Near occlusion	High, low or undetectable	Variable	Variable
	Total occlusion	Undetectable	Not applicable	Not applicable

*Peak diastolic velocity; [†]common carotid method.

the ICA PSV to CCA EDV ratio, shown in Table 8.3. An important factor that may affect the criteria selected for grading stenoses is whether ultrasound is to be used as a screening test before angiography, for which a high sensitivity is required (see Appendix B), or to select patients for surgery, without angiography, for which sensitivity and specificity should both be equally high, to keep the number of false-positive results as low as possible. The publications describing the criteria listed in Table 8.2 include details of the sensitivity and specificity obtained by these criteria. Each center should verify its criteria locally by comparing the ultrasound findings with angiography or MRA. If a department has more than one scanner, it is necessary to check the criteria used on each machine as different models of scanner may give different results. It is important for sonographers to understand how the results of their scans are used by the surgical or medical teams that have requested them and that these teams are aware of the method the sonographers use to define the degree of disease.

COMBINING B-MODE, COLOR IMAGING AND SPECTRAL DOPPLER INFORMATION

The information obtained from all three modalities should be used to estimate the degree of narrowing, as all modalities have their strengths and weaknesses. Figure 8.24 gives an example of how this can be done. Figure 8.24A shows a transverse image of a diseased ICA, with evidence of calcified atheroma (shown by arrow). This image suggests a diameter reduction of 50–70%. Figure 8.24B shows a longitudinal image of the vessel with an absence of flow seen in the proximal ICA. However, when the vessel is

Table 8.3 ICA peak systolic velocity to CCA end diastolic velocity criteria (after Nicolaides et al 1996 © International Society of Endovascular Specialists, with permission)

Angiographic percentage diameter stenosis		ICA PSV to CCA EDV ratio
NASCET	ECST	
≤11	≤50	<7
11–60	50–77	7–10
60–70	77–83	10–15
70–82	83–90	15–25
>82	≥90	>25

A

C

B

D

Figure 8.24 A combination of B-mode, color flow imaging and spectral Doppler can be used to assess carotid disease. A: A transverse image of a diseased ICA, with calcified atheroma (arrow) suggesting a 50–70% diameter reduction. B: A longitudinal image of the vessel with an absence of flow seen in the proximal ICA. C: When the vessel is imaged in a different plane, flow can be seen within the vessel. Although the vessel lumen looks to be only slightly narrowed in this plane, a velocity increase, demonstrated by aliasing, is seen. D: Spectral Doppler velocity measurement gives a peak systolic velocity of 200 cm/s and an end diastolic velocity of 75 cm/s in the ICA, indicating a 60–69% (NASCET) diameter reduction.

imaged in a different plane (Fig. 8.24C) the flow can be seen within the vessel. Although the vessel lumen looks to be only slightly narrowed on the color image, the presence of a velocity increase, demonstrated by aliasing, should alert the sonographer to the possible presence of a more significant narrowing. Spectral Doppler velocity measurement (Fig. 8.24D) gives a PSV of 200 cm/s and an EDV of 75 cm/s in the ICA. Using the velocity criteria of Filis et al (2002) (Table 8.2) these velocity measurements would indicate a narrowing of 60–69% (NASCET) diameter reduction. By using the appearance of both B-mode and color images in transverse and a variety of longitudinal imaging planes, along with velocity measurements, the sonographer is able to estimate the degree of narrowing. There will, however, be situations in which imaging and velocity measurement are limited and the sonographer is unable to make a judgment on the severity of the disease, and this should be made clear in the scan report.

NORMAL AND ABNORMAL APPEARANCES OF VERTEBRAL ARTERY FLOW

The vertebral artery and vein can be seen between the vertebral processes. The vein normally lies

Figure 8.25 A: Flow seen in a normal vertebral artery. B: Complete flow reversal. C: Partial flow reversal seen in the vertebral artery due to subclavian steal syndrome.

above the artery, and flow in the artery is normally seen travelling toward the head (cephaled flow) (Figs 8.12 and 8.25A). It is not uncommon to see a larger vertebral artery or higher velocities on one side, usually the left, compared with the other. Occasionally, it may only be possible to visualize one of the vertebral arteries. The Doppler spectrum obtained from the vertebral artery demonstrates a low-resistance waveform shape with high diastolic flow (Fig. 8.25A).

Reverse flow (i.e., flow away from the head) in one of the vertebral arteries would suggest subclavian steal syndrome (Figs 8.25B and 8.3). Doppler recordings obtained from the ipsilateral distal subclavian artery will appear damped (see Ch. 10), and sometimes it is possible to detect a stenotic jet in the proximal subclavian artery due to a stenosis. In some cases the appearance of the vertebral artery flow can be very confusing, showing flow away from the head during systole and toward the head during diastole, as shown in Figure 8.25C. Here, the pressure drop across the diseased subclavian artery is not sufficient to cause flow reversal in the vertebral artery throughout the whole cardiac cycle. To ensure this abnormal flow is due to subclavian steal, the patient should be asked to exercise the arm ipsilateral to the abnormal vertebral flow, by bending the forearm toward the shoulder once per second for 1 minute. Alternatively, a sphygmomanometer cuff can be used to induce hyperemia by inflating the cuff around the upper arm to a pressure above systolic pressure for 2–3 minutes and then deflating. The exercise or hyperemia will increase the blood flow to the arm and cause the flow in the vertebral artery to reverse throughout the whole cardiac cycle. It is not possible to scan the entire length of the vertebral artery because sections of it are obscured by the vertebral processes; however, if indicated, it is sometimes possible to image the vertebral artery origins in the base of the neck, although this can be quite difficult.

PROBLEMS ENCOUNTERED IN IMAGING CAROTID ARTERY FLOW

Calcified atheroma

Extensive calcified plaque within the carotid bifurcation leading to significant shadowing on the

Figure 8.26 Calcification of the anterior arterial wall may prevent B-mode imaging, color flow imaging and spectral Doppler recordings within the calcified segment of vessel. A: Color flow imaging does not suggest a significant change in velocity across the calcified segment. B: Marked flow disturbance (increased velocity and flow recirculation) is seen beyond the area of calcification.

Figure 8.27 Color flow image of a tortuous ICA.

image can cause problems with grading the disease. Calcification may prevent any B-mode, color or spectral Doppler information from being obtained from within the vessel. The initial appearance of the absence of flow detected by the color flow imaging may mislead the sonographer into thinking that the vessel is occluded. However, the presence of bright echoes on the anterior wall and an absence of echoes below this should suggest calcification (Fig. 8.26). Images of the vessel distal to the calcification should be obtained and the presence of flow established. If the distal vessel can be seen clearly, with no evidence of further calcification, but no flow is detected even when the scanner is optimized to detect low-velocity flow, the vessel is probably occluded. If flow is detected distal to a calcified area, the spectral Doppler waveform may assist in grading the degree of stenosis present within the calcified area.

The presence of extensive calcified atheroma may not necessarily relate to a significant narrowing. If the calcified atheroma only extends a short way along the vessel wall, the presence of a normal Doppler waveform beyond it would suggest that it was not causing a severe stenosis. If, however, the calcification extends for more than 1 cm, a normal waveform beyond it cannot be used to indicate the absence of any significant narrowing as normal flow can be established within a short distance distal to a stenosis. If an abnormal waveform is detected beyond the calcification, the presence of a significant stenosis can be more confidently predicted. High peak systolic and end diastolic velocities (Fig. 8.17B) produced by a jet extending beyond a stenosis, post-stenotic flow turbulence (Fig. 8.21) or low-velocity, damped flow would all suggest the presence of a significant stenosis. If any doubt about the presence or absence of significant disease remains at the end of the examination, the sonographer should make this clear in the report, as angiography may be required to clarify the degree of narrowing. In cases of less severe calcification, the sonographer may be able to overcome poor imaging by viewing the vessels in a different plane (Fig. 8.24).

Vessel tortuosity

Imaging tortuous vessels can be a problem as the vessel may not appear in a single plane. Its path may run parallel to the ultrasound beam, thus producing poor images of the vessel walls. Color Doppler imaging can be used to assist in following tortuous arteries (Fig. 8.27), but the changing direction of the vessel may require regular changes in the steering angle of the color box to allow the flow to be visualized. Poor Doppler angles may limit the color flow imaging and, in this situation, power Doppler may help to image the vessel and assist in ruling out filling defects in the vessel due to the presence of atheroma.

Figure 8.28   A montage image of a postoperative carotid endarterectomy site. The small arrows demonstrate the length of the endarterectomy site. The large arrow demonstrates the intima-media layer proximal to the endarterectomy site.

POSTOPERATIVE AND POST-ANGIOPLASTY CAROTID ARTERY APPEARANCE ON ULTRASOUND

Only a small percentage of patients develop severe recurrent stenosis or occlusion following surgery and, of these, only a few suffer from any symptoms. It has been shown that routine postoperative ultrasound surveillance does not significantly affect patient management, and patients are often rescanned only if symptoms recur. The scan procedure is the same as that already described, but the postoperative appearance differs slightly from the appearance of a normal carotid bifurcation. First, the vessel wall no longer has the double layer appearance where the plaque has been removed. It is often possible to see a step in the posterior CCA wall at the beginning of the site of the endarterectomy (Fig. 8.28). A vein or prosthetic patch may be used to close the site of the endarterectomy, as it is thought that this may reduce the risk of early postoperative thrombosis or late re-stenosis. If a patch has been used to widen the vessel, it will often produce a slightly dilated bifurcation compared to normal. A prosthetic patch produces a brighter echo than a vein patch or adjacent arterial wall, and it can therefore usually be seen quite easily on the image. Vein patches can be susceptible to rupture whereas prosthetic patches can be susceptible to infection. Ultrasound can be used to measure the dimensions of the endarterectomy site and investigate any recurrent disease. Ultrasound can also be used to follow up patients who have had a carotid stenosis treated by angioplasty and stenting. Figure 8.29 shows how the stent can be clearly seen within the carotid artery.

Figure 8.29   Color image showing a carotid artery that has been treated with angioplasty and stenting.

NONATHEROMATOUS CAROTID ARTERY DISEASES

Nonatheromatous extracranial carotid diseases include aneurysms, carotid body tumors and dissection, but all are relatively rare. Patients may have a pulsatile swelling in the neck, which can be investigated with ultrasound to rule out an aneurysm. The carotid arteries should be scanned along their length, especially in the area of the suspected swelling, and the cross-sectional diameter measured. Any unusual appearances relating to the arteries should be reported. In many cases, the 'pulsatile swelling' is due to a superficial brachiocephalic bifurcation or carotid bifurcation, often associated with tortuous vessels, leading to the vessel being easily palpated. Another possible cause of a pulsatile swelling is the presence of a carotid body tumor.

The carotid body is a small structure within the vessel wall, situated at the carotid bifurcation, and is responsible for detecting blood gases and pH. As a carotid body tumor grows, it causes the ICA and ECA to be splayed apart, and small tortuous vessels can often be seen within the tumor with color flow imaging (Fig. 8.30). However, further investigation is required to confirm any ultrasound findings. Carotid artery wall dissection, which can be due to trauma, can create a false lumen within the carotid arteries (Fig. 8.31). This may remain patent and be seen as a second flow lumen on color flow imaging. Alternatively, the false lumen may occlude, causing a reduction in the residual vessel lumen or possibly a complete occlusion of the vessel. An intimal flap may be seen on the image as a fine line within the lumen that may move due to the pulsatile blood flow; however, it may be difficult to image.

TRANSCRANIAL DOPPLER ULTRASOUND

Generally, ultrasound is not easily transmitted through bone, making imaging within the skull difficult. However, the temporal bone is thinner than the rest of the skull and, by using low-frequency ultrasound (e.g., 2 MHz), it is possible to obtain both color flow images and spectral Doppler recordings from segments of some of the intracranial vessels. Nonimaging transcranial Doppler has been used to monitor flow in the MCA during carotid surgery for many years. Carotid endarterectomy involves exposing the carotid bifurcation and clamping the CCA, ICA and ECA. This can lead to compromised cerebral circulation, and, where appropriate, a temporary plastic shunt can be used to maintain flow between the CCA and ICA while the plaque is surgically removed. Transcranial Doppler enables MCA blood velocity to be measured, allowing failure of the shunts to be detected. Air and particulate emboli generated at the site of the endarterectomy can be detected, using Doppler ultrasound, as they travel through the MCA. Emboli give a characteristic 'chirp' on the audible Doppler signal and may appear as a brighter line on the spectral Doppler waveform.

Transcranial color flow imaging is performed using low-frequency phased array transducers and can provide a color map of part or all of the MCA, ACA, PCA and circle of Willis (Fig. 8.32).

Figure 8.30   Transverse image of a carotid body tumor lying between the ICA and ECA.

Figure 8.31   B-mode image of a carotid artery wall dissection showing a false lumen imaged in transverse section (A) and in longitudinal section (B).

However, views can sometimes be limited by attenuation caused by the temporal bone. Transcranial color flow imaging requires an in-depth understanding of possible collateral pathways and, as yet, does not have a clear role in routine ultrasound

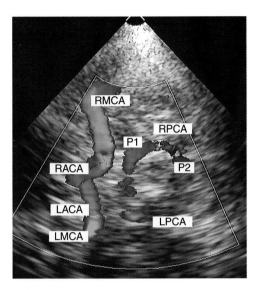

Figure 8.32 Transcranial color flow imaging can be used to investigate the intracerebral circulation (see Fig. 8.2A).

assessment of the cerebral circulation. The techniques used in transcranial Doppler assessment are beyond the remit of this book, and the reader is referred to the Further reading section at the end of this chapter.

REPORTING

The ultrasound report should describe the presence, locations and appearance of any atheroma seen within the CCA and ICA. Any significant velocity increases along the carotid arteries should be reported and interpreted to estimate the degree of narrowing present. Abnormal waveforms seen within the CCA, ICA or ECA should also be described, along with a suggestion as to what they may indicate. The presence and direction of vertebral artery flow should be noted. The report should make it very clear if there was any limitation of the carotid examination, such as the following:

- Inconclusive identification of an occlusion or subocclusion
- Calcification obscuring the vessel for more than 1 cm
- No visible endpoint to ICA disease
- Whether the scan was otherwise suboptimal.

> **Box 8.2   Information to include in a carotid scan report, especially when surgery is performed on the basis of ultrasound alone**
>
> - Locations and appearance of any atheroma seen within the CCA, bifurcation and ICA
> - Significant velocity increases seen in the carotid arteries and an estimation of the degree of narrowing present
> - Abnormal waveforms seen within the CCA, ICA and ECA
> - Endpoint of ICA disease
> - Presence and direction of vertebral artery flow
> - Level of the carotid bifurcation in relation to the angle of the jaw
> - Limitations of the examination

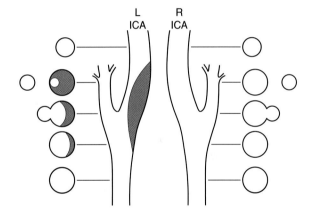

Figure 8.33 Example of a diagrammatic method of reporting a carotid ultrasound scan result.

When ultrasound is to be used to select patients for surgery, without the use of angiography, it is essential that the examination and report should cover the points listed in Box 8.2. The report can consist of a written report alone or may include images of atheroma and waveforms seen. Alternatively, a diagrammatic representation of the disease seen can be produced. Figure 8.33 is an example of a diagrammatic method of producing a report. It is important that the department has a written protocol, including the criteria used to interpret the Doppler findings and the method of reporting to be used.

References

Asymptomatic Carotid Atherosclerosis Study Group 1995 Carotid endarterectomy for patients with asymptomatic internal carotid artery stenosis. Journal of the American Medical Association 273:1421–1428

Bluth E I, Stavros A T, Marich K W, et al 1988 Carotid duplex sonography: a multicenter recommendation for standardized imaging and Doppler criteria. Radiographics 8:487–506

Bock R W, Lusby R J 1992 Carotid plaque morphology and interpretation of the echolucent lesions. In: Labs K H, Jager K A, Fitzgerald D E (eds) Diagnostic vascular ultrasound. Edward Arnold, London, pp 225–236

de Bray J M, Baud J M, Dauzat M 1997 Consensus concerning the morphology and the risk of carotid plaques. Cerebrovascular Disease 7:289–296

Donnan G A, Davis S M, Chambers B R, Gates P C 1998 Surgery for prevention of stroke. Lancet 351:1372–1373

European Carotid Plaque Study Group 1995 Carotid artery plaque composition—relationship to clinical presentation and ultrasound B-mode imaging. European Journal of Endovascular Surgery 10:23–30

European Carotid Surgery Trialists' Collaborative Group 1998 Randomised trial of endarterectomy for recently symptomatic carotid stenosis: final results of the MRC European Carotid Surgery Trial (ECST). Lancet 351:1379–1387

Filis K A, Arko F R, Johnson B L, et al 2002 Duplex ultrasound criteria for defining the severity of carotid stenosis. Annals of Vascular Surgery 16:413–421

Fraught W E, Mattos M A, van Bemmelen P S, et al 1994 Color-flow duplex scanning of carotid arteries: new velocity criteria based on receiver operator characteristic analysis for threshold stenosis used in the symptomatic and asymptomatic carotid trials. Journal of Vascular Surgery 19:818–828

Grant E G, Benson C B, Moneta G L, et al 2003 Carotid artery stenosis: gray-scale and Doppler US diagnosis. Society of Radiologists in Ultrasound Consensus Conference. Radiology 229:340–346

Hunink M G M, Polak J F, Barlan M M, O'Leary D H 1993 Detection and quantification of carotid artery stenosis: efficacy of various Doppler velocity parameters. American Journal of Roentgenology 160:619–625

Malaterre H R, Kallee K, Giusiano B, et al 2001 Holodiastolic reversal flow in the common carotid: another indicator of the severity of aortic regurgitation. International Journal of Cardiovascular Imaging 17:333–337

Mathiesen E B, Bonaa K H, Joakimsen O 2001 Echolucent plaques are associated with high risk of ischemic cerebrovascular events in carotid stenosis. Circulation 103:2171

Merrit C R B, Bluth E I 1992 Ultrasound identification of plaque composition. In: Labs K H, Jager K A, Fitzgerald D E (eds) Diagnostic vascular ultrasound. Edward Arnold, London, pp 213–224

Moneta G L, Edwards J M, Chitwood R W, et al 1993 Correlation of North American Symptomatic Carotid Endarterectomy Trial (NASCET) angiographic definition of 70% to 99% internal carotid stenosis with duplex scanning. Journal of Vascular Surgery 17:152–159

Moneta G L, Edwards J M, Papanicolaou G, et al 1995 Screening for asymptomatic internal carotid artery stenosis: duplex criteria for discriminating 60% to 99% stenosis. Journal of Vascular Surgery 21:989–994

Naylor A R, Beard J D, Gaines P A 1998 Extracranial carotid disease. In: Beard J D, Gaines P A (eds) Vascular and endovascular surgery. WB Saunders, London, pp 317–350

Nicolaides A N, Shifrin E G, Bradbury A, et al 1996 Angiographic and duplex grading of internal carotid stenosis: can we overcome confusion? Journal of Endovascular Surgery 3:158–165

North American Symptomatic Carotid Endarterectomy Trial Collaborators (NASCET) 1991 Beneficial effect of carotid endarterectomy in symptomatic patients with high-grade carotid stenosis. New England Journal of Medicine 325:445–453

North American Symptomatic Carotid Endarterectomy Trial Collaborators 1998 The final results of the NASCET trial. New England Journal of Medicine 339:1415–1425

Pignoli P, Tremoli E, Poli A, et al 1986 Intimal plus medial thickness of the arterial wall: a direct measurement with ultrasound imaging. Circulation 74(6):1399–1406

Robinson M L, Sacks D, Perlmutter G S, Marinelli D L 1988 Diagnostic criteria for carotid duplex sonography. American Journal of Roentgenology 151:1045–1049

Rothwell P M 2000 Who should have carotid surgery or angioplasty? British Medical Bulletin 56(2):526–538

Sidhu P S, Allan P L 1997 Ultrasound assessment of internal carotid artery stenosis. Clinical Radiology 52:654–658

Staikov I N, Nedeltchev K, Arnold M, et al 2002 Duplex sonographic criteria for measuring carotid stenoses. Journal of Clinical Ultrasound 30:275–281

von Reutern G M, von Büdingen H J 1993 Ultrasound diagnosis of cerebrovascular disease. Thieme Verlag, Stuttgart

Further reading

Allan P L, Dubbins P A, Pozniak M A, McDicken W N
2000 Clinical Doppler ultrasound. Churchill
Livingstone, London

Babikan V, Wechsler L 1999 Transcranial Doppler
ultrasonography. Butterworth Heinemann, Woburn

Newell D W, Aaslid R 1992 Transcranial Doppler.
Raven Press, New York

von Reutern G M, von Büdingen H J 1993 Ultrasound
diagnosis of cerebrovascular disease. Georg Thieme
Verlag, Stuttgart

Chapter 9

Duplex assessment of lower limb arterial disease

CHAPTER CONTENTS

Introduction 111
Anatomy of the lower limb arterial system 111
  Collateral pathways and anatomical
    variations 113
Ankle–brachial pressure measurements and
  exercise testing 113
Symptoms of lower limb arterial disease 116
  Intermittent claudication 116
  Chronic critical lower limb ischemia 116
  Acute ischemia 117
Practical considerations for lower extremity
  duplex scanning 118
  Scanner setup 119
Starting the scan 119
  Assessment of the aortoiliac artery and CFA 119
  Assessment of the femoral and popliteal
    arteries 120
  Assessment of the tibial arteries 122
  Assessment of tibial arteries and the plantar
    arch prior to bypass surgery 123
  Commonly encountered problems 123
Scan appearances 124
  B-mode images 124
  Color flow images 125
  Spectral Doppler 126
Assessment of arterial stents 129
Other abnormalities and syndromes 129
  Popliteal entrapment syndrome 129
  Cystic adventitial disease of the popliteal
    artery 130
Reporting 130

INTRODUCTION

Duplex scanning of the lower limb arteries is a well-established technique and provides comparable results to arteriography (Legemate et al 1989, Pemberton & London 1997). In most cases, this allows the vascular surgeon or physician to formulate a management plan without the aid of diagnostic arteriograms, which are known to carry a complication rate of 1–2% (Egglin et al 1995). For instance, it may be decided to treat the patient by conservative methods without further investigations. Vascular radiologists can spend less time performing diagnostic arteriograms, concentrating their skills on therapeutic treatment by balloon angioplasty. In some centers the patient undergoes surgery on the basis of diagnostic duplex scanning alone (McCarthy et al 1999, Proia et al 2001). This chapter provides an overview of lower limb arterial disorders and offers practical advice on color duplex scanning of peripheral arteries.

ANATOMY OF THE LOWER LIMB ARTERIAL SYSTEM

The anatomy of the lower limb arterial system is demonstrated in Figure 9.1. The abdominal aorta has been included in this section, as it can be a source of lower limb symptoms.

The aorta lies slightly to the left of the midline in the abdomen, and its bifurcation is located at the level of the fourth lumbar vertebra in the region of the umbilicus. The aorta divides into the left and right common iliac arteries (CIA) at the

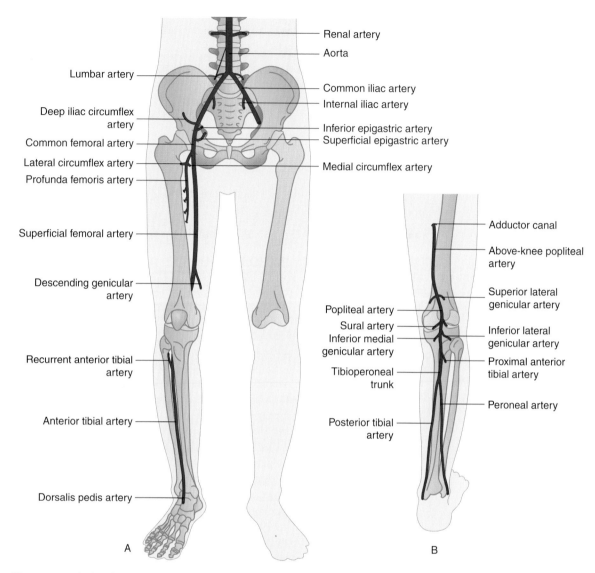

Figure 9.1 A: Arterial anatomy of the aortoiliac and lower limb arteries from an anterior view. B: Arterial anatomy of the lower limb from a posterior view.

aortic bifurcation. The CIA is variable in length (3.5–12 cm) and in some cases it is very short, with the iliac bifurcation occurring close to the aorta. The CIA divides into the external and internal iliac arteries at the iliac bifurcation, which lies deep in the pelvis. The internal iliac artery supplies blood to the pelvis and pelvic viscera. The external iliac artery varies in length (6–12 cm) and gives off the deep circumflex iliac artery and inferior epigastric artery, before becoming the common femoral artery (CFA)

at the level of the inguinal ligament. The aorta and iliac arteries lie behind the peritoneum, containing the bowel, which can make imaging of these vessels difficult due to overlying bowel gas. One branch of the CFA that can often be identified with ultrasound is the superficial epigastric artery.

The CFA divides into the deep femoral artery, also known as the profunda femoris artery, and the superficial femoral artery (SFA) at the level of the groin. The profunda femoris artery usually runs posterolateral to the SFA and supplies blood to the thigh. It also acts as an important collateral pathway in the presence of an SFA occlusion. The profunda femoris artery usually gives off the medial and lateral circumflex arteries just beyond its origin. The SFA follows a medial course down the thigh, becoming the popliteal artery at the level of the adductor canal above the knee. The SFA gives off relatively few major branches, although the descending genicular artery can act as an important collateral pathway. The popliteal artery then runs behind the knee, or popliteal fossa, and bifurcates below the knee into the anterior tibial (AT) artery and tibioperoneal trunk. The popliteal artery has a number of genicular and sural branches supplying blood to the knee joint and gastrocnemius and soleus muscles. The proximal AT artery runs in an anterolateral direction through the interosseous membrane to the anterolateral aspect of the upper calf. It then continues to run to the lower calf, becoming the dorsalis pedis artery over the dorsum of the foot. The tibioperoneal trunk can vary in length and bifurcates into the posterior tibial (PT) and peroneal arteries (Fig. 9.1B). The PT artery follows a medial course along the calf and runs behind the medial malleolus (or ankle bone) in its distal segment. The peroneal artery lies deeper than the PT artery against the border of the fibula and runs toward the lateral malleolus (outer aspect of the ankle) in its distal segment. It is important to note that the peroneal artery is often spared in the presence of tibial artery disease. This is why its identification can be useful if a distal bypass procedure is being considered.

The distal area of the foot is mainly supplied by the dorsalis pedis artery and the medial and lateral plantar arteries, which are terminal branches of the PT artery. The dorsalis pedis and plantar arteries anastomose to form the plantar arch, which supplies the arteries to the toes.

Collateral pathways and anatomical variations

If an arterial segment is severely diseased or occluded, there are often alternative pathways that are able to carry blood flow around the diseased segment, referred to as collateral vessels. In this situation, reverse flow is observed in major branches of arteries just distal to an area of severe disease, where they

Figure 9.2 An example of collateral flow. The CIA is occluded (O) and reverse flow (blue) is demonstrated in the internal iliac artery, as it supplies flow to the external iliac artery (red).

help to resupply blood flow to the main vessel. One such example is flow reversal observed in the internal iliac artery, supplying blood to the external iliac artery in the presence of a CIA occlusion (Fig. 9.2). It should be noted that it is actually very difficult to follow collateral vessels for any length using the duplex scanner, especially in the pelvis. This is not really a problem, as it is the length and severity of the disease in the main vessels that the sonographer is attempting to document. However, the quality of the collateral circulation is very important, and this can be determined by assessing the patient clinically and measuring the ankle–brachial pressure index (ABPI). Common collateral pathways are summarized in Table 9.1.

There are a number of anatomical variations in the lower limb arterial system that may be occasionally encountered during routine examinations. The most common variations are listed in Table 9.2.

ANKLE–BRACHIAL PRESSURE MEASUREMENTS AND EXERCISE TESTING

In the vascular laboratory the measurement of the ABPI using continuous wave Doppler is one of the simplest and commonest ways of detecting and grading arterial disease. The test normally takes 10–15 min and is performed as follows. The patient should be fully rested and lying supine to remove the effect of hydrostatic pressure. A blood pressure cuff is then placed around the ankle. A high-frequency

Table 9.1   Common collateral pathways of the lower limb arteries

Diseased artery	Distal normal artery	Common collateral pathway
Common iliac artery	External iliac artery	Lumbar arteries communicating with the iliolumbar arteries of the ipsilateral internal iliac artery, which supply the external iliac artery via retrograde flow; there can also be communication between the contralateral internal iliac artery and ipsilateral internal iliac artery
External iliac artery	Common femoral artery	Ipsilateral internal iliac artery via pelvic connections to the deep iliac circumflex artery or inferior epigastric artery
Common femoral artery	Femoral bifurcation	Ipsilateral pelvic arteries filling the profunda femoris artery via the femoral circumflex arteries, which supply the superficial femoral artery via retrograde flow
Superficial femoral artery	Above-knee popliteal artery	Flow via profunda femoris artery (or branches of the proximal superficial femoral artery if patent) to the descending or superior genicular arteries, depending on the length of the superficial femoral artery occlusion
Superficial femoral artery	Below-knee popliteal artery	Profunda femoris artery branches to inferior genicular branches of the popliteal artery
Popliteal artery	Distal popliteal artery	Flow via the superior genicular arteries to inferior genicular arteries, depending on the level of the occlusion
Proximal tibial arteries	Distal tibial arteries	There are numerous arterial collateral connections in the calf, but they may not be large enough to carry sufficient flow to the foot

Table 9.2   Anatomical variations of the lower limb arterial system

Artery	Variation
Common femoral artery bifurcation	The bifurcation can sometimes be very high; the proximal course of the profunda femoris artery can sometimes be variable and lies posterior medial to the superficial femoral artery in 5% of cases
Anterior tibial artery	High origin across the knee joint
Anterior tibial artery	May be small or hypoplastic
Peroneal artery	Origin from anterior tibial artery rather than the tibioperoneal trunk

(8–10 MHz) continuous wave Doppler probe is used to listen to the Doppler signals in the dorsalis pedis and PT arteries at the ankle, as shown in Figure 9.3. It is sometimes necessary to examine the peroneal artery, as it may be the only vessel supplying the foot in patients with severe arterial disease. The systolic blood pressure is measured at each of these points by briskly inflating the cuff to above the patient's systolic blood pressure, at which point the arterial flow signal disappears. The cuff should be inflated to at least 30 mmHg above the pressure that is required to occlude the artery. The cuff is then deflated, and the pressure at which the arterial signal reappears, corresponding to the systolic pressure at the position of the cuff, is recorded. The systolic brachial pressure is then measured in a similar way from both arms, in case there is upper extremity disease. The highest recorded ankle pressure is then divided by the highest brachial pressure to calculate the ABPI. This index is independent of the patient's systemic blood pressure and can be used to grade the severity of arterial disease as shown in Table 9.3 (AbuRahma 2000). The index is equal to, or greater than, 1 in normal subjects due to amplification of the arterial pulse wave along the limb. Conversely, an index of 0.25 would indicate a patient with severe ischemia and possible rest pain. Care

Figure 9.4   Color flow image of an anterior tibial artery taken from a diabetic patient. There is marked calcification of the vessel walls, demonstrated by the strong reflections (arrows). Note the beaded appearance of the color flow display due to vessel disease and attenuation caused by the calcification.

Figure 9.3   Measurement of the ABPI. Probe positions are shown to detect flow in the dorsalis pedis artery (probe) and the PT (large arrow). The peroneal artery is located on the outer aspect of the ankle (small arrow). The probe position has also been shown to detect flow from the plantar arch (curved arrow).

Table 9.3   Grading arterial disease using the ankle–brachial pressure index (ABPI)

ABPI	Comment
⩾1	Normal
>0.9 to <1	Mild disease
0.5–0.9	Claudication
0.3–0.5	Severe occlusive disease
<0.3	Ischemia

must be taken when interpreting ABPI measurements from diabetic patients as the arterial walls of the calf arteries are often calcified and rigid (Fig. 9.4). This means that the vessels may not collapse under the pressure of the cuff as it is inflated, leading to falsely elevated recordings. An example of such a measurement would be an ankle pressure of 280 mmHg and a brachial pressure of 120 mmHg (ABPI = 2.3). Abnormal ABPI measurements can confirm the presence of arterial disease but do not give any indication of the position of the disease in the leg. Segmental pressures can help to isolate the diseased segment with the use of multiple pressure cuffs placed at the ankle, below the knee, above the knee and at the top of the thigh. Significant pressure differences between cuffs would indicate disease between those segments.

Resting ABPI measurements may be normal in patients with mild to moderate claudication. However, ABPI measurements can be carried out before and after exercise on a treadmill to measure claudication distance and the degree of pressure reduction following exercise. This is because exercising muscles require increased blood flow. However, to increase flow an increase in the pressure gradient across the stenosis occurs, with a reduction in pressure distal to the stenosis. Eventually a point will be reached at which the stenosis limits any further increase in flow and the patient experiences the onset of claudication in the muscle groups distal to the disease. It is important to monitor patients closely during exercise testing as many with claudication have associated coronary artery disease. It is essential to have an emergency call system close at hand. In the absence of a treadmill it is possible to exercise the patient along the known length of a corridor. Another alternative is to use commercially available foot flexion devices to exercise the calf muscles while the patient sits on the examination table. This reduces cardiac stress. Exercise testing is also a particularly useful screening test, as some patients exhibiting symptoms of claudication may have other disorders producing their symptoms, such as spinal stenosis, sciatica or musculoskeletal problems. In these cases, the post-exercise pressures will be normal. Unfortunately, there is a wide range of exercise protocols used by vascular laboratories (e.g., speed 2–4 km/hour, exercise duration 2–5 min and treadmill incline 10–12%). This can make comparisons of results among units difficult. However, individual patients' performance can be measured on sequential visits to monitor their treatment or progress.

SYMPTOMS OF LOWER LIMB ARTERIAL DISEASE

Intermittent claudication

Atherosclerosis is a major health problem in developed countries where lifestyle factors, such as diet and smoking, can accelerate the progression of the disease. It is estimated that intermittent claudication affects approximately 4.5% of the population aged between 55 to 74 years, and there is evidence that persons with claudication have a significantly higher mortality rate from cardiac disease than non-claudicants (Fowkes et al 1991). Intermittent claudication is caused by arterial narrowing in the lower limb arteries, and symptoms may develop over a number of months or years. Claudication is typified by pain and cramping in the muscles of the leg while walking, which usually forces the patient to stop and rest in order to ease the symptoms. The severity of pain experienced and the distance a patient is able to walk can vary from day to day, but, generally, walking briskly or on an incline will produce rapid onset of symptoms. The location of pain (i.e. calf, buttock or thigh) is often associated with the distribution of disease. For instance, aortoiliac disease often produces thigh, buttock and eventually calf claudication whereas femoropopliteal

disease is associated with calf pain. There are sometimes physical signs of deteriorating blood flow in the lower limb, such as hair loss from the calf and an absence of nail growth. Claudication only occurs during exercise because, at rest, the muscle groups distal to a stenosis or occlusion remain adequately perfused with blood. However, during exercise the metabolic demand of the muscles increases rapidly, and the stenosis or occlusion will limit the amount of additional blood flow that can reach the muscles, so causing claudication.

Many patients with intermittent claudication are treated by conservative methods. This includes reduction or elimination of risk factors associated with atherosclerosis, such as smoking. Patients are also advised to undertake a controlled exercise program to build up the collateral circulation around the diseased vessel, which may ease symptoms over time. If necessary, serial ABPI measurements or exercise tests can be performed to monitor the patient's progress. Interventional treatment is mainly by angioplasty which involves the dilation of stenoses or occlusions with percutaneous balloon catheters (see Ch. 1). Arterial stents are sometimes used to prevent re-stenosis, although in-stent stenosis is known to occur in a proportion of cases due to the development of intimal hyperplasia (see Fig. 9.21). Sometimes the arterial lesion is so hard, the stent will not fully expand, leaving a residual stenosis. Duplex scanning can be used to detect and monitor in-stent stenosis. Surgical bypass is usually avoided, unless the patient is suffering from severe claudication, as there is a small but potential risk of complications occurring during or after surgery, which in extreme cases could lead to amputation or even death.

Chronic critical lower limb ischemia

Critical lower limb ischemia occurs when blood flow beyond an arterial stenosis or occlusion is so low that the patient experiences pain in the leg at rest because the metabolic requirements of the distal tissues cannot be maintained. This is frequently typified by severe rest pain at night, forcing the patient to sleep in a chair or to hang the leg in a dependent position over the side of the bed. This improves blood flow due to increased hydrostatic pressure. Ulceration and gangrene may also be present

Figure 9.5 The appearance of critical lower limb ischemia with gangrene of the small toe.

(Fig. 9.5). The European Working Group (1992) on critical limb ischemia (CLI) defined CLI as:

> … persistently recurring ischaemic rest pain requiring regular analgesia for more than two weeks, with an ankle systolic pressure of ≤50 mmHg and/or a toe systolic pressure of ≤30 mmHg; or ulceration or gangrene of the foot or toes, with ankle systolic pressure of ≤50 mmHg and/or a toe systolic pressure of ≤30 mmHg.

This may be a strict definition of CLI, as patients with ulceration are frequently seen in the vascular laboratory with ankle pressures above 50 mmHg. The treatment of lower limb ischemia includes angioplasty or arterial bypass grafting. Unfortunately some patients are not suitable candidates for any form of limb salvage, and amputation is the inevitable outcome.

Acute ischemia

Acute ischemia, as the name suggests, is due to sudden arterial obstruction in the lower limb arteries. The position of the obstruction can be variable. There are two main causes of acute ischemia.

First, acute thrombosis of an existing arterial lesion, a so-called acute-on-chronic occlusion, can occur when the blood flow across a diseased segment of an artery is so slow that it spontaneously thromboses. Long segments of an artery may occlude in this situation. Acute ischemia is more likely to occur if the collateral circulation around the disease is poorly developed. Occasionally, patients have predisposing coagulation disorders that lead to spontaneous arterial thrombosis.

Second, an embolus may be released from other areas of the body, such as the heart or from an aneurysm, which then blocks an artery in the extremity. An embolus frequently obstructs bifurcations such as the common femoral bifurcation or distal popliteal artery and tibioperoneal trunk. Another example is obstruction of the aortic bifurcation by an embolus projecting down both CIA origins, referred to as a saddle embolus. The body has very little time to develop collateral circulation around embolic occlusions, and the limb may be very ischemic.

The symptoms of acute ischemia are of rapid onset, and the patient classically presents with a cold, painful, pulseless, paresthetic leg. In this situation, emergency intervention by surgical embolectomy, bypass surgery or thrombolysis should be performed, provided that the patient is fit enough for treatment. Left untreated, acute ischemia can lead to muscle death or necrosis. This can cause swelling of the calf muscle, and eventually the sac, or fascia, surrounding the muscles will restrict any further swelling, leading to a pressure increase within the muscle compartments. This is known as a compartment syndrome, and the increased intra-compartmental pressure can further exacerbate the muscle ischemia. If limb salvage is possible, surgical splitting of the fascia, called a fasciotomy, may be required to release the excess pressure.

Severe muscle ischemia can produce toxins causing systemic symptoms that can lead to organ failure and death. An urgent amputation is usually performed if there is no viable option to restore blood flow to the limb. Acute ischemia can also occur due to microembolization to the foot, leading to occlusion of the small vessels. The microemboli can originate from the heart, from atherosclerotic plaques or from an aneurysm. In this situation it is not unusual for the patient to have a palpable popliteal pulse.

Microembolization into the foot is often called 'trash foot'. Localized tissue necrosis can occur and the outcome is sometimes poor when a large area of tissue is affected.

PRACTICAL CONSIDERATIONS FOR LOWER EXTREMITY DUPLEX SCANNING

The objective of the examination is to locate and grade the severity of arterial disease in the lower limb arterial system. The time allocated for the examination depends on the number of segments that need assessing. The femoropopliteal segment can normally be examined in both legs in half an hour. However, a bilateral aortoiliac to ankle scan may take up to an hour and a half, depending on experience. There is usually no special preparation required before a lower limb duplex scan. Nevertheless, some vascular units request patients to fast overnight prior to an examination of the aortoiliac arteries to improve imaging of this region. In our experience this is of little help, especially if patients require scans

Figure 9.6 The anatomy of the right femoral artery and vein at the groin, with corresponding transverse B-mode images at four different levels. Vessels shown on the diagram are: 1 common femoral artery, 2 common femoral vein, 3 saphenofemoral junction, 4 superficial femoral artery, 5 profunda femoris artery, 6 superficial femoral vein, 7 profunda vein. Vessels demonstrated on the images are the common femoral vein (V), common femoral artery (CFA), saphenofemoral junction (SFJ), superficial femoral artery (SFA), profunda femoris artery (PA), superficial femoral vein (SFV) and profunda vein (PV). Note that the femoral artery bifurcation is sometimes found above the level of the saphenofemoral junction. In addition, the superficial femoral artery tends to roll on top of the superficial femoral vein, as shown in the B-mode image.

at short notice. Bowel preparations have proved useful, although in practice they can be difficult to administer to elderly or diabetic patients and are impractical in a single visit clinic.

The patient should have an empty bladder prior to an aortoiliac scan as this improves the visualization of these segments and also causes less patient discomfort if transducer pressure has to be applied. The examination room should be at a comfortable ambient temperature (>20°C) to avoid peripheral vasoconstriction.

Scanner setup

A peripheral arterial scanning option should be selected before starting the examination, but adjustment of the control settings will often be required in the presence of significant disease (see Ch. 7). The color PRF is usually set in the 2.5–3 kHz range for demonstrating moderately high velocity flow.

STARTING THE SCAN

It is useful to start the assessment by examining the CFA at the groin, as the observed blood flow patterns at this level can reveal information about the condition of the aortoiliac arteries and also provide some clues to the condition of the superficial femoral artery (SFA) (i.e., origin occlusion or high resistance flow pattern due to proximal obstruction). It is important to have a good understanding of the anatomy of the arteries and veins at the level of the groin and to be able to identify the major branches and junctions and their relationship to each other (Fig. 9.6). A 5 MHz, or broad-band equivalent, linear array transducer is the most suitable probe for scanning the femoral, popliteal and calf arteries. A 3.5 MHz, or broad-band equivalent, curved linear array abdominal transducer is used for the aortoiliac segment. The segmental guidelines can be used in any order. A combination of B-mode imaging, color flow imaging and spectral Doppler recordings should be used throughout the examination. Color flow imaging is essential for identifying the aortoiliac and calf arteries. Spectral Doppler velocity measurements should be made at an angle of 60° or less (see p. 69).

Assessment of the aortoiliac artery and CFA

The patient should be relaxed and lying in a supine position with the head supported by a pillow. The patient should be asked to relax the abdominal muscles and to rest the arms by the sides. The scanning positions for assessing the inflow arteries are shown in Figure 9.7, and a color image of the arteries is shown in Figure 9.8. The procedure for assessment is as follows:

1. Using a 5 MHz, or broad-band equivalent, linear array transducer, the CFA is identified at the level of the groin in transverse section, where it lies lateral to the common femoral vein (Figs 9.6 and 9.7A). The CFA is then followed proximally in longitudinal section until it runs deep under the inguinal ligament and can no longer be assessed

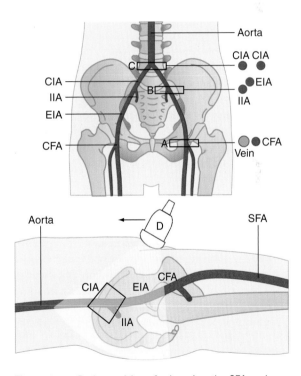

Figure 9.7 Probe positions for imaging the CFA and aortoiliac arteries. A: CFA transverse. B: Origin of external and internal iliac arteries transverse. C: Aortic bifurcation transverse. D: Arteries in the longitudinal plane. Starting at the groin and pushing bowel gas upward with the transducer (arrow) can help visualization. Positioning the color box to the edge of the scan sector can improve the angle of insonation with spectral Doppler.

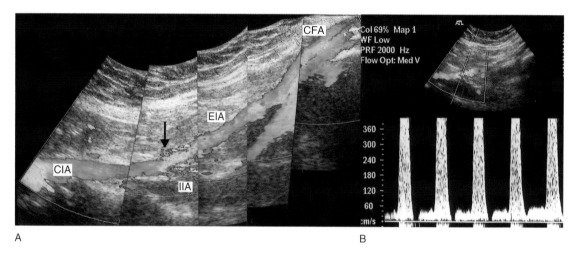

Figure 9.8   A: A color montage of the inflow arteries showing the CIA, external iliac (EIA) and internal iliac arteries (IIA) and the CFA. Note the stenosis at the iliac artery bifurcation (arrow), demonstrated by aliasing. B: Spectral Doppler demonstrates a high-grade stenosis of the EIA, indicated by high systolic velocity, aliasing and spectral broadening. The color box has been positioned to the edge of the sector to improve the angle of insonation.

with this probe. A 3.5 MHz curved array transducer should then be selected. Using the probe to push any gas upwards and driving the color box toward the edge of the sector can help in visualizing the aortoiliac region and in maintaining adequate spectral Doppler angles (Fig. 9.7D).

2. The external iliac artery is then identified in longitudinal section and followed proximally toward its origin using color flow imaging. Sometimes, tilting or rolling of the transducer and the use of oblique and coronal probe positions along the abdominal wall are useful in imaging around areas of bowel gas.

3. The common iliac bifurcation should be identified by locating the origin of the external iliac and internal iliac arteries. This can be achieved in the longitudinal plane, but transverse imaging is also helpful for confirmation if the image is adequate, as the internal iliac artery usually divides in a posteromedial direction (Fig. 9.7B). This area serves as an important anatomical landmark for localizing areas of disease in the aortoiliac system. Sometimes it is not possible to identify the internal iliac artery, and the position of the common iliac bifurcation has to be inferred, as it usually lies in the deepest part of the pelvis, as seen on the scan image.

4. The CIA is then followed back to the aortic bifurcation in longitudinal section (Fig. 9.7D). At this point, it is useful to confirm the level of the aortic bifurcation in transverse plane (Fig. 9.7C). The origins of the CIA are assessed in the longitudinal plane. The aorta should also be examined in transverse and longitudinal planes to exclude an aortic aneurysm or stenosis (see Ch. 11).

Assessment of the femoral and popliteal arteries

To start the examination, the patient should be lying reasonably flat with the leg rotated outward and the knee gently flexed and supported. A color image of the femoropopliteal and calf arteries is shown in Figure 9.9. The scanning positions for imaging the femoropopliteal arteries are shown in Figure 9.10. The procedure for assessment is as follows:

1. The CFA is identified in transverse section with a 5 MHz, or broadband equivalent, flat linear array transducer at the groin and followed distally to demonstrate the femoral bifurcation (Figs 9.6 and 9.10A). The CFA lies lateral to the common femoral vein (Fig. 9.6).

2. Turning to a longitudinal plane, the femoral bifurcation is examined (Fig. 9.10B). The profunda femoris artery usually lies posterolateral to the SFA, requiring a slight outward turn of the transducer. The profunda femoris artery can

Figure 9.9 A color montage of the femoropopliteal and calf arteries. The image shows the profunda femoris artery (PA), SFA, popliteal artery (POP), tibial peroneal trunk (TPT), PT, AT and peroneal artery (PER).

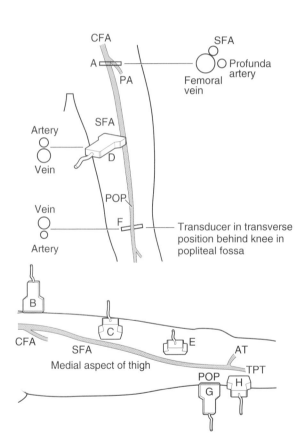

Figure 9.10 Probe positions for imaging the femoropopliteal arteries. A: Femoral artery bifurcation transverse. B: Femoral bifurcation longitudinal. C: SFA longitudinal. D: SFA transverse. E: Proximal popliteal artery above-knee longitudinal. F: Popliteal artery transverse. G: Popliteal artery longitudinal, from the popliteal fossa. H: Origin of the AT.

often be followed for a considerable distance, particularly if the SFA is occluded and it is supplying a collateral pathway to the lower thigh. The origin of the SFA is usually located anteromedial to the profunda femoris artery, requiring a slight inward turn of the transducer.

3. The SFA is then followed distally along the medial aspect of the thigh in a longitudinal plane, where it will lie above the superficial femoral vein (Fig. 9.10C). If the image of the SFA is lost it is easier to relocate in transverse section (Fig. 9.10D). In its distal segment the SFA runs deep and enters the adductor canal, becoming the popliteal artery. It is usually possible to image the proximal popliteal artery to just above the knee level from this position (see Fig. 9.10E). A 3.5 MHz transducer can help to image the artery in a large thigh.

4. The popliteal artery can be examined by rolling the patient onto the side. Alternatively, the patient can lie in a prone position, resting the foot on a pillow, although a lot of elderly patients are not able to tolerate this position. It is also possible to image the popliteal artery with the legs hanging over the edge of the examination table and the feet resting on a stool. Whichever method is used, it is important not to overextend the knee joint as this can make imaging difficult.

5. Starting in the middle of the popliteal fossa, the popliteal artery is located in transverse section and is seen posterior to the popliteal vein (Fig. 9.10F). Turning into a longitudinal plane, the popliteal artery is then followed proximally,

above the popliteal fossa, to overlap the area previously examined from the lower medial thigh (Fig. 9.10G).

6. The popliteal artery is then examined longitudinally across and below the popliteal fossa, where it is possible to continue directly into the tibioperoneal trunk. The tibioperoneal trunk can be imaged from a number of positions.

Assessment of the tibial arteries

The tibial arteries can be imaged from several different transducer positions, as demonstrated in Figure 9.11. It is often easier to locate the tibial arteries in the distal calf and follow them proximally to the top of the calf. However, for the purposes of this section, the description of the examination starts just below the knee. It should be noted that imaging of the distal tibial arteries at the ankle is often easier with a high-frequency 10 MHz, or broadband equivalent, flat linear array transducer.

Anterior tibial artery

1. With the leg rolled outward and the knee slightly flexed, the origin of the anterior tibial (AT) artery is imaged from a posteromedial position just below the knee, where it will be seen to drop immediately away from the popliteal artery (Fig. 9.10H). Often it is only possible to see the first 1–2 cm of the AT from this position. The tibioperoneal trunk is usually seen as a direct continuation of the popliteal artery distal to the AT artery origin.

2. The proximal AT artery is then imaged from the anterolateral aspect of the upper calf, just below the knee, where it will be seen to rise toward the transducer in a curve, through the interosseous membrane. The membrane can be identified as a bright echogenic line running between the tibia and fibula in cross section. The artery will lie on top of the membrane. The AT artery is then followed distally, along the anterolateral

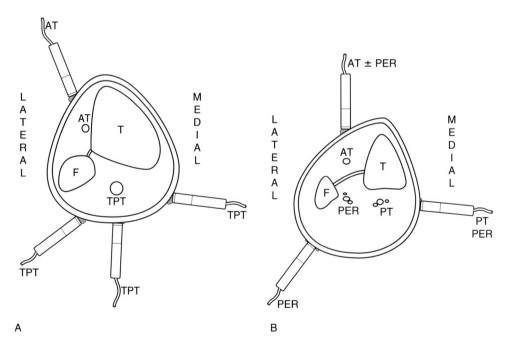

A   B

Figure 9.11 Cross-sections of the calf to show longitudinal transducer positions for imaging the tibial arteries and veins in the calf. A: Several positions can be used to image the vessels in the upper calf proximal to the bifurcation of the tibioperoneal trunk (TPT). B: Probe positions to image the PT, AT and peroneal artery (PER) in the mid- and lower calf. Note that it is possible to image two vessels from a similar position, as shown.

border of the calf, until it becomes the dorsalis pedis artery, over the top of the foot.

Posterior tibial artery

1. With the leg rolled outward and the knee flexed, the origin of the posterior tibial (PT) artery is imaged from a medial position, below the knee, where the tibioperoneal trunk divides into the PT artery and the peroneal artery. The proximal PT artery will gently rise toward the transducer, and the associated paired veins act as useful landmarks. The origin of the peroneal artery is often visible from this plane and will lie posterior to the PT artery origin.
2. The PT artery is then followed along the medial aspect of the calf toward the inner ankle or medial malleolus. The PT artery lies superficial to the peroneal artery when imaged from the medial aspect of the calf.
3. The origin and a short segment of the PT artery can often be visualized from a posterolateral position below the knee, where it will be seen to run deep as it divides from the tibioperoneal trunk.

Peroneal artery

Imaging of the peroneal artery may have to be performed from a number of different positions (Fig. 9.11B). The optimum position varies from patient to patient.

View 1   The peroneal artery can be followed from its origin along the calf using the same medial calf position as that described to image the PT artery. From this position, the peroneal artery will be seen lying deeper than the PT artery against the border of the fibula, surrounded by the larger peroneal veins. Slight anterior or posterior longitudinal tilting of the probe may be needed to follow the artery distally.

View 2   The peroneal artery can usually be followed distally from its origin using a posterolateral position, below the knee and along the calf.

View 3   The peroneal artery can sometimes be imaged from the anterolateral aspect of the calf, where it will be seen lying deep to the AT artery.

This is the most difficult position from which to obtain images of the peroneal artery.

Assessment of tibial arteries and the plantar arch prior to bypass surgery

Duplex scanning in combination with continuous wave Doppler recordings can be a useful method of determining which calf artery is supplying most blood to the distal region of the foot prior to distal bypass surgery (McCarthy et al 1999). In this way, it is possible to select a target vessel to position the distal anastomosis. This is important as there needs to be a low-resistance arterial pathway to the foot, distal to a graft, to ensure that the graft remains patent and the foot perfused. The three tibial arteries of the calf have connections to the plantar arch, which is located toward the end of the foot. The PT and dorsalis pedis arteries usually contribute most flow to the arch via plantar arteries. The plantar arch supplies blood to the plantar metatarsal arteries and digital arteries of the toes. The patient should be assessed with the leg in a dependent position to maximize blood flow distal to the diseased part of the vessel. Using the duplex scanner, it is possible to assess the patency and quality of each of the tibial arteries to ankle level. A continuous wave Doppler probe is then used to assess the Doppler signals from the plantar arch. The probe position for recording flow at the plantar arch is demonstrated in Figure 9.3. Selective digital pressure is then applied over the most suitable tibial artery, as previously demonstrated by duplex scanning of the target vessel, to occlude it at the ankle. A substantial reduction or cessation of flow at the plantar arch during compression would suggest that the arch is in continuation with the selected tibial artery. This type of assessment can be complex, as there may be more than one patent tibial artery supplying the plantar arch. The peroneal artery can also supply the distal AT artery or dorsalis pedal artery via branches, which in turn may supply the plantar arch.

Commonly encountered problems

There are a number of problems and pitfalls associated with lower limb duplex scanning. Table 9.4 lists some of the more frequently encountered problems.

Table 9.4   Common problems encountered during duplex evaluation of the lower limb arteries

Segment	Problem	Solutions
Aortoiliac arteries	Bowel gas obscuring part or all of the image	Try different probe positions (medial, lateral or coronal positions); leave the segment and try again in a few minutes
Aortoiliac arteries	Tortuous arteries	Use the color display to follow the artery; considerable adjustment of the probe position is often needed
Femoropopliteal arteries	Severe calcification of the artery producing color image dropout	Try different transducer positions to work around the calcification
Femoropopliteal arteries	Obese patient with large thigh	When using a broad-band transducer, lower the color and spectral Doppler transmit frequencies for better penetration; consider switching to a 3.5 MHz curved linear array transducer in very difficult situations
Tibial arteries	Large calf with gross edema	Start the scan at the ankle and work proximally; a 3.5 MHz linear array probe can be used to image these vessels proximally
Tibial arteries	Very low flow due to proximal occlusions	Lower the pulse repetition frequency and wall filters; place the leg in a dependent position to increase distal blood flow

SCAN APPEARANCES

B-mode images

Normal appearance

Like the carotid arteries, the lumen of a normal peripheral artery should appear clear, and the walls should be uniform along each arterial segment, although noise may cause speckle within the image of the vessel. The intima-media layer of the arterial wall is sometimes seen in normal femoral and popliteal arteries. In practice, it is frequently difficult to clearly image the vessels in the aortoiliac segment, abductor canal region and calf without the help of color flow imaging.

Abnormal appearance

Areas of atheroma, particularly if they are calcified, may be seen within the vessel lumen. The atheroma may be extensive and diffusely distributed, especially in the SFA (Fig. 9.12). Large plaques at the common femoral bifurcation are relatively easy to image, and

Figure 9.12   Calcified atheroma (arrows) is present in the SFA, leading to drop-out of the color flow signal in parts of the lumen.

these may extend into the proximal profunda artery or SFA. Calcification of the arterial wall, especially in diabetic patients, produces strong ultrasound reflections, and the walls of the calf arteries can appear particularly prominent (Fig. 9.4). When an arterial segment has been occluded for some time, the vessel may contract and appear as a small cord adjacent to the corresponding vein. This appearance

Figure 9.13 An acute occlusion of the popliteal artery. The vessel is patent to the level of the two arrows. The occlusion is demonstrated by the relatively low level echoes in the lumen distally. Note some intimal detail is still visible in the occluded section (curved arrow).

Figure 9.14 Two severe stenoses are demonstrated in the SFA by areas of color flow disturbance and aliasing (arrows).

is most frequently seen in the SFA and popliteal artery. B-mode imaging in combination with color flow imaging is also very useful for identifying acute occlusions of the SFA or popliteal artery, where there may be fresh thrombus present in the vessel lumen. The lumen will appear clear or demonstrate minimal echoes on the image, because thrombus has a similar echogenicity to blood (Fig. 9.13). However, color flow imaging reveals an absence of flow in the occluded segment of the vessel. The start of the occlusion can often be very abrupt, with little disease seen proximally.

Abnormal dilatations or arterial aneurysms should be measured using the B-mode image, as described in Chapter 11.

Color flow images

Normal appearance

Normal arterial segments can be interrogated rapidly using color flow imaging. There should be color filling to the vessel walls. The color image normally demonstrates a pulsatile flow pattern, with the color alternating between red and blue due to flow reversal during the diastolic phase (see Ch. 5). There are situations in which flow in nondiseased lower limb arteries may have reduced pulsatility or even be continuous. Examples include increased flow (hyperemia) due to limb infection or the presence of arteriovenous fistulas. Hyperemic flow will be

demonstrated as continuous flow in one color scale but there should be no evidence of arterial stenosis.

Abnormal appearance

Utilizing the color controls as described in Chapter 7, arterial stenoses will be demonstrated as areas of color flow disturbance or aliasing. Severe stenoses frequently produce a disturbed color flow pattern extending 3 to 4 vessel diameters beyond the lesion (Figs 9.8 and 9.14). Any areas of color flow disturbance should be investigated with angle-corrected spectral Doppler to estimate the degree of narrowing. In addition, the color flow image of flow in a nondiseased artery distal to severe proximal disease may demonstrate damped low-velocity flow, which will be seen as continuous flow in one direction.

Occlusions of lower limb arteries most frequently occur in the SFA and popliteal artery. An occlusion is demonstrated by a total absence of color flow in the vessel. Occlusions can occur at the origins of arteries or in mid-segment. If an artery is occluded from its origin, at the level of a major bifurcation, flow will normally still be seen in the sister branch. For example, the profunda femoris artery is usually found to be patent when the SFA is occluded (Fig. 9.15). When an artery occludes in mid-segment, collateral vessels are normally seen dividing from the main trunk at the beginning of the occlusion. Similarly, collateral vessels resupply flow to the artery at the distal end of the occlusion (Fig. 9.16). Collateral vessels can follow tortuous routes as they divide from the main trunk, and they are sometimes only seen when the main artery is imaged in cross-section. It is therefore helpful to interrogate any suspected

Figure 9.15 A: Color flow image of the femoral bifurcation demonstrating an SFA origin occlusion (arrow). The profunda femoris artery (PA) is patent. B: Color flow image of an external iliac artery (EIA) occlusion (arrow). The CIA and internal iliac artery (IIA) are patent. The common iliac vein (CIV) is visible in this image.

Figure 9.16 A short mid-SFA occlusion is demonstrated by an absence of color flow in the vessel (large arrow). Large collateral vessels are seen at both ends of the occlusion (small arrows).

occlusion in both longitudinal and transverse imaging planes. The PRF often needs to be lowered (typically to 1 kHz) distal to an occlusion in order to increase the sensitivity of the scanner to lower flow velocities. The color flow image distal to an occlusion often demonstrates a continuous forward flow pattern with reduced pulsatility due to damping of the normal blood flow pattern. Blood flow in the main artery may also improve progressively over the first few centimeters distal to the occlusion as more collateral vessels join the main trunk. This effect can be observed on the color flow image (Fig. 9.17). High-velocity flow in a collateral vessel can produce an area of marked color flow disturbance in the main artery at the point where the collateral joins. This can be misinterpreted as a stenosis. Spectral Doppler should be used to interrogate this area carefully. It is possible

to misdiagnose a long stricture as an occlusion because of very slow flow through the stricture due to the development of good collateral flow around the diseased site. The PRF should be lowered to examine low-velocity flow across these lesions.

Spectral Doppler

Normal recordings

At rest, the normal spectral Doppler display of extremity arterial blood flow demonstrates a triphasic flow pattern with a clear spectral window (Fig. 9.18). It may even be possible to see four phases in young healthy adults. In elderly patients or patients with poor cardiac output, the waveform may be biphasic or even monophonic. The average

Figure 9.17 A color montage demonstrates flow in the popliteal artery distal to an occlusion (O). The flow becomes progressively higher distal to the occlusion, as more collateral vessels join the main artery (arrows). Marked areas of flow disturbance can occur at points where collateral vessels feed the main artery, and these can be mistaken for stenoses.

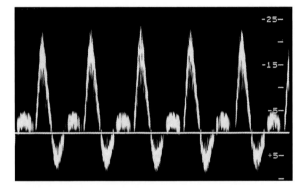

Figure 9.18 A normal triphasic Doppler waveform recorded from the SFA.

peak systolic velocity found in the external iliac, SFA and popliteal arteries are 119, 90 and 68 cm/s, respectively (Jager et al 1985). During the examination, spectral Doppler recordings should be taken at frequent intervals to confirm that the flow pattern is normal. Spectral Doppler recordings taken from patients with infections such as cellulitis may demonstrate hyperemic flow with reduced pulsatility.

Abnormal recordings and grading of stenoses

Areas of color flow disturbance should always be interrogated with spectral Doppler. The spectral Doppler sample volume should be small, and the measurements should be taken just proximal to, across and just beyond the lesion. In the presence of a significant stenosis, there will be an increase in flow velocity across the lesion associated with spectral broadening and turbulence just distal to the lesion. As demonstrated previously, a concentric

Figure 9.19 An SFA stenosis is assessed using spectral Doppler. A: Measurement of the peak systolic velocity just proximal to the stenosis. B: Measurement of the peak systolic velocity across the stenosis. The peak systolic velocity ratio is calculated by dividing B by A, producing a velocity ratio of 5. This would indicate a severe stenosis.

50% diameter reduction of the arterial lumen will produce a 75% reduction in cross-sectional area, leading to significant flow changes. The main criterion used to grade the degree of narrowing in a lower limb artery is the measurement of the peak systolic velocity ratio. The peak systolic velocity ratio is calculated by dividing the maximum peak systolic velocity recorded across the stenosis (V_s) by the peak systolic velocity recorded in a normal area of the artery just proximal to the stenosis (V_p), as demonstrated in Figure 9.19. Different protocols

Table 9.5 Suggested criteria for grading lower limb arterial disease using velocity ratios, based on several references (see text)

Diameter reduction	Velocity ratio (V_s/V_p)	Comments
0–49%	<2	Waveform is triphasic but mild spectral broadening and an increase in end diastolic velocities are recorded as the degree of narrowing approaches 49%
50–74%	≥2	Waveforms tend to become biphasic or monophasic; there is an increase in end diastolic velocity; spectral broadening is present; flow disturbance and some damping are recorded distal to the stenosis
75–99%	≥4	Waveform is usually monophasic with a significant increase in end diastolic velocity; marked turbulence and spectral broadening are demonstrated; flow is damped distal to the stenosis
Occluded	No flow detected	Doppler waveforms proximal to an occlusion often demonstrate a high-resistance flow pattern

have been published for defining a 50%, or greater, diameter reduction in the lower limb arteries. Many vascular units use a peak systolic velocity ratio of equal to or greater than 2 (Cossman et al 1989, Sensier et al 1996), although a ratio of 2.5 is used by other centers (Legemate et al 1991). It is important to audit and evaluate the criteria used by your unit against other imaging techniques such as angiography or MRA. Table 9.5 shows how the velocity ratio can be used to grade the severity of lower limb disease (Hennerici & Neuerburg-Heusler 1998). Velocity ratios can still be used to grade stenoses in the presence of multi-segment disease. Other methods of measurement, including pulsatility index (PI), have tended to be used with continuous wave Doppler but are probably less useful for duplex scanning where velocity changes can be measured directly.

Abnormal waveform shapes

The shape of the spectral Doppler waveform can provide considerable information about the condition of lower limb arteries. Damped monophasic waveforms with an increased systolic rise time are characteristic of disease proximal to the point of measurement (Fig. 9.20B). Conversely, high-resistance, low-volume flow waveforms often indicate severe disease distal to the point of measurement. One such example is the characteristic shoulder seen on the systolic downstroke of an SFA waveform recorded proximal to severe disease in the SFA (Fig. 9.20A). This is due to a reflected

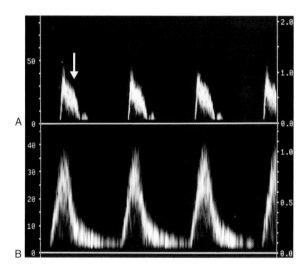

Figure 9.20 Waveform shapes can reveal useful information about the condition of proximal and distal arteries. A: Waveform recorded from the SFA just proximal to an occlusion. Note the high-resistance, low-volume waveform shape and characteristic shoulder on the systolic downstroke (arrow), due to pulse wave reflection from distal disease. B: Damping of the CFA waveform with an increased systolic acceleration time and loss of pulsatility indicates significant proximal disease.

wave from the distal disease or occlusion. Severe calcification of the arterial wall may also affect the shape of the recorded Doppler waveform due to changes in vessel compliance. This is commonly observed in the tibial vessels of diabetic patients, where the waveform shape may become monophasic.

Much debate has surrounded the shape of the CFA waveform as an indicator of iliac artery or inflow disease. A study by Sensier et al (1998) demonstrated that qualitative assessment of the CFA Doppler waveform has a sensitivity of 95%, a specificity of 80% and an accuracy of 87% for the prediction of significant aortoiliac artery disease. This study therefore suggests that observation of the CFA waveform shape is a useful technique for the investigation of inflow disease. The presence of triphasic flow with a short systolic rise time is an indicator of normal inflow. However, care should be exercised when investigating younger patients, who may have a very short proximal iliac stenosis, as the arterial waveform shape may have recovered at the level of the CFA, appearing normal. Marked damping of the CFA waveform with an increase in systolic acceleration time is a good indicator of severe inflow disease. Perhaps the most confusing situation occurs where the inflow arteries are normal but the SFA is occluded and the profunda femoris artery is severely stenosed. This can give rise to a monophonic waveform pattern in the CFA with a high end diastolic velocity, although the systolic acceleration time remains short. A great deal of care should be used in interpreting flow patterns in this situation.

Areas of aneurysmal dilation typically demonstrate a reduction in peak systolic velocity, frequently associated with disturbed flow patterns.

ASSESSMENT OF ARTERIAL STENTS

Arterial stents are used to prevent re-stenosis, although there is limited published evidence to demonstrate that they are any more effective than standard angioplasty at maintaining long-term vessel patency. Stents are mainly deployed in the aortoiliac arteries and proximal CFA, although they are also used in the SFA and popliteal artery. Stents are available in different lengths and sizes, and multiple stents can be deployed if the disease is very extensive. They are usually visible on the B-mode image, producing a stronger reflection compared to the arterial wall. The cross-hatched, or lattice, metal structure can often be identified. It is sometimes possible to see nipping of the stent if the atheroma in the artery is very calcified or fibrous and has not been completely compressed to the vessel wall. Color flow imaging

Figure 9.21   Color flow imaging demonstrates a long stricture in a CFA stent caused by intimal hyperplasia. The stent walls are clearly visible (arrows).

and spectral Doppler can be used to assess the flow across the stent (Fig. 9.21). It is not uncommon to find some localized flow disturbance in the region of the stent due to the step between the arterial wall and proximal and distal ends of the stent. Spectral Doppler should be used to grade the degree of any in-stent stenosis using the same criteria as used for grading lower limb disease. Stents placed in arteries close to joints, such as the CFA or popliteal artery, can be stressed by joint movement and may kink or bend. Localized aneurysms can be excluded by inserting a covered stent across the aneurysm; this is discussed in Chapter 11.

OTHER ABNORMALITIES AND SYNDROMES

Lower limb symptoms in younger patients are sometimes due to inflammatory or small vessel disorders, such as Buerger's disease. Flow recordings are normal in the larger arteries proximally, but the distal vessels in the calf may demonstrate low-flow, high-resistance waveforms.

Popliteal entrapment syndrome

Popliteal entrapment syndrome is also a rare but potential cause of claudication and possible distal embolization due to arterial wall damage. In this situation, the popliteal artery follows an anomalous course below the knee and is trapped by the heads of the gastrocnemius muscle during plantar flexion. The popliteal artery can also be trapped by fibrous bands in this area. To test for popliteal entrapment syndrome, the patient should lie prone with the legs gently flexed and the feet hanging over the end of the examination table. The below-knee popliteal artery should be imaged at the level of the gastrocnemius muscle heads. The patient should point the foot down (plantar flex) against a counterpressure, typically by having a colleague apply moderate pressure against the foot. Narrowing or occlusion of the popliteal artery during this maneuver may indicate popliteal entrapment syndrome. However, there is evidence to suggest that significant compression of the popliteal artery can occur in normal volunteers during this investigation, casting some doubt on the usefulness of this test (Erdoes et al 1994).

Cystic adventitial disease of the popliteal artery

This rare disease is caused by cystic swelling of the arterial wall, which impinges into the lumen of the popliteal artery, leading to eventual occlusion. The location of the lesion is often found across the knee joint. It should be considered as a potential cause of symptoms in the young patient, especially in the absence of any other pathology. Treatment is by excision and local repair or bypassing.

REPORTING

In our experience, the use of diagrams demonstrating the position of disease and corresponding velocity measurements and ratios is the simplest method of reporting results, as shown in Figure 9.22. Areas that were impossible to assess can be hatched out on the diagram. Surgeons and physicians also find this method of reporting helpful when reviewing results in a busy outpatient clinic, as reading pages of text can be very time-consuming. Copies of the report can be sent to the radiology department with a request card if the patient requires an angiogram or angioplasty, thus allowing the radiologist to pre-plan puncture sites. In many situations an angioplasty can be performed without a diagnostic arteriogram.

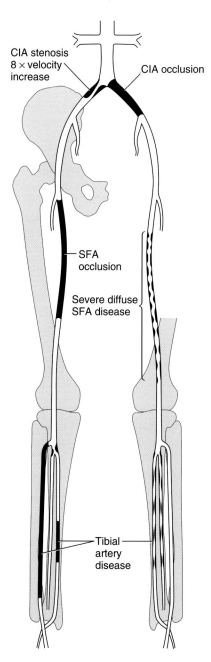

Figure 9.22 The easiest method of reporting lower limb scans is by the use of diagrams. Areas of narrowing can be drawn onto the map and the corresponding velocity recordings indicated. Occlusions are demonstrated by blocking out the appropriate regions.

References

AbuRahma A F 2000 Segmental Doppler pressures and Doppler waveform analysis in peripheral vascular disease of the lower extremities. In: AbuRahma A F, Bergan J J (eds) Noninvasive vascular diagnosis. Springer, London, pp 213–229

Cossman D V, Ellison J E, Wagner W H, et al 1989 Comparison of contrast arteriography to arterial mapping with color-flow duplex imaging in the lower extremities. Journal of Vascular Surgery 10(5):522–529

Egglin T K, O'Moore P V, Feinstein A R, et al 1995 Complications of peripheral arteriography: a new system to identify patients at increased risk. Journal of Vascular Surgery 22(6):787–794

Erdoes L S, Devine J J, Bernhard V M, et al 1994 Popliteal vascular compression in a normal population. Journal of Vascular Surgery 20(6):978–986

European Working Group on Critical Leg Ischaemia. Second European consensus document on chronic critical leg ischaemia 1992. European Journal of Vascular Surgery 6(5)[Suppl A]:1–32

Fowkes F G, Housley E, Cawood E H, et al 1991 Edinburgh Artery Study: prevalence of asymptomatic and symptomatic peripheral arterial disease in the general population. International Journal of Epidemiology 20(2):384–392

Hennerici M, Neuerburg-Heusler D 1998 Vascular diagnosis with ultrasound. Thieme, Stuttgart, pp 179–180

Jager K A, Ricketts H J, Strandness D E Jr 1985 Duplex scanning for the evaluation of lower limb arterial disease. In: Bernstein E F (ed) Noninvasive diagnostic techniques in vascular disease. C V Mosby, St Louis, pp 619–631

Legemate D A, Teeuwen C, Hoeneveld H, et al 1989 The potential of duplex scanning to replace aortoiliac and femoro-popliteal angiography. European Journal of Vascular Surgery 3(1):49–54

Legemate D A, Teeuwen C, Hoeneveld H, et al 1991 Spectral analysis criteria in duplex scanning of aortoiliac and femoropopliteal arterial disease. Ultrasound in Medicine and Biology 17(8):769–776

McCarthy M J, Nydahl S, Hartshorne T, et al 1999 Color-coded duplex imaging and dependent Doppler ultrasonography in the assessment of cruropedal vessels. British Journal of Surgery 86(1):33–37

Pemberton M, London N J 1997 Color flow duplex imaging of occlusive arterial disease of the lower limb. British Journal of Surgery 84(7):912–919

Proia R R, Walsh D B, Nelson P R, et al 2001 Early results of infragenicular revascularization based solely on duplex arteriography. Journal of Vascular Surgery 33(6):1165–1170

Sensier Y, Hartshorne T, Thrush A, et al 1996 A prospective comparison of lower limb color-coded duplex scanning with arteriography. European Journal of Vascular and Endovascular Surgery 11(2):170–175

Sensier Y, Bell P R, London N J 1998 The ability of qualitative assessment of the common femoral Doppler waveform to screen for significant aortoiliac disease. European Journal of Vascular and Endovascular Surgery 15(4):357–364

Further reading

AbuRahma A F, Bergan J J 2000 Noninvasive vascular diagnosis. Springer, London

Polak J F 1992 Peripheral vascular sonography. Williams & Wilkins, Baltimore

Zwiebel W J 1992 Introduction to vascular ultrasonography, 3rd edn. W B Saunders, Philadelphia

Chapter **10**

Duplex assessment of upper extremity arterial disease

CHAPTER CONTENTS

Introduction   133
Anatomy of the upper extremity arteries   133
Symptoms and treatment of upper limb
   arterial disease   135
Practical considerations for duplex assessment
   of upper extremity arterial disease   135
Scanning techniques   136
   Subclavian and axillary arteries   136
   Brachial artery   137
   Radial and ulnar arteries   137
   Palmar arch and digital arteries   138
   Commonly encountered problems   138
Ultrasound appearance   138
   Normal appearance   138
   Abnormal appearance   138
Thoracic outlet syndrome (TOS)   139
   Maneuvers for assessing TOS   140
   Duplex assessment of TOS   141
Aneurysms   142
Ultrasound assessment of hemodialysis
   access grafts and arteriovenous
   fistulas (AVF)   142
Other disorders of the upper extremity
   circulation   143
Reporting   143

INTRODUCTION

In contrast to lower limb arteries, atherosclerotic disease in the upper extremities is rare and accounts for approximately 5% of all extremity disease (Abou-Zamzam et al 2000). The most commonly affected sites are the subclavian (SA) and axillary arteries. The disorder is sometimes associated with extracranial carotid artery disease. Radiotherapy in this region, resulting in fibrosis and scarring, can also cause damage to the SA and axillary arteries. Compression of the SA in the area of the thoracic outlet, known as thoracic outlet syndrome (TOS), can produce significant upper limb symptoms.

Acute obstruction of the axillary or brachial arteries may also occur due to embolization from the heart or SA aneurysms. In this situation, duplex scanning is useful for demonstrating the length and position of the occlusion. Microvascular disorders, such as Raynaud's phenomenon, can produce significant symptoms in the hands, which may be confused with atherosclerotic disease.

ANATOMY OF THE UPPER EXTREMITY ARTERIES

The anatomy of the upper extremity arteries is illustrated in Figures 10.1 and 10.2. The left SA divides directly from the aortic arch, but the right SA originates from the innominate or brachiocephalic artery. The thoracic outlet is the point where the SA, subclavian vein and brachial nerve plexus exit the chest. The SA runs between the anterior and middle scalene muscles and passes

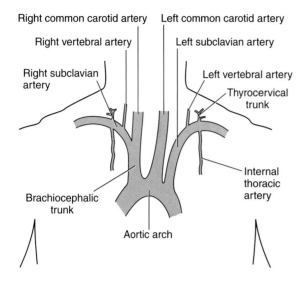

Figure 10.1 The arterial anatomy of the aortic arch and subclavian artery.

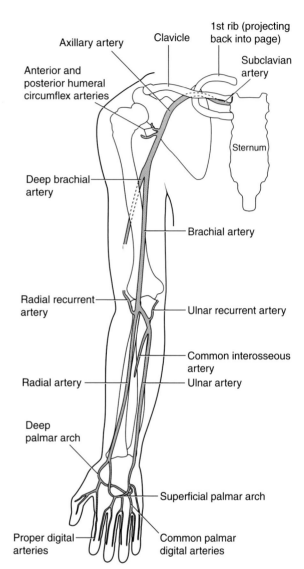

Figure 10.2 The arterial anatomy of the arm and hand.

between the clavicle and first rib to become the axillary artery. The diameter of the SA ranges from 0.6 to 1.1 cm. The SA has a number of important branches, including the vertebral artery and internal thoracic artery (also referred to as the mammary artery), which is frequently used for coronary artery bypass surgery.

The axillary artery becomes the brachial artery as it crosses the lower margin of the tendon of the teres major muscle, at the top of the arm. The diameter of the axillary artery ranges between 0.6 and 0.8 cm. The brachial artery then runs distally on the medial or inner side of the arm in a groove between the triceps and biceps muscles. The deep brachial artery divides from the main trunk of the brachial artery in the upper arm and acts as an important collateral pathway around the elbow if the brachial artery is occluded distally. The brachial artery runs in a medial to lateral course over the inner aspect of the elbow (cubital fossa) and then divides, 1–2 cm below the elbow, into the radial and ulnar arteries. The ulnar artery dives deep beneath the flexor tendons in the upper forearm. The radial artery runs along the lateral side of the forearm toward the thumb and is palpable at the wrist. The ulnar artery runs along the medial side of the forearm and is sometimes the dominant vessel of the forearm. The common interosseous artery is an important branch of the ulnar artery in the upper forearm as

it can act as a collateral pathway if the radial and ulnar arteries are occluded. The radial artery supplies the deep palmar arch in the hand, and the ulnar artery supplies the superficial palmar arch. There are usually communicating arteries between the two systems. In some people only one of the wrist arteries will supply the palmar arch system. The fingers are supplied by the palmar digital arteries. There are a number of anatomical variations in the arm, which are shown in Table 10.1. The arms

Table 10.1 Anatomical variations of the upper limb arteries

Artery	Variation
Left subclavian artery	Common origin with common carotid artery from aortic arch
Brachial artery	High bifurcation of brachial artery
Radial artery	High origin from axillary artery
Ulnar artery	High origin from axillary artery

Table 10.2 Major collateral pathways of the upper arm

Diseased segment	Normal distal artery	Possible pathways
Proximal subclavian artery	Distal subclavian artery	Vertebral artery, internal thoracic artery and thyro-cervical trunk
Distal subclavian or proximal axillary artery	Distal axillary artery	Collateral flow to the circumflex humeral arteries
Brachial artery	Distal brachial artery or proximal radial and ulnar arteries	Deep brachial artery to the recurrent radial and ulnar arteries
Radial and ulnar arteries	Distal radial and ulnar arteries	Interosseous artery and branches of the recurrent radial and ulnar arteries

Box 10.1 **Common causes of symptoms involving the arterial and microvascular circulation of the arms and hands**

- Atherosclerotic disease
- Acute obstruction due to emboli from the heart
- Aneurysms
- Fibrosis of the subclavian and axillary arteries due to radiotherapy
- Shoulder and arm dislocation
- Trauma or stab wounds
- Damage caused by arterial access and invasive blood pressure lines
- Thoracic outlet syndrome
- Raynaud's phenomenon
- Reflex sympathetic dystrophy
- Vibration white finger disease
- Takayasu's arteritis

normally develop good collateral circulation around diseased segments. The major collateral pathways of the arm are summarized in Table 10.2.

SYMPTOMS AND TREATMENT OF UPPER LIMB ARTERIAL DISEASE

The main causes of upper limb disorders are shown in Box 10.1. Many patients with chronic upper limb arterial disease experience few symptoms because of the development of good collateral circulation in the arm. However, some patients complain of aching and heaviness in the arm following a period of use or exercise. Patients with significant chronic symptoms can be treated by angioplasty, provided that the lesion is suitable for dilation. Arterial bypass surgery is rarely performed in the upper extremities. Acute obstructions can produce marked distal ischemia, and the forearm and hand may be cold and painful. In many cases of acute ischemia the condition of the arm and hand improves with appropriate anticoagulation. However, embolectomy, thrombolysis or bypass surgery may be performed if there is persistent distal ischemia. Trauma, due to injury or stab wounds to the arm or shoulder, can result in arterial damage, requiring local repair or bypass surgery. SA or axillary artery aneurysms can be bypassed with grafts, although in some cases a covered stent can be deployed to exclude flow in the aneurysm sac. Occasionally, patients with arteriovenous fistulas will be encountered. These fistulas range in size and distribution and can affect the hand as well as the arm.

PRACTICAL CONSIDERATIONS FOR DUPLEX ASSESSMENT OF UPPER EXTREMITY ARTERIAL DISEASE

The objective of the scan is to identify and grade the severity of arterial disease in the upper limb arteries. In addition, the thoracic outlet can be investigated for possible compression of the SA. A minimum of half an hour should be allocated for the examination.

There is no special preparation required prior to the scan, although the patient will have to expose the shoulder and upper arm for scanning of the distal SA and axillary arteries. The examination room should be at a comfortable ambient temperature ($>20°$ C) to prevent vasoconstriction of the distal arteries. The patient should lie supine with the head supported on a thin pillow for comfort. The SA and proximal axillary artery can be scanned by sitting behind the patient. This is usually a more comfortable position than scanning from the side of the patient. To image the distal axillary and brachial arteries, the patient should be examined from the side of the examination table and the arm should be abducted, be externally rotated and be resting on an arm board or a suitable rest. The distal brachial, radial and ulnar arteries are imaged with the hand in a palm-up position, resting on a support. The scanner should be configured for a peripheral arterial examination, and in the absence of a specific upper limb preset, a lower limb arterial option should be selected.

SCANNING TECHNIQUES

A 5 MHz, or broad-band equivalent, flat linear array transducer is the most suitable probe for scanning the SA and axillary arteries. A 10 MHz, or broad-band equivalent, flat linear array transducer produces the best images of the brachial, radial and ulnar arteries, particularly as the radial and ulnar arteries are very superficial at the wrist. In addition, a 5–7 MHz curved linear array transducer can be useful for imaging the proximal SA at the level of the supraclavicular fossa, as it fits more easily into the contour of this region. The transducer positions for imaging the upper extremity arteries are shown in Figure 10.3. A color flow montage of the upper extremity arteries is shown in Figure 10.4.

Subclavian and axillary arteries

The SA is initially located in a transverse plane in the supraclavicular fossa, where it will lie superior

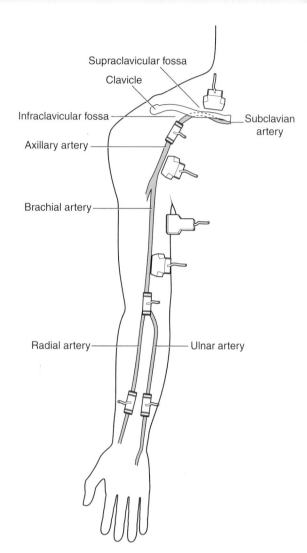

Figure 10.3 Transducer positions for scanning the upper extremity arteries.

to the subclavian vein. The transducer is turned to image the artery in longitudinal section and followed proximally toward its origin. The left SA origin is usually impossible to image, as the vessel arises from the aortic arch. It can sometimes be tracked toward its origin with a 2–2.5 MHz phase array transducer. This type of transducer can also be useful for imaging the brachiocephalic artery. Sometimes the origin of the right SA can be difficult to image, especially if the patient has a large or short neck. Extra gel may be needed to fill the depression of the supraclavicular fossa to enable

Figure 10.4 A color flow montage of the left upper extremity arteries demonstrating the subclavian artery (SA), axillary artery (AA), brachial artery (BA), deep brachial artery (DB), radial artery (RA), common interosseous artery (I) and ulnar artery (UA).

below the clavicle (see Fig. 10.12). A mirroring artifact of the SA is often seen due to the chest wall beneath the artery (see Fig. 7.7).

The SA reappears from underneath the clavicle and is followed distally, where it becomes the axillary artery. Two positions may be used to image the length of the axillary artery. The first is the anterior approach, in which the axillary artery will be seen to run deep beneath the shoulder muscles. A 3.5 MHz curved array transducer can sometimes be useful for following the distal axillary artery from this position. The second approach images the axillary artery from the axilla (armpit), where it can be followed distally to the brachial artery.

It is worth noting that the proximal segment of the internal thoracic artery, a proximal branch of the SA, can often be imaged. This artery is frequently used in coronary bypass surgery and is surgically grafted to the heart. It divides at a 90° angle from the inferior aspect of the SA to run down the chest wall. It is possible to confirm graft patency by identifying flow in the proximal thoracic artery just beyond its origin. The flow pattern in the artery supplying the heart will exhibit an unusual waveform shape, as most of the flow occurs in the diastolic phase of the cardiac cycle.

Brachial artery

The brachial artery is followed as a continuation of the axillary artery along the inner aspect of the arm to the elbow, where it curves around to the cubital fossa and lies in a superficial position.

The distal brachial artery is scanned across the elbow to the point where it divides in the upper forearm into the radial and ulnar arteries.

Radial and ulnar arteries

The bifurcation of the brachial artery into the radial and ulnar arteries is easier to locate in a transverse plane. The two arteries are then followed distally to the wrist in a longitudinal plane. In its proximal segment, the ulnar artery runs deep to the radial artery before becoming more superficial in the mid-forearm. It is often easier to locate the radial and ulnar arteries at the wrist and then to follow them back to the elbow.

good contact with a flat linear array transducer. The SA should then be followed laterally in longitudinal section, where it will disappear underneath the clavicle. There will be a large acoustic shadow

Palmar arch and digital arteries

Duplex scanning can be used to image the palmar arch and digital vessels, although continuous wave Doppler can be considerably quicker and easier to use for the detection of arterial signals, especially in the digital arteries. The radial artery is sometimes used as a graft for coronary artery bypass surgery. It is possible to listen to the digital arteries and palmar arch flow signals with continuous wave Doppler, while the radial artery is being manually compressed, to ensure that perfusion to the hand and fingers is being maintained by the ulnar artery. If this is not the case, removal of the radial artery could result in hand ischemia.

Commonly encountered problems

Most problems occur due to poor imaging, especially in large or obese patients, in whom the proximal arteries may be very difficult to image. In particular, the SA in the area of the supraclavicular fossa can be difficult to locate. Color flow imaging can present a confusing display as there are often strong signals from the adjacent subclavian vein, which may appear pulsatile due to the proximity to the right side of the heart. Imaging of the axillary artery can be difficult where the artery runs deep under the shoulder muscles. Scanning from the axilla or selecting a lower frequency probe may help.

ULTRASOUND APPEARANCE

Normal appearance

The normal appearance of upper extremity arteries is the same as that described for the duplex scanning of lower limb arteries (see Ch. 9). The spectral Doppler waveform is normally triphasic at rest but becomes hyperemic with high diastolic flow following exercise. Changes in external temperature can have marked effects on the observed flow patterns in the distal arteries. There is a cyclical effect on the appearance of the flow patterns in the distal arteries related to factors such as body temperature control. This cyclical effect can cause the waveform shape to change from high-resistance flow to hyperemic flow over a period of a minute or two (Fig. 10.5). Peripheral vasodilation will cause a reduction in peripheral resistance and an increase in

Figure 10.5   A cyclical change in the appearance of the blood flow patterns in the radial and ulnar arteries can be observed, relating to factors such as the control of body temperature.

flow. In this situation, the waveform in the radial and ulnar arteries can become hyperemic. Vasoconstriction increases peripheral resistance, producing a reduction in flow, and the waveform becomes biphasic. The range of normal peak systolic velocities in the SA has been reported as 80–120 cm/s (Edwards & Zierler 1992). It is often assumed that the radial artery is the dominant vessel in the forearm because it is easier to palpate at the wrist, but in many cases there is higher flow in the ulnar artery.

Abnormal appearance

In the absence of any specific criteria for grading upper limb arterial stenoses, we would advocate the use of the same criteria as for grading lower limb disease. Therefore, a doubling of the peak systolic velocity across a stenosis compared with the proximal normal adjacent segment indicates a ≥50% diameter reduction. However, many upper limb lesions are located at the origin to the SA, making proximal measurements from the aortic arch or brachiocephalic artery unreliable or impossible due to vessel depth, size and geometry. In this situation the diagnosis is usually made by indirect signs, such as high-velocity jets, turbulence or post-stenotic damping (Fig. 10.6). In addition, the ipsilateral vertebral artery should be examined for evidence of flow changes, indicated by damping or flow reversal (see Ch. 8). It can also be very difficult to visibly identify plaques at the origin to the SA. Occlusions of the proximal SA can be difficult to differentiate from severe stenoses (von Reutern & von Büdingen 1993), and any uncertainty should be highlighted in the report. Dissection of the radial, brachial or axillary arteries can occur due to trauma of the vessel wall following catheter access. It may

Figure 10.7 An embolus from the heart has acutely obstructed the brachial artery at the elbow. The arterial lumen appears clear, as the embolus has a similar echogenicity to blood, but there is a sudden cessation of flow at the start of the occlusion (arrow).

Figure 10.6 A severe high-grade stenosis of the proximal SA (arrow) is demonstrated by marked color flow disturbance and aliasing, high peak systolic velocity (389 cm/s), abnormal waveform shape and spectral broadening.

be possible to see flaps, dual lumens or acute obstruction.

Acute occlusions of upper extremity arteries are frequently caused by embolization from the heart and occur most commonly in the brachial, radial and ulnar arteries. The arterial lumen may appear relatively clear, but there will be an absence of flow in the vessel as demonstrated by color flow imaging (Fig. 10.7). Some acute occlusions occur as a result of embolization from the SA due to damage caused by TOS.

Large arteriovenous malformations will be immediately obvious with color flow imaging as a region of high vascularity. Spectral Doppler will demonstrate low-resistance, high-volume flow waveforms within the malformation.

THORACIC OUTLET SYNDROME (TOS)

The vascular laboratory is frequently asked to assess patients with suspected TOS. The thoracic outlet is

the region where the SA and brachial plexus leave the chest and pass in between the anterior and middle scalene muscles over the first rib and underneath the clavicle (Fig. 10.8). This is a compact anatomical area, and compression on the nerves or arteries by a number of mechanisms can produce sensory symptoms in both the hand and arm. Compression can occur in three main areas. The first is at the point where the SA passes between the scalene muscles and can be caused by muscle hypertrophy or fibrous bands or may be due to the presence of an additional accessory rib originating from the seventh thoracic vertebra, termed a cervical rib (Fig. 10.9). Accessory ribs occur in less than 1% of the population (Makhoul & Machleder 1992). The second area of compression occurs as the artery runs between the first rib and clavicle. Fibrous bands or fibrosis due to injuries in this region, such as fractures of the clavicle, can also cause compression. The third, less common area of compression occurs in the subcoracoid region, where the axillary artery runs under the pectoralis minor muscle and close to the coracoid process of the scapula.

Typically, the vessels and nerves are compressed when the arm is placed in specific positions. The symptoms include sensory changes, such as pain, pins and needles in the hand, hand weakness and other neurological disorders. TOS can be purely neurogenic, due to compression of the brachial plexus alone (this accounts for approximately 90% of cases). Neurogenic TOS often produces abnormal nerve conduction recordings and can be associated

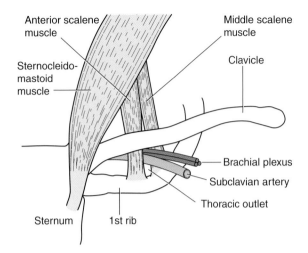

Figure 10.8   The anatomy of the thoracic outlet.

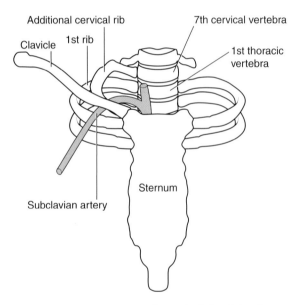

Figure 10.9   The presence of a cervical rib originating from the seventh thoracic vertebra can cause compression of the brachial nerve plexus and subclavian artery.

with muscle weakness and wasting in the lower arm or hand.

Arterial and venous TOS is less common and accounts for approximately 10% of cases, although there is sometimes a combination of neurogenic and vascular compression. Aneurysmal dilations of the SA are sometimes seen just distal to the point of compression due to post-stenotic dilation.

These aneurysms can be the source of distal emboli in the fingers, which can be the initial presentation of a patient with TOS. There is still considerable debate about the assessment and treatment of TOS, which often involves surgical resection of a cervical rib and sometimes the first rib, with the division of any fibrous bands to relieve the compression. Although the majority of patients who have undergone surgery show improvement in symptoms, a few show no signs of improvement and may return to the vascular laboratory for further assessment.

Maneuvers for assessing TOS

Continuous wave Doppler recording of the radial artery signal, performed with the arm in a range of positions, can be a useful prelude to the duplex examination (Fig. 10.10). There are a range of provocation maneuvers that can be used, but the most common include the following.

Hyperabduction test

The patient should be sitting comfortably, and the arm should then be slowly extended outward (abducted). With the arm fully abducted, the forearm is rotated so that the palm faces upward and the elbow downward (external rotation). The arm should be raised and lowered in this position and the patient's head turned away from the side under investigation. This test can indicate compression between the clavicle and first rib or coracoid region.

Costoclavicular maneuver

The patient is asked to push the chest outward while forcing the shoulders backward with deep inhalation, the so-called 'military position', as this may reveal arterial compression between the clavicle and first rib.

Deep inspiration maneuver

During deep inspiration the patient is asked to extend the neck and rotate the head to the affected side and then to the other side while the pulse is checked at the wrist. A positive test indicates

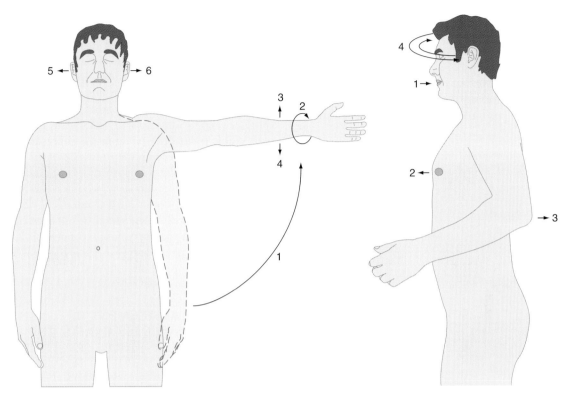

Figure 10.10 Provocation maneuvers used for the assessment of TOS. A: Hyperabduction test. The arm is abducted (1) and the arm externally rotated (2). The arm can also be raised or lowered during this test (3 and 4) and the head rotated to either side (5 and 6). B: Costoclavicular maneuver. During deep inspiration (1) the chest is pushed forward (2) and the arms backward (3). The head is turned from side to side (4).

possible compression between the scalene muscles or the presence of a cervical rib.

Finally, the patient should also be asked to place the arm in any position that provokes symptoms, such as raising it above the head. Any change to, or loss of, the Doppler signal during these maneuvers suggests compression of the SA. The patient should also be asked to indicate any symptoms that occur during arm maneuvers, as a normal Doppler signal in the presence of symptoms may indicate a nonvascular cause for the complaint.

Duplex assessment of TOS

To perform a duplex scan for TOS, the patient should lie supine on the examination table with the arms resting by the sides. Sometimes it may be necessary to image the arteries with the patient in a sitting position so that certain provocation tests can be performed. The SA is initially imaged from the supraclavicular and infraclavicular positions. The flow velocities are recorded and any abnormalities, such as tortuosity or aneurysmal dilations, noted. The SA can then be imaged using any of the provocation maneuvers that were found to reduce or obliterate the radial artery signal with pencil Doppler. One very useful maneuver involves scanning of the SA from the infraclavicular position while the arm is fully abducted (Fig. 10.11). The hand can be drawn toward the back of the patient's head and eventually placed behind the head. Pressure is then gently applied to the arm to push it backward. Any changes in the flow pattern or areas of significant velocity increase along the SA during provocation tests should be recorded. Typically, most high-velocity jets are recorded in the region of the clavicle (Fig. 10.12). There are no clearly defined criteria as to the point at which TOS is indicated, but a doubling of the peak systolic velocity at one location is indicative of a significant hemodynamic effect. Patients with severe vascular symptoms show complete occlusion of the SA during provocation maneuvers, posing less of a diagnostic dilemma.

Figure 10.11 Scanning for TOS. The SA should be examined from the supraclavicular and infraclavicular fossae while the arm is abducted; see text.

ANEURYSMS

Aneurysms involving the upper extremities are rare and are most frequently seen in the SA, associated with TOS. False aneurysms or pseudo-aneurysms are most commonly seen in the radial, brachial or axillary artery following arterial puncture for catheter access. Some patients present to the clinic with visible pulsatile swelling in the supraclavicular fossa, which is usually on the right side of the neck. This is invariably due to tortuosity of the distal brachiocephalic artery, proximal common carotid artery and proximal SA. Occasionally, pulsatile swellings are seen in the area of the radial or ulnar artery at the wrist, which can be due to a ganglion lying adjacent to the artery and distorting its path. The ganglion can be surgically removed.

ULTRASOUND ASSESSMENT OF HEMODIALYSIS ACCESS GRAFTS AND ARTERIOVENOUS FISTULAS (AVF)

Hemodialysis access grafts and arteriovenous fistulas (AVF) are surgically constructed for patients who require long-term dialysis. They provide a superficial high-volume, low-resistance pathway

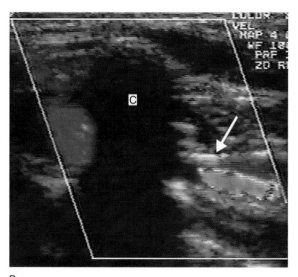

A   B

Figure 10.12 A: A normal color flow image of the SA (S) as it passes underneath the clavicle (C) with the arm at rest. B: Following arm abduction there is marked compression of the SA associated with color aliasing (arrow), indicating TOS. Note the large acoustic shadow below the clavicle.

to blood flow (Fig. 10.13) that can be regularly punctured. Usually they are located in the upper or lower arm, but they can also be created in the upper leg. It is imperative to minimize failure of these grafts as there are only a limited number of sites at which they can be placed. Ultrasound can be used to assess AVF or access grafts, especially when a clinical problem has been found, such as inadequate flow in the graft or fistula to allow adequate hemodialysis. Ultrasound can be used to measure volume flow in access grafts or in the access segment of AVFs. It can also be used to identify occlusions, stenoses, thrombus formation, aneurysms or false aneurysms in the fistula or graft. Preoperative assessment of the in-flow artery and vein can also be performed with ultrasound. In depth discussion of these scanning techniques is beyond the remit of this book, so we refer the reader to the work published by Landwehr (1995) and Deane & Goss (2001).

OTHER DISORDERS OF THE UPPER EXTREMITY CIRCULATION

Some hand and arm symptoms are due to microvascular or neurological disorders. Duplex scanning can exclude large vessel disease, but patients suffering from these types of abnormalities are best evaluated in specialist microvascular units.

Figure 10.13   A typical high-volume flow, monophasic waveform obtained from a hemodialysis graft. Note aliasing in the color image despite a PRF of 7000 Hz.

Raynaud's phenomenon is a microvascular disorder that can produce symptoms of digital ischemia in response to changes in ambient temperature and emotional state. This is observed as color changes of the fingers, causing blanching, or bluish discoloration due to cold. The blanching is followed by a period of rubor caused by hyperemia as the fingers warm. These signs may be mistaken for the presence of atherosclerotic occlusive disease, but pencil Doppler recordings will detect pulsatile flow signals in the radial and ulnar arteries, and the brachial systolic pressure should be equal in both arms.

Vibration white finger disease is a disorder caused by the use of drills and other vibrating machinery over a long period of time, leading to damage to the nerves and microvascular circulation in the fingers and hand. It can result in blanching of some or all of the fingers, loss of sensation and loss of dexterity. Again, Doppler signals may be normal to wrist level. However, Doppler recordings may demonstrate high-resistance flow patterns in the digital arteries due to the increased resistance to flow caused by the damaged arterioles and capillary beds. If the damage is severe, no flow may be detected with Doppler interrogation.

Reflex sympathetic dystrophy (RSD) is a poorly understood condition that usually occurs after local trauma, sometimes minor, to the hand or arm and results in severe pain, sensitivity and restricted movement of the affected area. Patients often report pain that is out of proportion to the severity of the injury, which might be a simple sprain or bruise. The condition can persist for many months, and intensive treatment is sometimes required to restore full use to the limb. This condition can affect young adults and children. The hand or arm may feel cold to the touch and appear discolored or cyanosed. However, Doppler recordings usually demonstrate pulsatile arterial signals in the brachial, radial and ulnar arteries. RSD can also affect the lower extremities.

REPORTING

The simplest form of reporting upper extremity investigations is with the use of diagrams, similar to the method used for lower limb investigations. This can be associated with a brief report. In the case of TOS, a written report may suffice.

References

Abou-Zamzam A M Jr, Edwards J M, Porter J M 2000 Noninvasive diagnosis of upper extremity disease. In: AbuRahma A F, Bergan J J (eds) Noninvasive vascular diagnosis. Springer, London, p 269

Deane C R, Goss D E 2001 Limb arteries. In: Meire H B, Cosgrove D, Dewbury K (eds) Clinical ultrasound, 2nd edn. Churchill Livingstone, Edinburgh, pp 1001–1034

Edwards J M, Zierler R E 1992 Duplex ultrasound assessment of upper extremity arteries. In: Zwiebel W J (ed) Introduction to vascular ultrasonography, 3rd edn. W B Saunders, Philadelphia, p 228

Landwehr P 1995 Hemodialysis shunt. In: Wolf K J, Fobbe F (eds) Color duplex sonography. Thieme, Stuttgart, pp 92–109

Makhoul R G, Machleder H I 1992 Developmental anomalies at the thoracic outlet: an analysis of 200 consecutive cases. Journal of Vascular Surgery 16(4): 534–545

von Reutern G M, von Büdingen H J 1993 Ultrasound diagnosis of cerebrovascular disease. Thieme, Stuttgart, pp 249–250

Further reading

Hennerici M, Neuerburg-Heusler D 1998 Vascular diagnosis with ultrasound. Thieme, Stuttgart

Chapter 11

Duplex assessment of aneurysms

CHAPTER CONTENTS

Introduction 145
Definition of an aneurysm 145
Anatomy of the abdominal aorta 146
Pathology of aneurysms 146
Aortic aneurysms: symptoms and treatment 146
    Surgical techniques for aortic aneurysm
        repair 147
Aneurysm shapes and types 149
Practical considerations for duplex scanning of
    aortic aneurysms 149
Scanning technique 150
Ultrasound appearance 150
    Normal appearance 150
    Abnormal appearance 151
Measurements 152
    Aorta diameter 152
    Distance between the renal arteries and the
        upper limit of the aneurysm 154
Limitations and pitfalls of aortic aneurysm
    scanning 154
Surveillance of endovascular aneurysm repair 154
    Scanning technique 154
    Types of endoleak 156
    Assessment of aneurysms excluded by covered
        stents 157
Other true aneurysms 157
    Iliac aneurysms 157
    Popliteal aneurysms 157
    Femoral artery aneurysms 158
False aneurysms 158
    Scanning false femoral aneurysms 159
    Treatment of false femoral aneurysms 160
Reporting 160

INTRODUCTION

True aneurysms are abnormal dilations of arteries. The term ectasia is often used to describe a moderate dilation of arteries. The abdominal aorta is one of the commonest sites for aneurysms to occur. Rupture of abdominal aortic aneurysm (AAA) is a common cause of death in men over the age of 65 years. Ultrasound is a simple noninvasive method of detecting aneurysms and can be used for serial investigations to monitor any increase in size. However, if surgical intervention is being considered, other imaging techniques, such as CT and MRI, may be required to demonstrate the relationship of an aneurysm to major branches and other structures within the body. There have been significant developments in the treatment of aneurysms over the last several years, with the introduction of endovascular devices to repair aortic aneurysms and covered stents to exclude flow in aneurysms in other areas of the body. This chapter concentrates on ultrasound scanning of aortic aneurysms but also considers the assessment of aneurysms in other areas of the peripheral circulation.

DEFINITION OF AN ANEURYSM

It has been suggested that an aneurysm is a permanent localized dilation of an artery having at least a 50% increase in diameter compared to the normal, expected diameter (Johnston et al 1991). Ectasia is characterized by a diameter increase <50% of the normal, expected diameter. It is worth remembering that there is considerable variability in the normal diameter of arteries among individuals, and this will be dependent on factors such as physical size, sex and age.

ANATOMY OF THE ABDOMINAL AORTA

The abdominal aorta commences at the level of the diaphragm and descends slightly to the left of the midline to the level of the fourth lumbar vertebra, where it divides into the left and right common iliac arteries (Fig. 11.1). It tapers slightly as it descends, owing to the large branches it gives off. Major branches of the aorta that can be easily identified with ultrasound include the coeliac axis, the superior mesenteric artery (SMA) and renal arteries. These can act as important reference points when determining the upper limit of an aneurysm.

PATHOLOGY OF ANEURYSMS

The mechanism of aneurysm development is still uncertain but may involve a multifactorial process leading to the destruction of aortic wall connective tissue. There is evidence that increased local production of enzymes capable of degrading elastic fibers as well as interstitial collagens are associated with AAA (Wassef et al 2001). The lumen of an aneurysm is often lined with large amounts of thrombus, which can be a potential source of emboli. This is also why arteriograms, which only demonstrate the flow lumen, are not accurate for estimating the true diameter of an aneurysm, as the flow lumen can be significantly smaller than the

diameter of the entire vessel. Dissection of an aneurysm can occur following a tear in the intima, and blood can leak into the space between the intima and media, sometimes creating a false flow lumen. Aortic aneurysms can also extend into the iliac arteries. Some aortic aneurysms are involved in an inflammatory process, with marked periaortic fibrosis surrounding the aorta making surgical resection difficult. Aneurysms can also be caused by a variety of infections, such as bacterial endocarditis, and are termed mycotic aneurysms. These can occur anywhere in the body.

Popliteal aneurysms may be the source of distal emboli. They can also occlude, leading to symptoms of acute lower limb ischemia. This should always be considered as a potential cause of the acutely ischemic leg, especially in patients with no other obvious risk factors.

False aneurysms occur predominantly in the femoral artery following puncture of the arterial wall for catheter access. In this situation, blood continues to flow backward and forward through the puncture site into a false flow cavity outside the artery.

AORTIC ANEURYSMS: SYMPTOMS AND TREATMENT

The normal size of the abdominal aorta varies between 1.4 and 2.5 cm in diameter (Johnston et al 1991) (Fig. 11.2). An aortic diameter slightly above 2.5 cm is considered mildly abnormal or ectatic.

Figure 11.1   Anatomy of the abdominal aorta and its major branches.

Figure 11.2   A transverse image of a normal abdominal aorta (A). The inferior vena cava (IVC) is seen to the right of the aorta (note that the probe orientation means that the right side of the patient is on the left of the image).

A small aortic aneurysm is generally regarded as an aorta having a diameter of 3–3.5 cm, and many surgeons will not request serial screening scans unless the aorta reaches this level. However, some vascular units monitor patients with slightly enlarged aortas, especially if the patient is young. As the aorta increase in size, there is a potential for rupture due to increased tension in the arterial wall. The UK Small Aneurysm Trial Participants (1998) demonstrated that the average annual growth rate of aneurysms measuring between 4 and 5.5 cm was 0.33 cm a year. However, rates will vary among individuals and are also dependent on the size of the aneurysm. The prevalence of aortic aneurysms is six times greater in men than women (Vardulaki et al 2000). In addition, there seems to be a strong familial link, with siblings of aneurysm patients having a higher risk of developing an aneurysm compared with the general population.

Clinically, there are usually no symptoms associated with the development of an aortic aneurysm and many are discovered incidentally, during routine examinations or on plain abdominal radiographs. Occasionally, patients present with symptoms of renal hydronephrosis. This is caused by compression of a ureter leading from one of the kidneys by the aneurysm sac and most frequently occurs on the left side. The symptoms associated with aneurysm leakage or rupture include back or abdominal pain and acute shock. Ultrasound is occasionally used to confirm the diagnosis in the emergency room, although the symptoms are usually so acute that emergency surgery is required. The mortality rate for acute rupture of an aortic aneurysm is very high, 65–85% (Kniemeyer et al 2000), and many patients do not reach hospital alive.

The risk of aortic aneurysm rupture increases with size. The UK Small Aneurysm Trial Participants (1998) found that the mean risk of rupture of aneurysms measuring 4–5.5 cm was 1% per year. However, larger aneurysms carry a higher rate of rupture, and a recent study demonstrated that the average risk of rupture in male patients with a >6 cm aneurysm was 14% per year (Brown et al 2003).

Clearly, there are benefits in detecting aneurysms at an early stage so that serial follow-up can be carried out and elective repair performed if the aneurysm becomes too large. The UK Small Aneurysm Trial Participants (1998) have shown no survival benefit for open repair of aneurysms measuring less than 5.5 cm in diameter compared to ultrasound surveillance. In this study, age, sex or initial aneurysm size did not modify the overall hazard ratio. Therefore, many surgeons will only carry out elective repair if the aneurysm has a diameter of equal to or greater than 5.5 cm, or if there are indications that smaller aneurysms are becoming symptomatic and are at risk of rupturing. There is now reliable evidence that aortic screening programs, involving a single ultrasound scan of men aged 65 years or over, is beneficial and cost-effective in reducing aneurysm-related mortality (Ashton et al 2002). Although aortic aneurysms are much more prevalent in men, there is some evidence that women with aneurysms in the 5–5.9 cm range may be up to four times more likely to undergo rupture compared to men with similar sized aneurysms (Brown et al 2003). Further research may prompt a lower threshold for repairing aneurysms in female patients.

Surgical techniques for aortic aneurysm repair

Open repair

Open repair of aortic aneurysms has been performed for over 20 years and involves a large incision in the abdomen and mobilization of the intestines to expose the aorta. Fortunately, the majority of abdominal aneurysms (approximately 95%) start below the level of the renal arteries (infrarenal aneurysms). This means that surgical clamps, to control the aneurysm, can be positioned below the renal arteries, ensuring that the kidneys are perfused during the operation. Aortic aneurysms that extend above the renal arteries (suprarenal aneurysms) carry a higher rate of perioperative and postoperative complication, as the aorta has to be clamped above the level of the renal arteries and reimplantation of the renal arteries is necessary. Patients can suffer from renal failure following this procedure. This is why it is important that the surgeon be aware of the level of the proximal neck before surgery is performed. Aortic aneurysms are repaired using straight tube grafts unless the aneurysm extends into the iliac arteries, where a bifurcating graft is used. The graft is sutured into position and the sac closed around the graft. Postoperatively, patients normally spend a day or two in intensive care and usually leave hospital 10–14 days after surgery. The elective mortality rate for open repair is in the region of 5% (Akkersdijk et al 1994). However, surgically unfit patients have a risk of much higher morbidity and mortality rates.

Endovascular repair

Endovascular repair of aortic aneurysms was described in the early 1990s. There have been significant technical developments in this field since that time, and several types of commercially manufactured grafts are now available. The prosthetic stent graft is introduced through an arteriotomy made in the femoral artery and deployed in the aorta to exclude flow into the aneurysm sac. The grafts are made of a synthetic material such as dacron and polytetrafluoroethylene (PTFE) and are supported on an expandable metal framework, or skeleton, of nitonol or stainless steel to prevent kinks and twisting. Nowadays, almost all endovascular grafts are bifurcating devices (Fig. 11.3). These are modular systems with the graft supplied in two parts. The bulk of the graft consists of the main body, one complete limb and the short stump of the second limb. The remaining modular limb is delivered separately via an arteriotomy in the contralateral common femoral artery. The grafts are prepacked onto the delivery catheter during the manufacturing process and retained in place by an outer sheath until deployment in the aorta. During the procedure the femoral artery is surgically exposed, and the catheter containing the main graft is inserted over a guide wire and positioned with the aid of an imaging intensifier so that the top of the graft lies just below the renal arteries in the proximal neck. Many of these devices have uncovered metal stents that extend across the renal arteries (suprarenal fixation) to hold the device in place. The graft is deployed by slowly withdrawing the outer covering sheath. A soft balloon is inflated to ensure the graft is fully expanded in the proximal neck, just above the sac. Some grafts have hooks at the top that anchor into the aortic wall for further security. The modular limb is then delivered on a separate catheter via the contralateral femoral artery. Under radiographic control it is positioned so that it fits into the stunted limb of the main body and then is fully expanded using a balloon to make a seal. The distal end is then anchored in the common iliac artery.

As the devices are modular, it is possible to add extensions to the limbs to exclude long iliac artery

Figure 11.3   An example of endovascular aortic aneurysm repair. Note that the left limb of the device is delivered on a separate catheter. Image supplied by courtesy of W L Gore & Associates (UK) Ltd.

aneurysms. Postoperative recovery is usually very quick, with some patients going home within 3 to 5 days. However, not all aneurysms are suitable for endovascular repair. This can be due to aneurysm tortuosity, excessive proximal neck diameter, limited proximal neck length, severe iliac artery disease and marked iliac artery tortuosity. Although endovascular repair appears much less traumatic for the patient, a number of complications are possible, including endoleak. An endoleak occurs when blood leaks into the aneurysm sac from the graft or from another source, such as a lumbar or inferior mesenteric artery. In this situation the aneurysm sac can continue to expand and rupture (van Marrewijk et al 2002). The different types of endoleak and their ultrasound appearances are discussed later in this chapter. Some devices have been withdrawn from use due to problems such as hook fractures and structural failure. At the time of writing, the long-term durability and outcome of endovascular repair compared to conventional open repair is unknown and is the subject of ongoing trials in Europe and the United States.

ANEURYSM SHAPES AND TYPES

Aneurysms vary considerably in shape and size (Fig. 11.4). Most aneurysms are fusiform in shape and there is uniform dilation across the entire cross-section of the vessel. Saccular aneurysms exhibit a typical localized bulging of the wall. Dissecting aneurysms occur due to a disruption of the intimal lining of the vessel, allowing blood to enter the subintimal space. This can result in the stripping of the intima, and sometimes of the media, from the artery wall. If the aorta partially dissects, large amounts of thrombus may be seen in the subintimal space (Fig. 11.4F). If there is a full dissection, a false flow lumen is created and the dissected layer of intima and media may be seen flapping freely in time with arterial pulsation (Fig. 11.4G). Some aortic dissections are not associated with aneurysms and can start in the chest, extending through the aorta into the iliac arteries. Occasionally, two aneurysmal dilations may be seen along the length of the abdominal aorta, separated by a normal segment of the aorta, which gives rise to a classic 'dumb-bell' shape when viewed in longitudinal section (Fig. 11.4H). As the aorta dilates, it also tends to increase in length, producing tortuosity that often shifts the aorta to the left of the midline or deflects it in an anterior direction.

PRACTICAL CONSIDERATIONS FOR DUPLEX SCANNING OF AORTIC ANEURYSMS

The purposes of the scan are to determine if there is an aneurysm involving the aorta or peripheral arterial system and, if appropriate, to monitor the

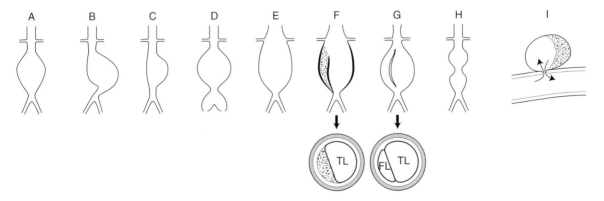

Figure 11.4   Aneurysms are very variable in shapes and types. A: Fusiform infrarenal aortic aneurysm. B: Tortuous elongated aortic aneurysm with the sac shifted to the left of the midline. C: Saccular aortic aneurysm. D: Infrarenal aortic aneurysm extending into the iliac arteries. E: Suprarenal aortic aneurysm involving the renal arteries. F: Dissecting aortic aneurysm with a tear between the intima and media allowing blood into the subintimal space. G: Dissecting aortic aneurysm in which the intima or media has fully dissected, creating a false flow lumen. H: Double aneurysm of the aorta producing a 'dumb-bell appearance'. I: False aneurysm of the common femoral artery following arterial puncture. (TL, true lumen; FL, false lumen.)

size of the aneurysm on a serial basis. A screening scan can be performed in 5 to 10 min, but more detailed scans or follow-up of endovascular grafts may take 20–30 min.

No special preparation is required, although some units use a bowel preparation to improve visualization of the aorta; however, for screening scans this is rarely necessary. The patient should be lying supine with the head supported on a pillow and the arms resting by the sides. Sometimes the patient may have to roll to one side to improve visualization. The scanner should be configured for an aortic investigation but, in the absence of a specific preset, a general abdominal examination setup should be selected. Ensure that the image depth setting is not too shallow or too deep. A depth setting of 10–12 cm is usually sufficient for the average-sized patient. A 3.5 MHz curved linear array transducer, or broad-band equivalent, is the most suitable probe for this investigation. Harmonic imaging can be useful for improving the image quality. In very obese patients a 2–4 MHz phased array transducer can help to identify the aorta.

Figure 11.5   Transducer positions for scanning the abdominal aorta. A: Transverse. B: Sagittal or longitudinal. C: Coronal. The coronal view is used for measuring the lateral diameter of the aorta (i.e., side to side).

SCANNING TECHNIQUE

The following description is for a comprehensive investigation of the aorta. However, some departments only perform screening scans and the maximum diameter of the aorta is the only measurement required. Measurements of diameter should be made from a number of different positions. In addition, the shape of the aneurysm and features such as tortuosity or dissection should be documented. The scanning technique for imaging the aorta is demonstrated in Figure 11.5. The procedure is as follows:

1. The aorta is usually easiest to identify by starting with the transducer in a transverse image plane, approximately 3–4 cm above the umbilicus. The aorta is then imaged throughout its visible length, from the upper abdomen above the celiac axis, or SMA, to the aortic bifurcation. Where appropriate, the level of the renal arteries can be identified using color flow imaging as described later in this chapter. However, it is frequently impossible to image these vessels in the presence of a large aneurysm.

2. The abdominal aorta is then imaged in a longitudinal or sagittal plane, from the midline along its length to the aortic bifurcation.
3. The aorta is then viewed from a coronal scan plane throughout its length in a longitudinal view to obtain more accurate measurements of the lateral diameter of the aorta (side to side).
4. It is good practice to assess the proximal iliac arteries in transverse and longitudinal scan planes (see Ch. 9) to exclude an isolated iliac artery aneurysm or to define the lower limit of an aneurysm if it extends into the iliac arteries (see Fig. 11.16).

ULTRASOUND APPEARANCE

Normal appearance

The aorta should measure less than 2.5 cm at its maximum diameter (Fig. 11.2) and there is usually slight tapering of the aorta from top to bottom. In

A 8.03 cm

B 7.47 cm
   7.52 cm

Figure 11.6 A large abdominal aortic aneurysm is shown from two different imaging planes. A: Transverse image. The anteroposterior diameter is measured from the outer wall to the outer wall (callipers). B: A sagittal image of the same aneurysm, demonstrating the calliper positions to measure the aneurysm in this plane. Note that in this example the diameter measured in the transverse image (A) is larger, due to obliquity.

the longitudinal plane, the aorta is sometimes seen to curve gently in a slight convex direction as it lies on the lumbar spine.

Abnormal appearance

The aorta appears abnormally enlarged, as seen on the B-mode image in Figure 11.6. The shape of the aneurysm can vary (Fig. 11.4). Marked kinking of the posterior wall at the level of the proximal neck can occur due to elongation of the aorta, which can be mistaken as an atherosclerotic stenosis. If the aneurysm deflects in an anterior direction, it can be very difficult to demonstrate the level of the renal arteries, and the proximal segment of the

Figure 11.7 A transverse image of an aortic aneurysm demonstrates a localized area of thrombus liquefaction (L), which may be confused with a dissection. Large areas of thrombus (arrows) separate the area of liquefaction from the flow lumen (FL).

abdominal aorta may become tortuous, which is sometimes described as a 'swan neck' appearance.

Thrombus may be imaged as concentric layers with differing degrees of echogenicity depending on the age and organization. Sometimes localized liquefaction of the thrombus can occur, which appears as hypoechoic areas within the thrombus. This appearance can be confused with a dissection, although there is usually a thick layer of thrombus separating the liquefied region and the flow lumen (Fig. 11.7). A dissection may be undetected, as blood that has leaked into the wall may be mistaken for mural thrombus. In a full dissection, flow will be observed in the false flow lumen, which is separated from the true lumen by a flap of intima and, sometimes, media (Fig. 11.8).

Inflammatory aneurysms demonstrate a hypoechoic area of ill-defined fibrosis around the aorta on the B-mode image, but this appearance can be confused with the presence of periaortic lymph nodes. The ultrasound diagnosis of a leaking aneurysm is extremely difficult, although it is sometimes possible to identify areas of fresh blood or hematoma as hypoechoic areas associated with the aneurysm in the retroperitoneal space. This type of assessment should be carried out by an experienced sonographer; however, other imaging techniques, such as CT and MRI, are better suited for this investigation.

A

B

C

Figure 11.8 A: B-mode image of a dissecting aortic aneurysm. In this example the true (T) and false (F) lumens are seen. B: Color flow imaging demonstrates flow in the false flow lumen (arrow). C: In this example, a dissection into the thrombus and the vessel wall has occurred (arrow).

MEASUREMENTS

It is important to make accurate diameter measurements of the aorta, especially if a patient is having serial follow-up scans to monitor the size of an

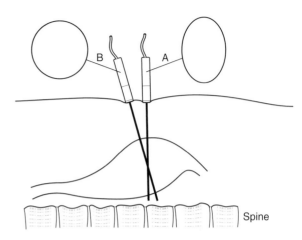

Figure 11.9 The anteroposterior diameter of a tortuous aorta may be overestimated because of measurement in the wrong scan plane. In this example, the aorta is deflecting in an anterior direction. Scanning in a transverse plane along line A will result in an oblique image of the aorta, and the anteroposterior diameter will be overestimated. The transducer should be tilted to obtain the correct line of measurement along line B. An example of this problem is shown in Figure 11.6.

aneurysm. The UK Small Aneurysm Trial Participants (1998) showed that the error between operators was in the region of 0.2 cm for aneurysms measuring 4–5.5 cm in diameter. This section explains how to make diameter measurements of the aorta and identifies the potential pitfalls that may be involved. It should be noted that some of these measurements may not be necessary for screening scans.

Aorta diameter

Transverse scanning plane

The maximum diameter of the aorta should be measured in the anteroposterior (AP) direction from the outer anterior wall to the outer posterior wall (Fig. 11.6). If an aneurysm is present, overestimation of its size can occur if oblique measurements are made, due to tortuosity or folding of the aorta (Figs 11.6 and 11.9). Measurements of the lateral diameter of the aneurysm (i.e., from lateral wall to lateral wall) in a transverse scan plane are prone to error as the lateral vessel walls are parallel to the ultrasound beam, which therefore produces a very poor image (see Ch. 2). The thickness of any thrombus can also

Figure 11.10 The positions of the left (LR) and right (RR) renal arteries are shown in this transverse image of the aorta (A). The diameter of the aorta is normal at the level of the renal arteries. The left renal vein (V) can be seen crossing over the aorta at the same level as the renal arteries. The SMA (S) is also seen in this image.

be measured in the AP plane. It is possible to assess whether the aneurysm starts below the level of the renal arteries by measuring the diameter of the aorta at this level with the aid of color flow imaging. With the transducer in a transverse plane, positioned at the upper abdomen, the right renal artery is normally seen dividing from the aorta at a 10 o'clock position and the left renal artery from a 4 o'clock position (Fig. 11.10). In practice, they can be very difficult to image, especially if the aneurysm is tortuous or projecting upward or kinked.

Longitudinal scan plane, from sagittal and coronal positions

Estimates of aortic diameter in sagittal and coronal scan planes are often more accurate than measurements in the transverse plane. This is because it is easier to avoid measurement errors due to oblique views of the aorta. To find the maximum diameter of the aorta, the transducer should be swept laterally across the aorta until the widest point can be seen (Figs 11.6 and 11.11). The coronal imaging plane should also be used for measuring the lateral diameter of the aneurysm, as some aneurysms are larger in the lateral than in the AP dimension. The length of the aneurysm sac should also be measured in the

Figure 11.11 Measurements of an aortic aneurysm made in the longitudinal plane. The maximum diameter of the aorta is measured across line A. The length of the aneurysm sac is measured along line B. The distance from the SMA origin to the approximate level of the renal arteries is measured along line C. The left renal vein (RV) can also be seen in transverse section as it crosses over the aorta at the level of the renal arteries. The distance from the SMA origin to the aneurysm sac is measured along line D. The diameter of the aorta between the aneurysm and the level of the renal arteries is measured across line E.

longitudinal scan plane (Fig. 11.11). The presence and thickness of thrombus can sometimes be difficult to assess on a poor B-mode image. Color flow imaging can be useful for demonstrating the lumen, which may be small in the presence of a large thrombus load.

Distance between the renal arteries and the upper limit of the aneurysm

When requested, the distance between the renal arteries and upper limit of the aneurysm can be measured. In practice, this can be an extremely difficult or virtually impossible assessment to make. First, the presence of the aneurysm may obscure views of the upper abdominal aorta. Second, the renal arteries cannot usually be imaged with the probe in the longitudinal direction required to make this measurement. However, the position of the renal arteries can be estimated by identifying the SMA in the longitudinal plane, as the renal arteries should lie approximately 1.5 cm below the SMA origin (Fig. 11.11). Accessory renal arteries may arise well below this point. The left renal vein can act as another useful landmark, if it is found to be at the level of the renal arteries in a transverse image (Fig. 11.10). Turning the transducer into a longitudinal plane, it is possible to identify the renal vein as it crosses over the top of the aorta (Fig. 11.11). Other imaging techniques, such as CT, MRI or arteriography, are generally used to identify the position of the renal arteries in large aneurysms, especially with the increasing use of endovascular devices to repair aneurysms.

LIMITATIONS AND PITFALLS OF AORTIC ANEURYSM SCANNING

The main limitation of aortic scanning is poor visualization due to bowel gas or obesity. It can sometimes be difficult to define the posterior wall of an aneurysm, when the tissue between the lumbar spine and posterior wall appears to merge, making placement of the calliper difficult. Any limitations or doubts should be documented. A major pitfall is to set the image depth too deep when scanning thin patients and misinterpret the lumbar spine as the aorta (Fig. 11.12).

Figure 11.12 In this image, the scanning depth has been set too deep in a thin patient, and the lumbar spine (S) has been mistaken for an aneurysm. The aorta (A) is of normal diameter. The vena cava (V) can be seen to the right of the aorta.

SURVEILLANCE OF ENDOVASCULAR ANEURYSM REPAIR

Duplex ultrasound is an accurate method for the detection of endoleaks following endovascular repair (McLafferty et al 2002). It is important to optimize the scanner controls so that the system is sensitive to detecting low-velocity flow. This can be achieved by reducing the PRF to 1–1.5 kHz and increasing color sensitivity. The wall filter should be set to a minimum level and write zoom used to image the area of interest to maintain frame rate. This can produce a noisy color image, but without optimization it is possible, in our experience, to miss endoleaks.

Scanning technique

1. It is easiest to start the scan by imaging the aorta in transverse section in the middle of the sac using B-mode imaging alone. At this level it is usual to see the two limbs of the graft, which usually lie adjacent to each other (Fig. 11.13A). In some circumstances they can be seen to spiral around each other as the probe is moved in a superior or inferior direction.
2. The graft is then followed proximally through the sac in transverse section. The bifurcation of

A   B

Figure 11.13   A: A transverse color flow image of a successfully deployed aortic endovascular graft taken below the level of the graft bifurcation. Flow is demonstrated in both graft limbs, but there is no flow in the aneurysm sac. B: Longitudinal color flow image of an endovascular graft. In this example the limbs are lying on top of each other, but in many cases they lie side by side, as shown in example A, where use of a coronal scan plane would be needed to demonstrate both limbs in the same image.

the graft should be clearly seen, and it is usually possible to see the upper extent of the graft and sometimes the aorta at the level of the renal arteries.

3. Next, the aneurysm and graft are followed distally to the aortic bifurcation, where the two graft limbs should be seen to run down the common iliac arteries. Anechoic areas in the aneurysm sac should be noted, as these could represent areas of blood flow, and should be scrutinized carefully with color flow imaging. Some devices can appear very pulsatile, with considerable movement of the graft walls.

4. The aorta is then scanned in transverse section using color flow imaging. There should be color filling of the graft but no flow visible in the sac outside the device (Fig. 11.13A). The maximum diameter of the aneurysm sac should be recorded so that any changes in size can be assessed on serial scans. A progressively expanding scan could indicate an undetected endoleak or endotension. A variety of scan planes, including a coronal plane, may be required to obtain the maximum diameter. Some units also measure proximal neck diameter to monitor any increase in size due to progression of aneurysmal disease. Other measurements may be taken for research purposes.

Figure 11.14   A diagram of the different types of endoleak that can occur following endovascular repair of an aortic aneurysm (see text for description). A: Type I, failure of proximal or distal anastomotic seals. B: Type II, perfusion of the sac via patent lumbar or inferior mesenteric arteries. C: Type III, failure of the modular limb seal or perforation and tears in the graft material. Type IV endoleak cannot be demonstrated in this example.

5. Color flow imaging in longitudinal section using sagittal and coronal planes is used to examine flow through the device and to identify any areas of flow disturbance or stenosis that could be caused by kinking of the graft,

Figure 11.15 Color flow and B-mode images of different types of endoleak. A: Longitudinal image showing a type I endoleak (arrow) from the distal end of the graft into the sac. B: A transverse image of a type II endoleak demonstrating perfusion of the sac via a patent inferior mesenteric artery (arrow). C: A transverse image of a type II endoleak from a patent lumbar artery. D: There is failure of the junction between the modular limb and main body of the graft (arrow), indicating a type III endoleak.

especially of the limbs as they run through the common iliac arteries (Fig. 11.13B). Endoleaks can also be examined in longitudinal section as this may help to identify their source.

Types of endoleak

Endoleaks have been categorized into the types described below (Veith et al 2002) and are demonstrated in Figure 11.14. The ultrasound appearance of some types is shown in Figure 11.15. Remember

it may be possible for a patient to have more than one type of endoleak.

Type I   Attachment site leaks. This occurs at the top or bottom of the graft when there is an inadequate seal between the device and the aortic or iliac artery wall, respectively. Color flow imaging demonstrates a jet of flow at the point of the leak, filling part of the aneurysm sac (Fig. 11.15A). The amount of flow in the sac can be variable and in some cases the entire sac may be perfused.

Type II   Collateral endoleaks involve some filling of the sac via lumbar vessels or the inferior mesenteric artery or accessory renal arteries (Fig. 11.15B and C). They can be difficult to detect with ultrasound. Many type II endoleaks will seal spontaneously after a month or two (Veith et al 2002). Persistent leaks may require embolization.

Type III   Leaks between the modular limb and main body of the graft or tears in the graft (Fig. 11.15D). These types of leaks are less commonly seen.

Type IV   Thought to occur due to graft porosity or 'sweating' of graft material, leading to progressive increase in sac size within the first month. It is not possible to image this type of leak in real-time, but serial surveillance scans may show a progressive increase in the diameter of the aneurysm sac.

In addition, the concept of endotension has been defined. This is described as a persistent or recurrent pressurization of the sac without a visualized endoleak. This can lead to expansion of the sac and potential rupture. The causes of endotension are uncertain, but it has been suggested that the sac is pressurized by mechanisms such as excessive pulsation of the graft, osmosis into the sac or transmission of pressure through the thrombus. In practice, some cases of endotension could be due to a very small, undetected endoleak.

The management of endoleaks remains unclear, but there is evidence to suggest that type I and III endoleaks should be treated, as they are more likely to be associated with an increase in sac size and potential rupture.

Assessment of aneurysms excluded by covered stents

Flow can be excluded in aneurysms involving other areas of the arterial circulation by inserting a covered stent across the region of the aneurysm. The proximal and distal ends of the stent are positioned above and below the aneurysm. These types of stents are most commonly used in the iliac arteries to exclude true aneurysms. They can also be used to exclude flow into false aneurysms following vessel perforation or rupture during angioplasty. They are occasionally used in the subclavian arteries.

The stent is usually visible on the ultrasound image. Flow should be assessed across the stent and then the aneurysm should be scanned, using low-flow settings, to detect any possible filling of the aneurysm sac.

OTHER TRUE ANEURYSMS

Iliac aneurysms

The normal diameter of the common iliac artery ranges between 1.1 and 1.4 cm (Johnston et al 1991). Iliac aneurysms usually occur as an extension of, or in association with, aortic aneurysms. Isolated iliac aneurysms are relatively rare, but rupture can be fatal, and elective repair should be considered for aneurysms measuring 3.5 cm or larger (Santilli et al 2000) (Fig. 11.16). The technique for scanning the iliac arteries is described in Chapter 9. The measurement of iliac aneurysms is more accurate in a longitudinal plane, as it is difficult to avoid oblique planes if imaging in transverse section. Iliac aneurysms are clinically difficult to diagnose, and ultrasound, CT and MRI are the methods used for diagnosis.

Popliteal aneurysms

Patients with an aortic aneurysm have a higher incidence of popliteal aneurysms compared to patients

Figure 11.16   This longitudinal image of a distal aortic aneurysm (A) and right common iliac artery (I) demonstrates two large iliac artery aneurysms (seen between arrows).

without such aneurysms. The normal diameter of the popliteal artery ranges between 0.4 and 0.9 cm, and a popliteal aneurysm is frequently classified as a vessel diameter of greater than 1.5 cm (Fig. 11.17). The complications associated with popliteal aneurysms include embolization, acute occlusion or, occasionally, rupture. The symptoms of popliteal aneurysms can include pain or a feeling of fullness in the popliteal fossa. Sometimes patients present with a deep vein thrombosis due to compression of the popliteal vein by the aneurysm. Ultrasound is the primary technique for the diagnosis of popliteal aneurysms. However, a major diagnostic pitfall is the misdiagnosis of a Baker's cyst as a popliteal aneurysm.

Scanning of popliteal aneurysms

Using a 5 MHz, or broad-band equivalent, flat linear array transducer, the popliteal artery is examined in transverse and longitudinal planes from the popliteal fossa and from the medial aspect of the lower thigh in the adductor canal, as some aneurysms can be located above the knee. B-mode imaging is used to assess the size, length and amount of thrombus within the aneurysm. Color flow imaging is used to demonstrate the size of the flow lumen if the B-mode imaging is poor. Occluded popliteal aneurysms are demonstrated by an absence of color flow in the lumen. The popliteal vein should also be assessed for patency. Baker's cysts have a typical appearance of a tail trailing from the main body of the cyst to the joint capsule, and they have a hypoechoic appearance due to the synovial fluid inside (see Ch. 13).

Femoral artery aneurysms

True femoral artery aneurysms occur less frequently and are usually associated with aneurysmal disease elsewhere. However, aneurysmal dilations can occur where graft anastomoses have been performed.

FALSE ANEURYSMS

False aneurysms, also known as pseudo-aneurysms, primarily occur following arterial puncture for catheter access, due to poor control of arterial bleeding following the procedure. This is usually due to insufficient pressure being applied over the puncture site or pressure being applied for too short a time. They may also occur following trauma. Blood flows

Figure 11.17   A: A transverse image of a popliteal artery aneurysm (PA) containing thrombus (T) below the arrow. The popliteal vein (V) is compressed in this example. B: A longitudinal image demonstrating thrombus in the lumen. The popliteal vein is seen superficial to the artery.

backward and forward through a hole in the arterial wall into the surrounding tissue, forming a flow cavity in the tissue adjacent to the artery. The false lumen often contains thrombus, which may be layered. False aneurysms can increase in size over time. Color flow imaging should be used to confirm flow in the false lumen. The color flow image typically demonstrates a high-velocity jet originating from the defect in the artery wall, which is associated with a swirling pattern inside the false lumen, similar to the 'yin-yang' sign. Spectral Doppler usually demonstrates an equal forward flow and reverse flow component to the arterial jet as flow enters the false aneurysm during systole and exits during diastole (Fig. 11.18). The audible Doppler signal is very characteristic, with high-frequency Doppler shifts heard in the forward and reverse phases across the neck.

The common femoral artery is the main vessel in which false aneurysms occur, as it is the commonest site for catheter access. False femoral aneurysms may be very large, and bleeding into the retroperitoneal cavity can be a serious complication, leading to shock and death.

Scanning false femoral aneurysms

The patient should lie as flat as possible. The procedure should be started by scanning the common femoral artery in transverse section. A midfrequency 5 MHz, or broad-band equivalent, flat linear array transducer will usually provide an adequate image. However, in some cases an abdominal curved array transducer may be required, especially if the patient is obese or if the puncture has been very high. In addition, areas of hematoma lying over the vessel, associated with the puncture site, can make the imaging difficult. The common femoral artery should be identified and scanned along its length in transverse section using color flow imaging. The proximal few centimeters of the superficial femoral artery and profunda femoris artery should also be examined, as low punctures can result in false aneurysms of these vessels. A potentially confusing situation can occur if the inferior epigastric artery, a superficial branch of the common femoral artery, runs close to an area of hematoma or swelling, as this might be mistaken for a small leak. Spectral Doppler recordings taken from the superficial epigastric

A

B

Figure 11.18   A: A transverse image of a false femoral artery aneurysm and corresponding spectral Doppler waveform from the communicating jet. The arrow indicates the arterial jet between the femoral artery (A) and the false lumen (FL). There is marked perivascular tissue vibration associated with the arterial jet in this example. B: The false aneurysm was successfully thrombosed (T) by ultrasound guided compression.

artery will demonstrate a peripheral arterial type waveform with overall flow in the forward direction as opposed to the high forward and reverse flow components seen in the necks of false aneurysms (Fig. 11.18).

Treatment of false femoral aneurysms

Traditionally, false aneurysms were repaired surgically, but ultrasound compression of pseudo-aneurysms has been demonstrated as a safe and effective technique for thrombosing false aneurysms. The patient should be lying supine, and some form of analgesia or sedation should be administered as the procedure can be uncomfortable. The distal ankle artery signals should be assessed with continuous wave Doppler to ensure there is good distal perfusion of the leg before beginning the procedure. Firm transducer pressure is applied over the point of communication between the true lumen and false lumen to occlude the arterial jet. Compression is maintained for 10 min intervals

with a brief release of pressure to allow for distal perfusion. It may take over an hour to successfully thrombose the aneurysm.

More recently, ultrasound guided human thrombin injection into the false lumen has proved to be a highly effective method of treating false aneurysms. Blood in the false lumen clots within 1 to 2 seconds of the injection, and this can be observed on the ultrasound image. Thrombin injection may become the main method of treating false femoral aneurysms (Olsen et al 2002).

REPORTING

Reporting is usually in the form of a written report accompanied by appropriate images recorded from the scanner. It is important to note any limitations of the scan and to state clearly what measurements were made and from what positions. Situations have occurred in which the points of measurement have been ambiguously reported and the overall length of an aneurysm has been mistakenly interpreted as its diameter.

References

Akkersdijk G J, van der Graaf Y, van Bockel J H, et al 1994 Mortality rates associated with operative treatment of infrarenal abdominal aortic aneurysms in The Netherlands. British Journal of Surgery 81(5):706–709

Ashton H A, Buxton M J, Day N E, et al 2002 The Multicentre Aneurysm Screening Study (MASS) into the effect of abdominal aortic aneurysm screening on mortality in men: a randomised control trial. Lancet 360:1531–1539

Brown P M, Zelt D T, Sobolev B 2003 The risk of rupture in untreated aneurysms: the impact of size, gender, and expansion rates. Journal of Vascular Surgery 37(2):280–284

Johnston K W, Rutherford R B, Tilson M D, et al 1991 Suggested standards for reporting on arterial aneurysms. Subcommittee on Reporting Standards for Arterial Aneurysms, Ad Hoc Committee on Reporting Standards, Society for Vascular Surgery and North American Chapter, International Society for Cardiovascular Surgery. Journal of Vascular Surgery 13(3):452–458

Kniemeyer H W, Kessler T, Reber P U, et al 2000 Treatment of ruptured abdominal aortic aneurysm, a permanent challenge or a waste of resources? Prediction of outcome

using a multi-organ dysfunction score. European Journal of Vascular and Endovascular Surgery 19:190–196

McLafferty R B, McCrary B S, Mattos M A, et al 2002 The use of color-flow duplex scan for the detection of endoleaks. Journal of Vascular Surgery 36(1):100–104

Olsen D M, Rodriguez J A, Vranic M, et al 2002 A prospective study of ultrasound scan-guided thrombin injection of femoral pseudoaneurysm: a trend towards minimal mediation. Journal of Vascular Surgery 36(4):779–782

Santilli S M, Wernsing S E, Lee E S 2000 Expansion rates and outcomes for iliac artery aneurysms. Journal of Vascular Surgery 31(1):114–121

The UK Small Aneurysm Trial Participants 1998 Mortality results for randomised controlled trial of early elective surgery or ultrasonographic surveillance for small abdominal aortic aneurysms. Lancet 352(9141):1649–1655

van Marrewijk C, Buth J, Harris P L, et al 2002 Significance of endoleaks after endovascular repair of abdominal aortic aneurysms: The EUROSTAR experience. Journal of Vascular Surgery 35(3):461–473

Vardulaki K A, Walker N M, Day N E, et al 2000 Quantifying the risks of hypertension, age, sex and smoking in patients with abdominal aortic aneurysm. British Journal of Surgery 87(2):195–200

Veith F J, Baum R A, Ohki T, et al 2002 Nature and significance of endoleaks and endotension: summary of opinions expressed at an international conference. Journal of Vascular Surgery 35(5):1029–1035

Wassef M, Baxter B T, Chisholm R L, et al 2001 Pathogenesis of abdominal aortic aneurysms: a multidisciplinary research program supported by the National Heart, Lung, Blood Institute. Journal of Vascular Surgery 34(4):730–738

Further reading

Hennerici M, Neuerburg-Heusler D 1998 Vascular diagnosis with ultrasound. Thieme, Stuttgart

Tooke J E, Lowe G D O (eds) 1996 A textbook of vascular medicine. Arnold, London

Zwiebel W J 1992 Introduction to vascular ultrasonography, 3rd edn. W B Saunders, Philadelphia

Chapter **12**

Anatomy of the lower limb venous system and assessment of venous insufficiency

CHAPTER CONTENTS

Introduction 164
Anatomy 164
　Deep venous system of the lower limbs 164
　Anatomy of the superficial vein
　　system 165
　Anatomical variations 168
　Venous valves 168
　Flow patterns in the venous system 169
Venous disorders of the lower limbs 169
　Varicose veins 169
　Treatment of superficial venous
　　disorders 170
　Skin changes and venous ulcers 170
Practical considerations for duplex scanning
　of varicose veins 171
Augmentation maneuvers and venous
　reflux 172
　Calf compression 172
　Valsalva maneuver 172
Grading of superficial and deep venous
　reflux 173
　Problems with reflux classification 175
Scanning protocol for the lower limb venous
　system 176
　Assessment of the LSV and deep veins of the
　　thigh and knee 177
　Assessment of the SSV 178
　Concluding the scan 181
　B-mode appearance of varicose veins and
　　perforators 181

Investigation of recurrent varicose veins 182
　Possible causes of LSV recurrences 182
　Possible causes of SSV recurrences 184
Assessment of patients with skin changes and
　venous ulceration 185
Other disorders of the venous system 186
　Superficial thrombophlebitis 186
　Klippel-Trenaunay syndrome (KTS) 186
　Venous hemangioma 187
Reporting 187

INTRODUCTION

Venous disorders are a common problem and consume a significant proportion of the resources available to health care systems. Approximately 20–25% of women and 10–15% of men have visible varicose veins (Callam 1994). Significant venous disease can lead to venous ulceration, resulting in a marked loss in quality of life. Duplex scanning has had a dramatic impact on the noninvasive assessment of the venous system, and it is now the most commonly performed procedure for the detailed investigation of lower limb venous insufficiency. Lower limb venous duplex imaging can be used for the assessment of patients with primary or secondary varicose veins or for the investigation of patients with skin changes and venous ulceration. In comparison with arterial duplex scanning, venous duplex investigations can be technically challenging due to the wide range of anatomical variations in the venous system. This chapter covers the basic anatomy of the venous system and scanning techniques used for the assessment of lower limb venous insufficiency.

ANATOMY

The lower limb venous system can be divided into the deep and superficial veins, located in two main compartments. The deep compartment contains all the deep veins and is bounded by the muscular fascia. The superficial veins lie in the superficial compartment and are bounded deeply by the muscular fascia and superficially by the dermis (Caggiati et al 2002) (Fig. 12.1). The muscular fascial layer is usually visible on an ultrasound image (Fig. 12.2). There are numerous interconnections between the deep and superficial veins via perforating veins.

Deep venous system of the lower limbs

The anatomy of the deep veins is shown in Figure 12.3. The main deep veins of the thigh and calf are the following:

- common femoral vein
- profunda femoris vein
- superficial femoral vein

Figure 12.1   A diagram of the deep and superficial vein compartments. The main trunk of the saphenous vein lies in the saphenous compartment (SC), located within the superficial compartment; see text.

- above-knee popliteal vein
- below-knee popliteal vein
- posterior tibial veins
- peroneal veins
- anterior tibial veins
- gastrocnemius veins
- soleal veins and sinuses.

The posterior tibial and peroneal veins are usually paired and are associated with their respective arteries, which frequently lie in between the paired veins. The paired veins join into common trunks in the upper calf before forming the below-knee popliteal vein. The soleal veins are deep venous sinuses and veins of the soleus muscle that drain into the popliteal vein. They are an important part of the calf muscle pump mechanism (see Ch. 5). The gastrocnemius veins drain the medial and lateral sides of the gastrocnemius muscle and are usually larger in the medial side. The main trunk of the gastrocnemius vein drains into the popliteal vein below the level of the saphenopopliteal junction. The anterior tibial vein is paired and associated with the anterior tibial artery. It drains to the popliteal vein. The above-knee popliteal vein runs through the adductor canal and becomes the superficial femoral vein in the lower medial aspect of the thigh. The name is misleading as it is not a superficial vein but part of the deep venous system. The superficial femoral vein runs toward the groin, where the profunda femoris vein, also known as the deep femoral vein, joins to form the common femoral vein. This junction lies below the level of the saphenofemoral junction and common femoral artery bifurcation (see Fig. 9.6). The common femoral vein lies medial to the

Figure 12.2 The main trunks of the superficial veins are shown in cross section. A: The long saphenous vein (V) lies in the superficial compartment, bounded by the deep muscular fascia (upward arrows) and the saphenous fascia (downward arrows). B: The short saphenous vein (V) is also bounded by the deep fascia (upward arrows) and saphenous fascia (downward arrows). The medial gastrocnemius muscle (MG) and lateral gastrocnemius muscle (LG) are shown on this image of the right leg.

artery, becoming the external iliac vein above the inguinal ligament (Fig. 12.3). The external iliac vein runs deep and is joined by the internal iliac vein, which drains blood from the pelvis, forming the common iliac vein. The left common iliac vein runs underneath the right common iliac artery to drain into the vena cava, which lies to the right of the aorta.

Anatomy of the superficial vein system

The main superficial veins in the lower limbs are the long saphenous vein (LSV) and short saphenous

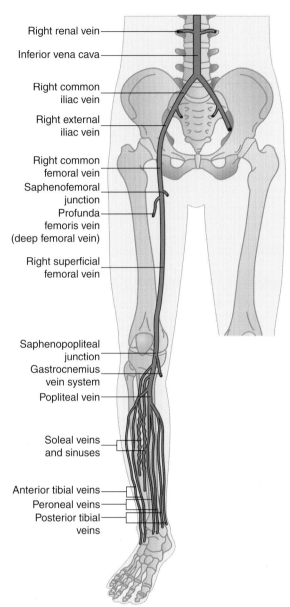

Figure 12.3 Anatomy of the deep venous system, including the iliac veins and vena cava.

vein (SSV) (Fig. 12.4) (sometimes referred to as the greater saphenous vein and lesser saphenous vein, respectively). It should be noted that within the superficial compartment there is a separate saphenous compartment which is bounded superficially by the hyperechoic saphenous fascia and deeply by the muscular fascia. The saphenous compartment contains the main trunks of the LSV or SSV and accompanying nerves. Branches, tributaries and cross-communicating veins lie external to this compartment (Caggiati et al 2002) (Fig. 12.1). The saphenous compartment and fascial layers can often be seen on the ultrasound image (Fig. 12.2). The distal LSV is located in front of the medial malleolus (inner ankle bone), runs up the medial aspect of the calf and thigh and has a number of superficial tributaries. There are a number of major perforating veins in the LSV system that can sometimes be identified by ultrasound. It is worth noting that many perforators do not connect directly to the main trunks of the LSV or SSV, but communicate via side branches of the main trunks. Crocket's perforators are located in the lower medial calf, at distances of approximately 6, 13 and 18 cm above the medial malleolus, and connect branches of the LSV to the posterior tibial veins. Boyd's perforator lies in the upper calf, approximately 10 cm below the knee joint, and runs between the LSV, or branches of the LSV, to the posterior tibial vein system. Finally, Dodd's perforator is located in the middle third of the thigh and runs between the LSV, or branches of the LSV, to the superficial femoral vein. The LSV drains into the common femoral vein approximately 2.5 cm below the inguinal ligament at the saphenofemoral junction. It is important to have a detailed understanding of the anatomy in this area, as there are at least six other tributaries draining to the LSV at the level of the saphenofemoral junction (Fig. 12.5). These tributaries can be the source of primary or recurrent varicose veins. It should be noted that it

Figure 12.4 Anatomy of the superficial veins. A: The long saphenous vein. B: The short saphenous vein.

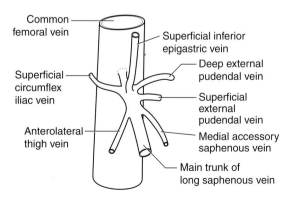

Figure 12.5 The anatomy of the saphenofemoral junction.

is not usually possible to identify all of these tributaries by ultrasound. The anterolateral thigh vein, sometimes called the anterior accessory saphenous vein, drains flow from the lateral aspect of the knee and runs obliquely across the anterior aspect of the thigh into the saphenofemoral junction (Fig. 12.5). However, it can sometimes join the LSV at a variable level below the junction. The anterolateral thigh vein is usually easy to identify with ultrasound (see Fig. 12.20B). The posteromedial thigh vein drains flow from the posteromedial and posterior regions of the lower thigh and usually joins the main trunk of the LSV in the upper thigh. There are sometimes connections between the proximal SSV (or its branches) and the posteromedial vein in the lower thigh, or upper calf.

The distal SSV arises behind the outer aspect of the ankle (lateral malleolus) and runs superficially up the posterior calf in the saphenous compartment (see Fig. 12.2B). There are usually a number of perforating veins associated with the SSV, especially from the gastrocnemius veins in the mid-calf. The SSV perforates the muscular fascia in the upper calf and passes between the heads of the gastrocnemius muscle. It drains to the popliteal vein via the saphenopopliteal junction at the popliteal fossa, superior to the origin of the gastrocnemius vein. Approximately 60% of all SSVs join the popliteal vein in the popliteal fossa within 8 cm of the knee joint (Browse et al 1999). However, the anatomy of the SSV can be extremely variable, and the saphenopopliteal junction may be found well above the popliteal fossa, draining to the above-knee popliteal vein or superficial femoral vein. Alternatively, the SSV can arise directly from the gastrocnemius vein or share a common origin (Fig. 12.6). In addition, some people have a vein that runs as a continuation of the SSV, along the posterior thigh above the saphenopopliteal junction, as shown in Figure 12.6. This vein is called the Giacomini vein, but it is not commonly referred to in surgical text books (Georgiev et al 2003). It is also sometimes referred to as the proximal thigh extension of the SSV. The termination of the Giacomini vein is variable, and it may drain to the LSV in the thigh or groin via a posteromedial thigh vein. It can course up the back of the thigh and drain directly to the femoral vein or branches of the internal iliac vein system, such as the inferior

gluteal vein (Fig. 12.6). There is sometimes confusion as to whether a posterior thigh vein is the Giacomini vein or merely a posteromedial branch of the LSV. Generally, the Giacomini vein appears to remain in a superficial fascia compartment (similar to the LSV and SSV) in the lower thigh, whereas posteromedial branches of the LSV tend to lie above the saphenous fascia. Finally, there are

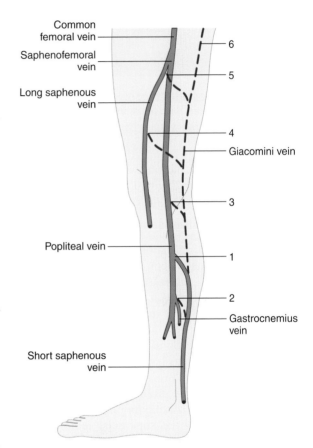

Figure 12.6 The level of the SSV origin can be highly variable, and potential positions are shown by numbers. The SSV normally drains to the popliteal vein in the popliteal fossa at the saphenopopliteal junction (position 1). It can arise from the gastrocnemius vein (GV) (position 2). It sometimes has a high origin from the popliteal vein (position 3). The Giacomini vein, when present, runs above the level of the saphenopopliteal junction and has a variable origin. It may drain to the LSV, femoral vein or branches of the internal iliac vein (positions 4, 5 and 6). Note it is possible to confuse the posteromedial branch of the LSV with the Giacomini vein; see text.

Figure 12.7 A transverse image of a duplicated or bifid superficial femoral vein with the artery (A) lying adjacent to the paired veins (V).

Figure 12.8 An image of a venous valve site in the long saphenous vein. The two valve cusps are demonstrated by the arrows.

usually cross-communicating veins in the upper calf, running between the LSV and SSV.

Anatomical variations

There are numerous anatomical variations in the lower limb venous system, and even experienced sonographers will encounter new variations from time to time. Duplicated, or bifid, vein systems are relatively common and mainly involve the LSV, superficial femoral vein and popliteal vein (Fig. 12.7). A potentially confusing anatomical variation occurs in patients who have a large deep femoral vein in the thigh. This vein runs between the popliteal vein and the profunda femoris vein and lies deep to the superficial femoral vein. In this situation, the size of the superficial femoral vein may be small when compared with the size of the superficial femoral artery, and this appearance may be mistaken for evidence of venous obstruction. However, good flow augmentation, with a calf squeeze, will be demonstrated in the common femoral vein just below the saphenofemoral junction. Careful inspection by duplex will normally reveal the larger deep femoral vein. A low-frequency 3.5 MHz curved linear array transducer may be necessary to identify this vein. A very rare anomaly can occur toward the level of the saphenofemoral junction, with the LSV running between the superficial femoral artery and profunda femoris artery to drain into the saphenofemoral junction.

Venous valves

Veins contain valves to prevent the reflux of blood to the extremities. Venous valves are bicuspid. There is often a characteristic dilation of the vein at the valve site that can sometimes be seen on the ultrasound image (Fig. 12.8). Venous valves are able to withstand high degrees of back pressure, typically in excess of 250–300 mmHg. The number of valves in each venous segment varies among individuals, but there are more valves in the distal veins than in the proximal veins, as they have to withstand higher hydrostatic pressures. The inferior vena cava and common iliac vein have no valves, and the majority of the population have no valves in the external iliac or common femoral vein. There is usually a valve at the origin to the superficial femoral vein and an average of three to four valves along the length of the superficial femoral and popliteal vein to the level of the knee, although the number can be inconsistent. There is a valve in the below-knee popliteal vein in the majority of people that is sometimes referred to as the 'gatekeeper', as it prevents venous reflux into the proximal calf. The deep veins in the calf contain numerous valves. The LSV and SSV contain approximately 8–10 valves along their main trunks (Browse et al 1999). In addition, there are normally valves at the junctions between the superficial and deep veins, and valves protecting many perforating veins so that flow is directed from the superficial venous system to the deep system. In very rare cases, patients may have absent venous valves due to congenital valve aplasia (Eifert et al 2000). This can be the cause of deep venous reflux in the very young patient.

Flow patterns in the venous system

The flow patterns in normal deep veins are described in Chapter 5. The venous flow patterns in the superficial veins can vary, depending on patient position and external factors, such as ambient temperature. Normally there should be no, or very little, spontaneous flow in the LSV and SSV when the patient is standing or sitting. If the ambient temperature in the room is high, vasodilation may result in increased flow in the superficial veins. Evidence of high-volume spontaneous or continuous flow in the superficial veins at rest should be treated with suspicion, as this may indicate obstruction of the deep veins or could be due to infection, such as cellulitis (Fig. 12.9).

VENOUS DISORDERS OF THE LOWER LIMBS

Deep vein thrombosis is covered in Chapter 13.

Varicose veins

The cause of varicose veins is uncertain, but there is evidence that increased age, female gender and pregnancy are risk factors (Callam 1994). However, other studies have demonstrated that chronic venous insufficiency and mild varicose veins are more common in men than in women (Evans et al 1999). Varicose veins appear as dilated, tortuous, elongated vessels on the skin surface, especially in the calf. Abnormal superficial veins can be classified according to their size. The clinical-etiologic-anatomic-pathophysiologic (CEAP) classification

Figure 12.9 High-volume spontaneous flow is demonstrated in the LSV of a patient with popliteal and superficial femoral vein obstruction.

system is widely used by many clinicians for the classification and grading of chronic venous disease (Porter & Moneta 1995).

Minor cosmetic or spider veins (telangiectases) are not visible by ultrasound. Small dilated intradermal veins (reticular veins) can also be difficult to image. Larger varicose veins, which often involve the main superficial trunks, can be assessed with ultrasound. Varicose veins most commonly occur due to incompetence of the LSV or SSV, or to a combination of both systems. It is important to identify the supply to the varicose areas and the level of incompetence in the LSV or SSV. This can be highly variable but frequently involves reflux from the saphenofemoral or saphenopopliteal junctions. In some situations varicose veins may be independent of the LSV or SSV systems. Much debate has surrounded the development of varicose veins, but it appears that incompetence in the main trunks develops distally, in the lower leg, and progresses in an ascending direction over time. This is contrary to traditional teaching, which proposed that incompetence developed at the saphenofemoral junction, leading to progressive valve failure in a descending direction. The model of progressively ascending valve failure would also explain why it is possible to observe segmental LSV reflux in the lower thigh but competence of the vein in the upper thigh and at the saphenofemoral junction (Abu-Own et al 1994). Symptoms and conditions caused by varicose veins can include aching, throbbing, burning, venous eczema, bleeding and ulceration. Some patients complain of symptoms that appear out of proportion to the size of their veins, which may be only mildly varicose. Some patients with superficial varicose veins may also have coexisting deep venous insufficiency.

Treatment of superficial venous disorders

The treatment of abnormal veins varies, depending on the severity of the condition (Browse et al 1999). Thread veins can be treated by injection sclerotherapy, followed by local compression to occlude the vein. They can also be treated by laser. Larger varicose veins can be surgically removed or stripped. In the case of the LSV, the saphenofemoral junction and tributaries are ligated at the groin, and the main trunk stripped with a vein stripper to knee level or below. In the case of the SSV, ligation of the saphenopopliteal junction is performed. Some surgeons strip the vein, but others leave it intact to avoid injury to the sural nerve, which is closely associated with the vein. Some surgeons ligate large perforators, and these can be marked preoperatively with the aid of duplex scanning. The remaining veins are then removed or avulsed using small microincisions. It is worthwhile watching some varicose vein surgery as it gives a better appreciation of the anatomy seen during duplex examinations.

A relatively new treatment known as endovenous saphenous obliteration has been introduced with promising results. This technique uses radiofrequency heating of a catheter tip introduced into the vein, causing collapse of the vein wall. The procedure is carried out under duplex guidance to position the catheters.

Skin changes and venous ulcers

A serious complication of superficial or deep venous insufficiency is the development of chronic venous hypertension in the lower limb, resulting in venous ulceration (Fig. 12.10). Risk factors associated with ulceration include post-thrombotic syndrome, obesity, immobility and arthritic conditions,

Figure 12.10 A picture of a venous ulcer involving the lower aspect of the medial calf and ankle. Varicose veins are also seen in the LSV distribution of the mid-calf.

which cause reduced movement of the ankle joint, leading to failure of the calf muscle pump. It is important to note that some ulcers that may appear to be venous in origin are caused by other conditions, such as vasculitis, rheumatoid arthritis or skin disorders. The underlying cause of ulceration is still unclear but is thought to involve changes in the microcirculation of the skin and subcutaneous tissues in response to local venous hypertension. The venous hypertension causes an increase in venular and capillary pressure, leading to local edema and reduced reabsorption of proteins and fluid from the interstitial tissue spaces. This is combined with damage to the capillary walls, which may cause localized tissue hypoxia. Leakage of red blood cells across the damaged capillary wall and into the interstitial tissue spaces produces the brown pigmentation associated with many ulcers. This is due to hemosiderin deposition caused by the breakdown of the red blood cells. Venous ulcers are usually reasonably shallow and vary in size, and in some cases they may be circumferential, involving a large area of the lower calf. They frequently become infected with different types of bacteria and can be extremely painful.

Skin changes around the ankle or lower calf are the first physical signs of venous hypertension. This is typically seen as areas of venous eczema and pigmentation, frequently associated with local skin irritation or itching. There is often development of lipodermatosclerosis, typified as hardening of the subcutaneous tissues in the lower calf and ankle, giving a hard, 'woody' feel to the area. The development of an ulcer is sometimes initiated by a minor injury or abrasion that fails to heal. It is important to remember that some venous ulcers are also associated with arterial disease, and patients with mixed venous and arterial ulceration pose a challenging diagnostic problem for the vascular laboratory. It is therefore routine practice to measure the ankle–brachial pressure index (ABPI) in all patients with venous ulceration to exclude a significant arterial component. However, in some situations it may be impossible to measure the ABPI due to pain, and a subjective assessment of the pedal Doppler signals will have to suffice. A layer of cling film is ideal for wrapping around areas of ulceration to protect the ulcer and to keep the pressure cuff clean.

Historically, it was thought that venous ulceration was primarily due to deep venous insufficiency following valve failure, post-thrombotic syndrome or failure of the calf muscle pump, resulting in deep venous hypertension. However, more recent studies (Scriven et al 1997, Magnusson et al 2001) demonstrated that a significant number of patients with ulceration have superficial reflux alone, with the deep veins being competent. Therefore, ligation of the relevant superficial vein junction, with or without stripping of the superficial vein, results in the healing of the majority of ulcers due to the reduction in venous hypertension. The role of perforator ligation remains controversial, but there is evidence that chronic venous insufficiency is associated with an increase in the number and diameter of medial calf perforators (Stuart et al 2000). Some vascular laboratories are asked to mark the position of incompetent perforators with the aid of the duplex scanner prior to surgery.

Varicose ulcers caused by significant deep venous insufficiency are not usually treated by the ligation or stripping of superficial varicose veins, as the underlying deep venous hypertension will not be corrected. Instead, the use of compression bandaging, which reduces edema and venous hypertension, has proved to be an effective method of healing ulcers. Different grades of compression bandaging can be used depending upon the clinical situation (Lambourne et al 1996). However, an ABPI >0.8 is required for the application of four-layer compression dressings, in order to avoid arterial compromise in the tissues under the bandaging. This can be a serious complication and can lead to limb loss in extreme cases.

PRACTICAL CONSIDERATIONS FOR DUPLEX SCANNING OF VARICOSE VEINS

The purpose of the scan is to assess the competency of the superficial and deep veins and identify the cause of the varicose veins. At least half an hour should be allocated for a bilateral vein scan. Adopting a logical approach to the examination is useful, as this reduces the amount of time required for the assessment. The patient should be asked the following questions before starting the examination:

- *Have you had any previous varicose vein treatment, either by surgery or by injection sclerotherapy?* It is not uncommon to find that the request card has omitted previous clinical details, and the patient may have undergone some form of treatment in the past. This may be evident on the duplex scan.
- *Have you ever had a deep vein thrombosis or severe leg swelling?* If the patient has had a deep vein thrombosis, there may be chronic damage of the deep venous system, causing deep venous insufficiency or obstruction, which may be the cause of the current symptoms.

The sonographer should also visually examine the position and distribution of the varicose veins, as this can provide a clue to their supply. There is no preparation required before the scan, but the legs should be accessible from the groin to the ankles. It is necessary to position the patient so that the feet are substantially lower than the heart in order to generate sufficient hydrostatic pressure to assess the competency of the venous valves. If the patient is lying completely flat, there is very little pressure differential between the central venous system and the legs. Therefore, any reflux occurring after a distal calf squeeze may be of such low velocity that it is not detected. Common positions in which to assess a patient include the supine position on the examination table with the whole table tilted feet down by an angle of at least 30° (reverse Trendelenburg position). Alternatively, the patient can sit on the edge of the examination table with the feet resting on a stool. Many units perform the examination with the patient in a standing position. The leg under investigation should be non-weight-bearing, and the patient can use a hand rail, or suitable alternative, for support. It should be noted that it is not uncommon for patients to feel faint during the examination (especially younger patients). Let the patient lie down immediately if he or she feels unwell, and, if necessary, appropriate medical advice should be sought.

AUGMENTATION MANEUVERS AND VENOUS REFLUX

Before considering the practical techniques used for scanning the venous system, it is important to have an understanding of the methods most commonly employed for assessing venous valve competency. These are calf compression, to augment flow toward the heart, and the Valsalva maneuver for examining the competency of the veins in the groin. In addition, proximal compression can be used to assess flow in perforators.

Calf compression

To assess the competency of the valves, the flow in the veins toward the heart should be temporarily increased or augmented. The easiest way to produce flow augmentation is to place a hand around the back of the calf and give a firm squeeze that is then quickly released. In our experience flow augmentation should be sufficiently strong to produce a transient peak flow velocity of >30 cm/s in the main superficial vein trunks so that valve closure should be rapid on the squeeze release (Fig. 12.11). However, this velocity can be difficult to achieve in very small veins. If an inadequate calf squeeze is performed, flow augmentation may be very poor, and this can be a source of conflicting results among different sonographers. For this reason some units prefer to use a rapid cuff inflater to inflate cuffs placed around the calf or thigh. The system inflates the cuff to a preset pressure before rapid deflation to provide reproducible compression. The disadvantage of this method is that it can be time-consuming and cumbersome to apply the cuffs.

Valsalva maneuver

The competency of the proximal deep veins and saphenofemoral junction can be assessed with a Valsalva maneuver. The patient is told to inhale deeply and then to push out and expand the cheeks without breathing out, while at the same time bearing pressure down on the abdomen. This produces an increase in intra-abdominal pressure, thus increasing the venous blood pressure in the iliac and femoral veins. It is usual to see the common femoral vein distending during a Valsalva maneuver. Provided that the venous valves are competent, there should be no reflux across the saphenofemoral junction or proximal superficial femoral vein during Valsalva testing (Fig. 12.12). There should be a temporary cessation of the normal

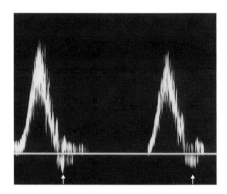

Figure 12.11 Augmentation of flow in the LSV following calf compression. There is a short duration of normal retrograde flow below the baseline (arrows) as the venous valves close.

Figure 12.12 The Valsalva maneuver demonstrates competency of the proximal superficial femoral vein. There is a cessation of normal phasic flow during the Valsalva maneuver followed by a surge of flow during expiration (END).

spontaneous phasic flow pattern in the superficial femoral and common femoral veins. If the sapheno-femoral junction is incompetent, venous back-pressure will produce significant reflux across the junction (Fig. 12.13). One potential pitfall of using the Valsalva maneuver for the assessment of proximal reflux can occur in patients who have a competent valve in the iliac vein system, which is usually valve-free. In this situation, the proximal valve will protect an incompetent saphenofemoral junction or proximal superficial femoral vein, and no reflux will be seen. The Valsalva maneuver is not used for the assessment of more distal veins.

GRADING OF SUPERFICIAL AND DEEP VENOUS REFLUX

Considerable debate surrounds the grading of venous reflux, especially as different patterns of reflux can be observed in the venous system. The following proto-col is used by our unit. With the relevant segment of vein imaged in longitudinal section, the color box is steered to obtain the best angle of insonation to the vein. A calf squeeze is performed and the augmenta-tion of flow demonstrated with color flow imaging. It is often possible to tell from the color flow display if the vein is normal or incompetent. A competent vein will display a burst of flow toward the heart dur-ing a calf squeeze, followed by an abrupt cessation of flow during squeeze release, although a very brief period of retrograde flow may be seen as the valves close. Significant venous reflux will be demonstrated by a sustained period of retrograde flow following calf release (Figs 12.14 and 12.15). However, the

Figure 12.13   Incompetence of the saphenofemoral junction is demonstrated by a large volume of reflux during a Valsalva maneuver (the arrow indicates the start of Valsalva).

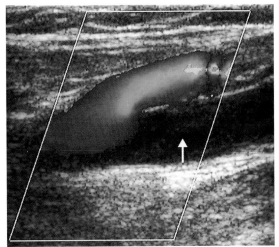

Figure 12.14   A: In this color flow image of the saphenopopliteal junction, flow in the SSV (S) and popliteal vein (coded blue) is toward the heart during distal augmentation. B: Following squeeze release there is significant retrograde flow (coded red) in the SSV and popliteal vein above the junction, due to saphenopopliteal junction incompetence. However, no retrograde flow is demonstrated in the popliteal vein below the level of the saphenopopliteal junction, indicating popliteal vein competency at this level (arrow).

Figure 12.15 Incompetence of the saphenofemoral junction and LSV is demonstrated with color flow imaging. Images 1 to 4 show flow across the junction (arrow) over a 3 s time interval at the end of distal augmentation. In image 1, flow (coded red) is toward the heart just before squeeze release. In images 2 and 3, there is increasing retrograde flow. In image 4, reflux (coded blue) is seen across the junction. Image 5 shows the LSV with flow toward the heart during augmentation. Image 6 demonstrates marked reflux following squeeze release.

grading of venous reflux on the basis of color flow imaging alone can lead to serious errors. This is because the color flow image may give very little impression of the flow volume or may not detect low-volume reflux at all. It is therefore always necessary to use spectral Doppler to grade the degree and duration of venous reflux (Fig. 12.16). The spectral Doppler sample volume should be large enough to cover the vein lumen, and the angle of insonation should be equal to or less than 60° to obtain a good spectral Doppler trace. Table 12.1 categorizes the degrees of venous reflux. The same criteria are used for grading venous reflux by calf compression or the Valsalva maneuver. Although the classification of venous reflux can sometimes be subjective, many contemporary scientific publications have used a reflux duration of >0.5 s to indicate abnormal valve function (Sarin et al 1994, Evans et al 1998, Ruckley et al 2002). In some cases, the reflux may be so severe that retrograde flow persists for more than 4 s.

Figure 12.16   Spectral Doppler is used to grade the duration of venous reflux. A: Moderate venous reflux of 0.55 s duration (R) is recorded across the saphenofemoral junction following distal augmentation. B: Severe venous reflux (R) of >2 s duration is demonstrated across the saphenofemoral junction.

Table 12.1   Grading of venous reflux

Grade	Reflux duration
Normal valve function	Reflux duration of <0.5 s, rapid closure of venous valves
Moderate reflux	Reflux duration of 0.5–1 s, mild to moderate retrograde flow
Significant reflux	Reflux duration of >1 s, large volume of retrograde flow

Figure 12.17   A: Partial incompetence of a venous valve is demonstrated by an area of retrograde flow (arrow) between the two valve cusps. B: Spectral Doppler demonstrates trickle or low-velocity reflux (R) in the popliteal vein following distal augmentation (S).

Finally, it may be possible to misinterpret a competent segment of a large vein as incompetent due to helical motion of flow during augmentation. This is especially true for the popliteal vein just above the knee, as the vein is large at this level, having been joined by a number of veins across and just below the knee.

Problems with reflux classification

Some patterns of reflux can be difficult to interpret, and attempts have been made to measure the volume of reflux using ultrasound volume flow measurements. In practice this is too time-consuming to be used routinely, but subjective assessment of the reflux volume can be useful. Trickle or low-velocity reflux can occur due to partially incompetent valves (Fig. 12.17). This can be observed in many veins but is common in the popliteal vein below the knee. It has

Figure 12.19   Venous stasis (S) is demonstrated as an echogenic speckle pattern in this B-mode image of a deep calf vein.

Figure 12.18   There can be problems in quantifying venous reflux. In this example the LSV was very large (8 mm diameter), but the duration of reflux (0.9 s) is shorter than that shown in Figure 12.16B. However, the volume of reflux is similar to that demonstrated during augmentation. In this example, the volume of blood flow during reflux is probably very significant due to the size of the vein. It should be noted that volume flow calculations are not routinely used in venous examinations.

been speculated that incipient deep venous reflux may occur due to gross superficial varicose veins causing overload of the deep venous system. This may cause some degree of dilation of the deep veins in the lower leg, which impairs normal valve function (Walsh et al 1994). Another problem of interpretation can occur when a vein is very large or dilated, as the duration of reflux may be relatively short. However, the volume of reflux can be high due to the large diameter of the vein. In this situation, significant reflux may be suspected if the shape of the spectral Doppler reflux pattern is the same as the augmentation pattern (Fig. 12.18). It may be difficult to augment flow in the veins of patients with gross venous stasis, and very little reflux will occur following distal release. However, the B-mode image often displays aggregation of the blood in the dilated vein as a speckle pattern (Fig. 12.19). Only a small amount of movement in the speckle pattern will be seen during calf compression. The deep venous sinuses in the calf

may be dilated and congested with blood, and this appearance can be mistaken for a deep vein thrombosis (see Ch. 13). Any problems of interpretation should be reported to the referring clinician, with a print taken of the relevant flow patterns. In some cases, it may be necessary to complement the duplex scan with other diagnostic tests, such as ambulatory venous pressures or plethysmography.

SCANNING PROTOCOL FOR THE LOWER LIMB VENOUS SYSTEM

A venous preset should be selected on the duplex scanner, which should typically set the PRF at a 1000 Hz. The color wall filter should also be set at a low level. A 10 MHz transducer, or broad-band equivalent, is normally used for scanning superficial varicose veins. However, a 5 MHz transducer, or broad-band equivalent, is usually required for imaging the deep veins and junctions. A combination of B-mode, color flow imaging and spectral Doppler is used throughout the examination. The assessment of venous reflux is performed with the transducer in a longitudinal plane to the vein. However, the assessment of perforator competency may require the probe to be orientated into other imaging planes to follow its course. It is necessary to perform an examination of the femoral and popliteal veins during any superficial vein assessment to assess the competency of these vessels. Also, the superficial veins can act as collateral pathways if the deep veins are obstructed, and surgery of the superficial veins would be contraindicated and potentially damaging. The technique for assessing varicose veins is described below, but it is often quicker to image the varicose veins distally and follow them back to their supply.

Assessment of the LSV and deep veins of the thigh and knee

1. The saphenofemoral junction is located by first identifying the common femoral vein in transverse section just below the level of the inguinal ligament. The anatomy in this region is demonstrated in Figure 9.6. The common femoral vein lies medial to the common femoral artery and is normally larger than the artery. The transducer is then moved distally, and the saphenofemoral junction will be seen on the medial anterior side of the common femoral vein (Fig. 12.20). It is usual to see other branches dividing from the saphenofemoral junction. Remember that these branches may be the main supply to the varicose veins.
2. The transducer should then be rotated so that the common femoral vein and saphenofemoral junction can be seen in longitudinal section (Fig. 12.21). The competency of the common femoral vein, saphenofemoral junction and proximal LSV can be assessed using distal compression and the Valsalva maneuver. The origin of the superficial femoral vein, which lies below the level of the saphenofemoral junction, should also be assessed for competency. Large visible branches dividing from the saphenofemoral junction can also be checked for competency, especially the anterolateral trunk, which can often supply varicose areas in the anterior thigh and calf. Medial branches of anterolateral vein in the upper and mid-thigh region can also supply varicose areas in the medial thigh. They can also run directly into the main trunk of the LSV. In this situation the main proximal trunk of the LSV may be competent.
3. The LSV is examined in transverse section along the medial thigh to the knee. In transverse section, it is often possible to see the LSV running directly into varicose areas. Large perforators, branches

Figure 12.20 A: A transverse image of the right common femoral vein demonstrating the position of the saphenofemoral junction (J), common femoral vein (V) and common femoral artery (A). This view is sometimes called 'Mickey Mouse' for obvious reasons. In this example, it is likely that the junction is incompetent as the LSV is very large. Note that some small branches are dividing from the junction (arrow). B: A transverse image taken in the upper thigh demonstrating the LSV (L), anterolateral branch (arrow), superficial femoral vein (V) and superficial femoral artery (A).

and bifid systems are relatively easy to identify on the transverse B-mode image. Large thigh perforators should be assessed for competency. The LSV is then followed in longitudinal section from the saphenofemoral junction to the knee and assessed for competency at frequent intervals.

A

B

Figure 12.21 A: A longitudinal image of the distal common femoral vein (CFV), saphenofemoral junction (J) and proximal LSV (S). A superior tributary is seen draining to the LSV, just proximal to the junction (arrow). It is often not possible to image the CFV distal to the SFJ in the same plane. B: An image of an abnormally large SFJ(J), which was found to be incompetent.

This is because the saphenofemoral junction and proximal LSV may be competent, but there may be segmental reflux in the upper, mid- or lower thigh, beyond incompetent valve sites, perforators or branches. It is even possible for the main trunk of the LSV to be competent, with isolated incompetence of side branches that supply superficial varicose areas in the thigh or calf. Another occasional finding is incompetence of the proximal LSV to the level of an incompetent superficial anterior or posterior thigh branch. Beyond the incompetent branch, it is possible for the main trunk of the LSV to be competent.

4. The SFV and proximal popliteal vein above the knee should be assessed for patency and competency. They are imaged from a medial thigh position in longitudinal section. The superficial femoral and popliteal veins lie deep to their respective arteries when imaged from this position.

5. The LSV is then followed in transverse section across the knee along the medial aspect of the calf to ankle. It is common to see large branches dividing from the main trunk of the LSV in the calf. Posteromedial varicose branches of the LSV in the upper calf sometimes interconnect to the SSV system in the posterior calf, causing SSV incompetence below this level (Fig. 12.22). The LSV and its major branches are then assessed in a longitudinal section using distal compression to augment flow. However, the varicose veins may be so obvious in the calf that little time need be spent on assessing the LSV at this level if it is the supply to the varicose areas. The LSV can also supply varicose areas on the lateral aspect of the calf, via incompetent branches that run over the front of the shin. There is considerable debate about the need to examine all calf perforators by duplex, and whether this is done may depend upon local protocols. In many cases perforators connect to side branches of the LSV and not to the main trunk.

6. The popliteal vein above and below the knee is examined from the popliteal fossa and assessed for patency and competency. The popliteal vein lies superficial to the popliteal artery when imaged from the popliteal fossa. Some clinicians request an assessment of the gastrocnemius veins. The investigation then continues with an assessment of the SSV.

Assessment of the SSV

1. The saphenopopliteal junction is usually located just above the skin crease in the popliteal fossa,

A   B

Figure 12.22   A: Posterior varicose branches (PB) of the LSV may interconnect to the SSV distribution in the posterior calf, causing SSV incompetence below the point of communication. (↑, competent veins; ↓, incompetent veins.) B: Medial varicose branches (MB) of the SSV can interconnect to the LSV in the calf, leading to segmental LSV incompetence.

Figure 12.23   A transverse B-mode image just below the popliteal fossa shows the position of the SSV lying in the superficial, saphenous compartment. The popliteal vein (PV) and gastrocnemius veins (GV) are seen below the fascia. The popliteal vein (PV) lies above the popliteal artery (PA) when imaged from this position.

although its position can be highly variable. The SSV is initially easier to locate just below the popliteal fossa in transverse section, where it will be seen lying within the superficial saphenous compartment (Figs 12.2B and 12.23). It is sometimes very small and easy to miss. The SSV is followed proximally into the popliteal fossa in transverse section, where it will be seen to perforate the muscular fascia and run deep to join the popliteal vein at the saphenopopliteal junction. It should be noted that the SSV can sometimes perforate the muscular fascia below the popliteal fossa. The proximal SSV sometimes curves medially or laterally toward the saphenopopliteal junction (Fig. 12.24). The actual junction can be located on the anterior, medial, lateral or, occasionally, posterior aspect of the popliteal vein when viewed from the popliteal fossa. In some situations, the junction

Figure 12.24   A transverse image of the left popliteal fossa showing an abnormally large saphenopopliteal junction (arrow), proximal SSV (S), popliteal vein (V) and popliteal artery (A). Note that the junction is located to the medial side of the popliteal vein in this example, but its position can vary.

and proximal SSV can be extremely tortuous, with the vein doubling back on itself in an S-shape pattern longitudinally, while following a tortuous path in either the medial or lateral direction. This leads to a very confusing image in which it is even possible to see different sections of the proximal SSV in the same scan plane. Slow, careful movement of the probe should be used to track the vein back to the popliteal vein. It is also possible to mistake branches of the gastrocnemius vein for the SSV if they run superficially within the gastrocnemius muscle. Care should be used when identifying the anatomy in this area. Finally, large perforators, separate from the SSV, can sometimes be found in the popliteal fossa, supplying superficial varicose areas.

2. The saphenopopliteal junction and proximal SSV are then imaged in longitudinal section (Fig. 12.25). In some cases, the junction is tortuous, and rotation of the probe is required to allow the junction to be visualized. The saphenopopliteal junction and proximal SSV should then be assessed for reflux with a strong calf squeeze. If not already performed previously, the competency of the above- and below-knee popliteal vein should be assessed.

3. Unlike the saphenofemoral junction, there is considerable anatomical variation in the position of the saphenopopliteal junction (Figs 12.6 and 12.26). In some cases it may be impossible to identify, owing to the height of the junction in the posterior thigh. The Giacomini vein, if present, can be the source of SSV incompetence. In this situation, it is possible to follow the Giacomini vein, which will be seen to run as a continuation of the SSV, in transverse section up the posterior thigh to its origin, which may be from a number of sources. These include the LSV, posterior thigh perforator or veins at the top of the posterior thigh. In the latter case, it may be impossible to identify the source, which

Figure 12.25 A longitudinal image of the popliteal fossa demonstrating a dilated saphenopopliteal junction and proximal SSV. There is a small deep vein (arrow) joining the SSV at the level of the junction (J) to the popliteal vein (PV). The popliteal artery (PA) lies below the vein. It is not always possible to see the junction in this plane or this clearly, especially if it lies to the medial or lateral side of the popliteal vein as shown in Figure 12.24.

Figure 12.26 An anatomical variation involving the proximal SSV. In this image the SSV (S) continued to run up the posterior thigh as the Giacomini vein (G). A gastrocnemius vein (GV) also drains to the SSV just proximal to the saphenopopliteal junction (J). The popliteal vein (PV) is demonstrated in this image.

may be from the internal iliac vein distribution. The Giacomini vein tends to run in a layer of fascia, which can aid its identification. It is possible to misidentify very superficial posterior thigh branches of the LSV as the Giacomini vein.

4. In transverse section, the SSV is followed distally from the popliteal fossa along the posterior aspect of the calf, where it runs toward the posterolateral aspect of the ankle. The SSV is then assessed for reflux along its length in longitudinal section. However, sometimes the vein is so small that it is difficult to demonstrate flow during compression. Large perforators can be assessed for competency. It is sometimes possible to see varicose branches from the LSV interconnecting to the SSV system. Conversely, medial varicose branches of the SSV may also interconnect to the LSV system (Fig. 12.22). The SSV can also supply varicose areas on the lateral and anterior aspects of the calf via branches.

5. The origin of the saphenopopliteal junction is sometimes marked preoperatively with the aid of duplex scanning, owing to its highly variable position. Some surgeons ask for a mark to be made on the skin corresponding to the position of the junction. However, others prefer a mark over the SSV just distal to the junction, so that the vein can be identified and followed back to the junction. Alternatively, a cross can be placed over the junction with a line drawn indicating the path of the SSV to the point where it becomes superficial. It is important for the surgeon and sonographer to agree on a system of marking to avoid any misunderstandings.

Concluding the scan

In some circumstances, the varicose veins may lie in more unusual distributions, such as the anterior aspect of the calf or lateral aspect of the thigh. In these situations, it is important to follow the varicose areas proximally in transverse section to identify the supply. The supply is frequently from varicose branches of the LSV or SSV, depending on the location of the varicose areas. One such example is incompetence of the anterolateral vein from the saphenofemoral junction. This vein often supplies varicose areas on the anterior aspect of the thigh and lateral calf. The main proximal trunk of the LSV can be competent or incompetent

in this situation. In certain circumstances, varicose veins running along the lateral aspect of the thigh and calf can be related to isolated perforators located on the lateral aspect of the upper thigh. Varicose veins in the lower posterior and posteromedial thigh can be supplied by the Giacomini vein. In this unusual situation, blood flows in a loop, across an incompetent saphenopopliteal junction and up the Giacomini vein, which then feeds the superficial varicosities running down the leg. This is a 'paradoxical' situation, in which the thigh veins are filled by 'antigravitational' flow, but in fact the flow will eventually make its way down into the calf via the incompetent veins, in the correct gravitational direction (Georgiev et al 2003). The main trunk of the SSV can be competent or incompetent in this situation. In some patients, it may be impossible to clearly define the source of the varicose veins, especially if they are very small, are diffusely distributed and generally run into very small superficial tributaries.

B-mode appearance of varicose veins and perforators

Varicose veins are relatively easy to identify on the B-mode image. They appear as single or multiple dilated tortuous vessels that vary randomly in diameter as the probe is swept across the varicose area (Fig. 12.27). They are superficial and may be located in the thigh as well as the calf. The main trunk supplying varicose areas, such as the LSV in the thigh, may be dilated but often has a reasonably even caliber and is frequently not visible on

Figure 12.27   A transverse image of tortuous dilated varicose veins.

A

B

Figure 12.28 A: A venogram demonstrating a perforator (P) running between the deep veins (DV) and superficial varicose veins (VV). B: A B-mode image demonstrating a large perforator (P). The fascia is demonstrated by the arrows, and there is a clear break in the fascia as the perforator runs between the deep vein (DV) and superficial vein (SV).

the skin surface. Occasionally a large localized dilation can be seen in the main trunk, called a varix. Sometimes the supplying vein may appear reasonably small, but reflux is demonstrated with color and spectral Doppler. The easiest way of locating perforators is to run the transducer steadily along the trunk of the superficial vein in transverse section. A break in the fascia will be seen on the B-mode image as the perforator runs between the subcutaneous and subfascial areas (Fig. 12.28).

INVESTIGATION OF RECURRENT VARICOSE VEINS

Some patients develop secondary or recurrent varicose veins over a variable time period following surgery. The scanning technique for the investigation of recurrent varicose veins is very similar to that used for the investigation of primary varicose veins. However, it is important to keep an open mind as to the source of the recurrent veins, as their supply can be unpredictable. It is often easier to begin the examination at the level of the varicose areas in transverse section and work proximally to the point of supply. The use of color flow imaging during calf augmentation can allow smaller varicose veins to be followed proximally if the B-mode imaging is poor. Some of the main causes of recurrent varicose veins are summarized below. However, it may be some considerable time before the trainee sonographer is familiar with all the variations.

Possible causes of LSV recurrences

Incomplete ligation of the saphenofemoral junction

Normally the junction should be ligated and any tributaries divided (Fig. 12.29A). However, due to misidentification or inadequate dissection, it is possible to ligate only a small tributary during surgery, rather than the main junction. The level of the saphenofemoral junction should be examined in transverse section, where it is easy to identify a large patent junction. Sometimes the scan demonstrates that the main trunk of the LSV has been ligated just distal to the saphenofemoral junction but a tributary has been left intact. This tributary then supplies the varicose veins or intact LSV trunk, if it has not been stripped. This is often the case when the anterolateral saphenous vein is found to be intact at the level of the saphenofemoral junction. It frequently supplies varicose areas in the anterior and medial aspects of the thigh, which in turn run into the calf (Fig. 12.30). Occasionally, there may be a very small recurrent junction that can be difficult to identify without the aid of color flow imaging (Fig. 12.29B).

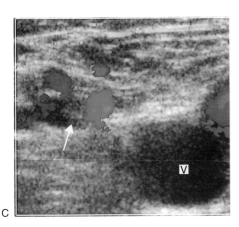

Figure 12.29   Three examples of ultrasound findings at the level of the saphenofemoral junction following surgery. The femoral vein (V) is seen in all three images. A: The saphenofemoral junction (arrow) has been completely ligated by surgery. B: A small recurrent junction (arrow) is seen to supply a diffuse network of small veins. C: The SFJ has been ligated but a diffuse web of small veins are seen adjacent to the vein (arrow).

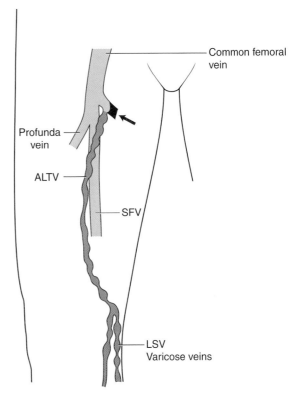

Figure 12.30   Incomplete ligation of the saphenofemoral junction can be the cause of recurrent varicose veins. In this example the anterolateral thigh vein (ALTV) has been left intact following incomplete ligation of the junction (arrow). The ALTV now supplies the varicose areas shown on the diagram.

Incompetent tributaries

In some cases, the saphenofemoral junction has been ligated, but small tributaries from the inner aspect of the groin supply varicose areas in the LSV distribution or the main LSV trunk, if it has not been stripped. These tributaries are often supplied from pudendal and perineal veins. Typically, the scan will demonstrate varicose veins, or an intact trunk if this has not been stripped in the upper thigh, breaking up into small tributaries before disappearing toward the inner aspect of the groin. These tributaries are usually seen as a fine, diffuse web of veins on the color flow image. Sometimes these tributaries may run close to the femoral vein, but no direct connection will be identified (Fig. 12.29C). It is also possible for recurrent varicose

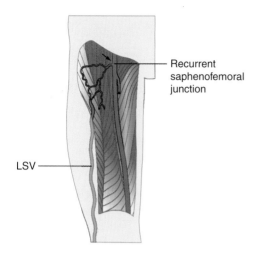

Recurrent
saphenofemoral
junction

LSV

Figure 12.31   A diagrammatic representation of neovascularization. There is a small recurrent connection between the femoral vein and a diffuse network of veins in the groin and upper thigh. In this example the main trunk of the LSV has not been stripped and is supplied by the small diffuse veins. The ultrasound appearance at the level of the femoral vein will be similar to that shown in Figure 12.29B.

veins to be supplied from veins running from the lower abdominal wall.

Neovascularization

It has been suggested that neovascularization or 're-growth' can occur between the femoral vein and superficial varicose veins at the groin following ligation of the saphenofemoral junction (Jones et al 1996) (Fig. 12.31). These small veins then supply the LSV, if it had not been stripped, or proximal secondary varicose veins. Duplex scanning will reveal a diffuse web of small tortuous veins in the groin, with a small connection to the femoral vein that may be impossible to follow without the aid of color flow imaging.

Thigh or calf perforators

Recurrent varicose veins can be supplied by thigh or calf perforators (Fig. 12.28). Large thigh perforators are relatively easy to identify by following the varicose trunk up the medial thigh in transverse section, where it will be seen to connect directly, or via side branches, to the perforator. Perforators to the deep veins can have very tortuous courses. If a mid-thigh perforator is the main supply to the varicose areas, there may be only small, or no, varicose veins seen above the level of the perforator. Duplex scanning can be used to mark the location of perforators preoperatively.

Incomplete stripping of the LSV trunk in the thigh

Sometimes the saphenofemoral junction has been ligated, but the vein stripper has been passed down a bifid trunk of the LSV or a branch, leaving the majority of the main trunk intact. The image will demonstrate the presence of an incompetent LSV trunk that breaks into small tributaries toward the groin with a variable supply, as described in some of the examples above.

Secondary varicose veins

Over time, it is not uncommon for secondary varicose veins to develop in the thigh and calf that were not visible when the original surgery was performed. These are often imaged as numerous tortuous varicose veins that may lie very superficially in the LSV distribution. They often have a diffuse supply, sometimes involving superficial tributaries in the groin.

Incompetence of the SSV

Varicose veins in the LSV distribution of the calf can occur due to incompetence of the SSV. In this situation, posteromedial varicose branches of the SSV interconnect to the LSV distribution (Fig. 12.22B).

Possible causes of SSV recurrences

Incomplete ligation of the saphenopopliteal junction

Recurrence can occur if there has been incomplete ligation or misidentification of the saphenopopliteal junction during surgery. With the transducer in transverse section, the SSV can be followed proximally, where it will be possible to see the saphenopopliteal junction clearly.

Incompetent Giacomini vein

In some circumstances a large incompetent Giacomini vein may run directly into the SSV, or varicose areas, at the popliteal fossa. Starting in a transverse section just below the popliteal fossa, the SSV is identified and followed proximally. The saphenopopliteal junction should not be seen if it has been correctly ligated. However, the SSV continues to course up the posterior thigh as the Giacomini vein. Alternatively, the superficial varicosities may be supplied directly by the Giacomini vein. The Giacomini vein can have a variable supply, as described previously.

Incompetent perforators

These perforators may arise from variable positions and can be found above the popliteal fossa, at the popliteal fossa or from the gastrocnemius vein in the proximal or mid-calf. Perforators arising in the region of the popliteal fossa can follow very tortuous routes. Perforators supplying varicose areas in the SSV distribution are easiest to identify in transverse section.

LSV incompetence

Varicose veins in the SSV distribution can occur due to LSV incompetence. Incompetent posterior veins in the LSV distribution, which are not prominent on the skin surface, may run into the SSV system in the upper posterior calf, where the veins become more prominent. The surgeon performing the original surgery may have assumed that these varicose veins were related to saphenopopliteal junction incompetence and ligated the junction, but in fact the SSV was competent above the point of communication between the LSV and the SSV. Therefore, ligation of the saphenopopliteal junction will not have controlled the varicose veins (Fig. 12.22A).

Diffuse varicosities in the popliteal fossa

Diffuse varicosities in the popliteal fossa may resupply the SSV. In this situation, although the saphenopopliteal junction has been ligated, the SSV

trunk is supplied by numerous small superficial tributaries that are difficult to follow.

ASSESSMENT OF PATIENTS WITH SKIN CHANGES AND VENOUS ULCERATION

Many patients with venous ulcers have never had varicose vein surgery, whereas others may have had a number of previous operations. However, the basic technique for assessing patients with venous ulceration is similar to the technique for the assessment of varicose veins. Many patients are elderly and are unable to stand during the examination, but the leg should be in a dependent position to assess for reflux. This is best achieved by hanging the leg over the side of the examination table with the feet resting on a stool. It is necessary to remove any pressure or compression dressings, as these may reduce venous reflux, leading to false results. Patients with venous ulceration are more likely to have deep venous incompetence or obstruction than patients with simple varicose veins. Therefore, it is important to assess the deep veins carefully. It is often easier to start the scan by examining the popliteal vein from the popliteal fossa, as many surgeons will not perform superficial surgery if there is gross reflux in the popliteal vein above and below the knee, and a less detailed scan of the superficial vein system may be possible.

There are a number of problems associated with the assessment of patients with venous ulcers. It can be difficult to image the deep veins in obese patients with large legs. In this situation, it may be worth trying a 3.5 MHz abdominal transducer to image the deep veins. Sometimes the calf is too ulcerated or sore to perform calf compression for the assessment of reflux. In such cases, try squeezing the upper portion of the calf, where there may be less ulceration or skin change. If in doubt, warn the patient that the test could be uncomfortable, as many patients are willing to cooperate but may be distressed if no prior warning of discomfort is given. In rare cases, some analgesia may be required. It can be difficult to assess the competency of veins in patients with continuous high-volume flow (hyperemic flow) in the superficial and deep veins due to infection. The high-volume flow toward the heart can lead to a reduction in reflux duration (Fig. 12.32). Under these circumstances it is very difficult to examine the function of the veins, but it may be an indication that the leg is infected. Appropriate action, such as antibiotic therapy and leg elevation, may need to be taken to reduce the infection or cellulitis. The leg can be reassessed when the hyperemia subsides.

OTHER DISORDERS OF THE VENOUS SYSTEM

Superficial thrombophlebitis

Superficial thrombophlebitis is an inflammatory process that involves the superficial veins (see Ch. 13). The superficial vein may become partially or fully thrombosed. Typically, the area around the phlebitis is reddened, tender and hot, and the superficial vein may be swollen and hard. Phlebitis is normally treated with analgesia and anti-inflammatory drugs, but superficial vein stripping may be required, especially if there is a thrombus tip extending to the saphenofemoral junction or saphenopopliteal junction.

Klippel–Trenaunay syndrome (KTS)

Klippel-Trenaunay syndrome is a congenital condition and consists of a range of abnormalities

that can involve the skin capillaries, often causing nevi (birthmarks or port wine stains), bone and soft tissue hypertrophy (excessive limb growth) and venous varicosities. Each case of KTS is unique, and often only one limb is affected, but other areas of the body may also be involved. Abnormalities of the venous system range in severity (Browse et al 1999). Visible varicose veins vary from very minor to severe and can be widely distributed throughout the leg. Varicosities are commonly seen on the lateral aspect of the thigh and calf. In some cases of KTS, the deep veins may be abnormal. Abnormalities can include absence of parts of the deep venous system, unusually small deep veins or large, dilated deep veins with nonfunctioning valves. It is therefore very important to scan the deep venous system in all patients with

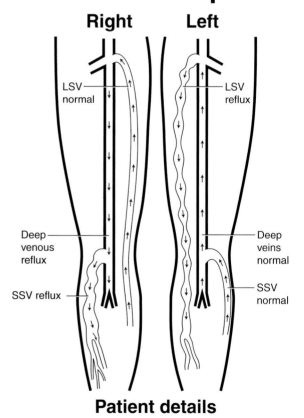

Figure 12.33   The use of diagrams makes it easier for the clinician to interpret the findings of a venous duplex examination (see text).

Figure 12.32   An example of hyperemic flow patterns in the superficial femoral artery and vein due to infection in the lower leg. The arterial signal, above the baseline, demonstrates high-volume flow throughout the cardiac cycle. There is continuous high-volume flow in the vein, shown below the baseline.

KTS, to detect any deep venous abnormalities, before treating any large superficial varicosities by surgery (Eifert et al 2000).

Venous hemangioma

Venous malformations can occur anywhere in the body and consist of an abnormal network of veins. Venous hemangiomas vary in size and can be very extensive. They can occur in the superficial tissues, muscles or organs. They can cause pain and swelling and may be disfiguring when they are superficial. Duplex scanning can be useful for imaging venous malformations to exclude evidence of arteriovenous fistulas, but it can be difficult to define the full extent of the lesion, especially if it is deep or involves joints. When imaging very superficial lesions, it is important not to apply too much pressure with the transducer, as this may occlude the veins. Other imaging techniques, such as MRI, are often used to investigate the extent of the malformation, especially if it is diffusely distributed in muscles.

REPORTING

Duplex assessment of varicose veins is a dynamic technique, and it can be difficult to demonstrate this quality on hard copy, although recordings of reflux patterns, as seen on the spectral Doppler display, may be useful. It is therefore easier to provide a functional map of the venous system, as shown in Figure 12.33. The superficial veins can be drawn onto the diagram, and black arrows pointing toward the heart indicate normal competent veins. Red arrows pointing toward the feet indicate venous reflux. This diagram can be accompanied by a brief report outlining any limitations of the scan. This type of report is easy for the surgeon to interpret in a busy outpatient clinic and is also useful to show to the patient, as it provides a clear explanation of the problem.

References

Abu-Own A, Scurr J H, Coleridge Smith P D 1994 Saphenous vein reflux without incompetence at the saphenofemoral junction. British Journal of Surgery 81(10):1452–1454

Browse N, Burnand K G, Irvine A T, et al 1999 Diseases of the veins, 2nd edn. Arnold, London, pp 191–248

Caggiati A, Bergan J J, Gloviczki P, et al 2002 Nomenclature of the veins of the lower limbs: an international interdisciplinary consensus statement. Journal of Vascular Surgery 36(2):416–422

Callam M J 1994 Epidemiology of varicose veins. British Journal of Surgery 81(2):167–173

Eifert S, Villavicencio J L, Kao T C, et al 2000 Prevalence of deep venous anomalies in congenital vascular malformations of venous predominance. Journal of Vascular Surgery 31(3):462–471

Evans C J, Allan P L, Lee A J, et al 1998 Prevalence of venous reflux in the general population on duplex scanning: the Edinburgh Vein Study. Journal of Vascular Surgery 28(5):767–776

Evans C J, Fowkes F G, Ruckley C V, et al 1999 Prevalence of varicose veins and chronic venous insufficiency in men and women in the general population: Edinburgh Vein Study. Journal of Epidemiology and Community Health 53(3):149–153

Georgiev M, Myers K A, Belcaro G 2003 The thigh extension of the lesser saphenous vein: from Giacomini's observations to ultrasound scan imaging. Journal of Vascular Surgery 37(3):558–563

Jones L, Braithwaite B D, Selwyn D, et al 1996 Neovascularisation is the principal cause of varicose vein recurrence: results of a randomised trial of stripping the long saphenous vein. European Journal of Vascular and Endovascular Surgery 12(4):442–445

Lambourne L A, Moffatt C J, Jones A C, et al 1996 Clinical audit and effective change in leg ulcer services. Journal of Wound Care 5(8):348–351

Magnusson M B, Nelzen O, Risberg B, et al 2001 A colour Doppler ultrasound study of venous reflux in patients with chronic leg ulcers. European Journal of Vascular and Endovascular Surgery 21(4):353–360

Porter J M, Moneta G L 1995 Reporting standards on venous disease: an update. An international consensus committee on chronic venous disease. Journal of Vascular Surgery 21(4):635–645

Ruckley C V, Evans C J, Allan P L, et al 2002 Chronic venous insufficiency: clinical and duplex correlations. The Edinburgh Vein Study of venous disorders in the general population. Journal of Vascular Surgery 36(3):520–525

Sarin S, Sommerville K, Farrah J, et al 1994 Duplex ultrasonography for assessment of venous valvular function of the lower limb. British Journal of Surgery 81(11):1591–1595

Scriven J M, Hartshorne T, Bell P R, et al 1997 Single-visit venous ulcer assessment clinic: the first year. British Journal of Surgery 84(3):334–336

Stuart W P, Adam D J, Allan P L, et al 2000 The relationship between the number, competence, and diameter of medial calf perforating veins and the clinical status in healthy subjects and patients with lower-limb venous disease. Journal of Vascular Surgery 32(1):138–143

Walsh J C, Bergan J J, Beeman S, et al 1994 Femoral venous reflux abolished by greater saphenous vein stripping. Annals of Vascular Surgery 8(6): 566–570

Further reading

Bellard G, Nicolaides A N, Veller M 1995 Venous disorders. W B Saunders, London

Browse N, Burnand K G, Irvine A T, et al 1999 Diseases of the veins, 2nd edn. Arnold, London

Greenhalgh R M (ed) 1995 Vascular imaging for surgeons. W B Saunders, London

Chapter 13

Duplex assessment of deep venous thrombosis and upper limb venous disorders

CHAPTER CONTENTS

Introduction 189
Epidemiology and pathology of DVT 189
  Signs, symptoms and treatment of DVT 190
  Investigations for diagnosing DVT 191
Practical considerations for duplex assessment of DVT 192
Deep vein examination for acute DVT 192
Scan appearances for the assessment of acute DVT 195
  B-mode images 195
  Color flow images 196
  Spectral Doppler 197
  Diagnostic problems 197
Accuracy of duplex scanning for the detection of DVT 198
Natural history of DVT 198
  Recurrent thrombosis 199
Other pathologic conditions that can mimic DVT 199
  Thrombophlebitis 200
  Hematoma 200
  Lymphedema 200
  Cellulitis 201
  Edema 201
  Baker's cysts 201
  Enlarged lymph nodes 202
  Other pathologic lesions 202
Upper limb veins 202
  Anatomy of the deep upper limb veins 202
  Anatomy of the superficial upper limb veins 203
  Thrombosis of the upper limbs 203
Technique for assessing the brachial, axillary and subclavian veins 204
  Other upper limb venous disorders 204
Reporting 205

INTRODUCTION

Deep venous thrombosis (DVT) is a common disorder that can lead to fatal pulmonary embolism (PE). Duplex scanning is considered to be the method of choice for the imaging of DVT, with venography reserved for technically incomplete or difficult duplex examinations. Duplex scanning can be used for serial investigations to monitor the progression and outcome of thrombosis. In addition, duplex scanning can be useful for assessing the long-term damage to veins and valve function as a result of chronic post-thrombotic syndrome (Haenen et al 2002). This can lead to the development of lower limb venous hypertension and possible leg ulceration. This chapter provides a description of duplex scanning techniques for the diagnosis of DVT and also considers other pathologic conditions that may mimic the symptoms of venous thrombosis.

EPIDEMIOLOGY AND PATHOLOGY OF DVT

DVT usually affects the lower limb veins, but it can also occur in the upper limbs, especially in conjunction with catheter access or malignancy. The published data on the epidemiology of DVT and PE demonstrate some variability, and reported rates of DVT and thromboembolism appear to be partly dependent upon methods of data collection (autopsy records, discharge diagnoses, and so forth) and the patient population studied. A recent systematic review by Fowkes et al (2003) indicated an incidence of DVT in the whole general population of approximately 5 per 10 000 per annum. However, the incidence was highly dependent upon age and increased from 2–3 per 10 000 person years at age 30–49 years to 20 per 10 000 person years at age 70–79 years. Around 40% cases of DVT were found to be idiopathic (of unknown cause). The annual rate of PE is somewhere in the region of 6 cases per 10 000 in the general population (Nicolaides et al 1994). A review by White (2003) indicated that death occurs in approximately 12% of PE cases within 1 month of diagnosis. Open or healed venous ulceration occurs in around 1% of the general adult population, with a proportion attributed to post-thrombotic syndrome (Fowkes et al 2001). The early detection and treatment of DVT can therefore reduce the subsequent risk of mortality or long-term morbidity.

Virchow (1846) described the association between thrombosis in the legs and emboli in the lung. The factors predisposing to thrombosis are described by his famous triad of coagulability of the blood, damage to the vein wall or endothelium and venous stasis. Venous thrombi are believed to originate in valve cusp pockets (Fig. 13.1) or in the deep venous muscular sinuses, such as the soleal veins. DVT most commonly occurs in the calf veins and can propagate to the proximal veins. It is not necessary for all the calf veins to be affected in order for proximal propagation to occur. It is believed that approximately 10–20% of calf vein thrombi propagate to the deep veins across and above the knee (Khaw 2002, Labropoulos et al 2002). This is thought to be associated with an increased risk of PE. Isolated thrombosis of the proximal veins, such as the femoral or iliac veins, is less common and can occur due to trauma, surgery, pregnancy or malignancy. Proximal and distal propagation of thrombus can occur in this situation. Venous stasis can also lead to DVT, and this is why patients undergoing long periods of bed rest or immobility are at greater risk of developing thrombosis. There is also increasing evidence to suggest that long-haul air travel is associated with an increased risk of DVT. The main risk factors associated with the development of venous thrombosis are shown in Box 13.1. In the early stages of a DVT, it is possible for a large proportion of the clot to be nonadherent to the vein wall. This is termed a free-floating thrombus. In this situation there is a risk of detachment, leading to PE. As free-floating thrombus becomes older (7–10 days), it becomes more organized and adherent to the vein wall.

Signs, symptoms and treatment of DVT

The clinical diagnosis of DVT is unreliable and inaccurate in up to 50% of cases (Cranley et al 1976). However, typical symptoms include the development of acute calf pain associated with localized tenderness, heat and swelling. The superficial veins may also be dilated. If the thrombosis involves the proximal veins, there may be significant swelling of the thigh. Unfortunately, other

Figure 13.1 A longitudinal B-mode image of the below-knee popliteal vein. An area of thrombus (arrow) is seen to extend from the valve site on the posterior wall.

Box 13.1   Risk factors for the development of deep vein thrombosis

- Coagulation disorders
- Immobilization
- Surgery and trauma
- Malignancy
- Septicemia
- Oral contraceptives
- Increasing age
- Stroke
- Heart failure
- Previous history of deep vein thrombosis
- Long-haul air travel

conditions, such as cellulitis and edema, can mimic the symptoms of DVT. In some cases of DVT the patient may be asymptomatic, especially if the thrombus is small. In extreme cases of DVT the outflow of the limb is so severely reduced that the arterial inflow may become obstructed, leading to venous gangrene. This condition is called phlegmasia cerulea dolens. The foot may appear blackened and the limb swollen and blue, even when elevated.

PE occurs when a segment of clot breaks loose, travels through the right side of the heart and lodges in branches of the pulmonary artery. This leads to a perfusion defect in the arterial bed of the lungs. The symptoms of PE include the following:

- sudden breathlessness
- pleuritic chest pain
- coughing up of blood
- right-sided heart failure or cardiovascular collapse
- death.

Radioisotope studies are frequently used for investigating perfusion and ventilation defects in the lungs.

The prevention of DVT includes the use of elastic support stockings, which increase venous return and therefore reduce the risk of venous stasis. Patients at high risk may be advised to take aspirin or be given low molecular weight heparin if they are undertaking any activity or treatment that may increase the risk of DVT. Treatment of DVT is usually with anticoagulation drugs. The initial treatment is by an intravenous infusion of heparin, which is then converted to long-term therapy with oral anticoagulants, such as warfarin. Occasionally, devices called vena caval filters are positioned in the vena cava to catch clots, when there is a high risk of embolization to the lungs. Surgery is sometimes performed to remove thrombus from the femoral and iliac veins.

The investigation and treatment of isolated calf vein thrombosis remain a contentious issue (Lohr et al 1991, Meissner et al 1997). It is beyond the scope of this book to consider the debate in any detail, but sonographers should be aware of the controversies surrounding this area. Some clinicians will always investigate and treat calf DVT, whereas others will not specifically ask for the calf veins to be examined. Some units perform serial scans of the popliteal vein over a period of 3–5 days to identify any propagation of calf vein thrombi to the popliteal vein.

Investigations for diagnosing DVT

Traditionally, x-ray venography was the main test used for the diagnosis of DVT. It involves an injection of a contrast agent into the venous system via a dorsal foot vein. In some cases it proves impossible to cannulate a foot vein, and in some situations patent deep calf veins do not fill with contrast agent (Bjorgell et al 2000). Currently, duplex scanning is the main method of imaging DVT, but it is often combined with pre-imaging tests, in a defined management pathway or protocol. The development of these protocols has occurred as a result of the increased workload and financial costs experienced by most ultrasound departments. These protocols may be complex; an example of one such pathway is shown in Figure 13.2. The process often begins with a clinical assessment, including a risk probability score derived from a set of standard questions. The lower the score, the lower the probability of DVT. The next stage usually involves a biochemical assay to measure D-dimer levels in the blood. D-dimers are products that are formed by

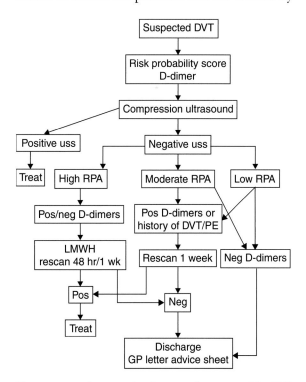

Figure 13.2 An example of a screening protocol for DVT. RPA, risk probability assessment; LMWH, low molecular-weight heparin. (After Khaw 2002, with permission.)

the interaction of fibrin, contained in thrombus, and plasmin. Increased levels of D-dimer are associated with the presence of DVT. Unfortunately, increased levels of D-dimer are also found in other conditions, such as malignancy, infection and trauma. Therefore, the D-dimer test has a high sensitivity but low specificity for the presence of DVT. Despite low specificity, negative predictive values as high as 98% have been reported (Bradley et al 2000). A negative predictive value indicates the probability that the patient will not have the disease in those who have a negative test outcome. It has been suggested that a combination of a low risk probability score and negative D-dimer test may be useful pre-selection tools to avoid unnecessary duplex examinations (Aschwanden et al 1999). Most ultrasound examinations use compression of the vein to confirm patency. This normally involves full examination of the deep veins from the groin to the calf. However, there is evidence that a limited compression test involving two- or three-point compression at the common femoral vein, popliteal vein and distal popliteal vein (third point) is a safe and rapid method of excluding DVT (Cogo et al 1998, Khaw 2002).

Magnetic resonance imaging and CT scanning are used for imaging the iliac veins and vena cava when other imaging tests are inadequate or impossible. However, because of their cost, they are unlikely to be used for routine DVT screening in the outpatient clinic in the immediate future.

PRACTICAL CONSIDERATIONS FOR DUPLEX ASSESSMENT OF DVT

The objective of the scan is to assess the deep venous system for patency and exclude the presence of a DVT. It is also important to locate the proximal position of a thrombosis, as this can influence subsequent treatment. Other conditions that mimic DVT can be identified with ultrasound. The main diagnostic criterion used to exclude DVT is complete collapse of the vein under transducer pressure. Color flow imaging and spectral Doppler can also be used during the assessment. At least 30 min should be allocated for a full scan, including the calf veins.

The legs should be accessible and the patient made as comfortable as possible. In very rare situations, the patient may require some sedation or analgesia before the examination if the limb is extremely painful. It is helpful to ask the patient to point to any areas of discomfort or tenderness, especially in the calf, as this can often be located over the site of the thrombosis. This region should be carefully examined by duplex scanning. The examination room should be at a comfortable ambient temperature to prevent vasoconstriction ($>20\,°C$). Wherever possible, the legs should be examined in a dependent position in order to fill and distend the veins. Ideally, the patient should be examined with the legs tilted downward from the head by at least 30° (reverse Trendelenburg position). Alternatively, the patient can be examined in a standing position, with the leg to be examined not bearing weight and the patient holding a hand rail or equivalent for support. The calf veins and popliteal fossa are easier to scan with the legs extended, hanging over the side of the examination table, and the feet resting on a stool. It is important not to overextend the knee when examining the popliteal vein, as this can lead to collapse or occlusion of the vein. Wherever possible, immobile or sick patients should be tilted into a reverse Trendelenburg position, although there may be situations in which the patient cannot be moved, such as in the intensive care unit.

DEEP VEIN EXAMINATION FOR ACUTE DVT

A 5 MHz, or broad-band equivalent, flat linear array transducer should be used for examining the femoral, popliteal and calf veins. The iliac veins are examined using a 3.5 MHz curved linear array transducer. The scanner should be configured for a venous examination. The color PRF should be low, typically 1000 Hz, to detect low-velocity flow. The color wall filter should also be set at a low level, and the spectral Doppler sample volume should be increased in size to cover the vessel, so that flow is sampled across the lumen.

Ultrasound compression is the main method of confirming vein patency. If direct transducer pressure is applied over a vein it will collapse, as the blood pressure in the deep veins is low, unlike the pressure in the adjacent artery, and the walls will be seen to meet (coapt). The adjacent artery should demonstrate little or no distortion. In contrast, if there is thrombus in the vein it will not collapse. This technique is demonstrated in Figures 13.3 and 13.4. It should be noted that fresh thrombus, which is soft, can partially deform. Compression should be applied at frequent intervals along the length of a vein to confirm patency. Partial collapse of the vein suggests the presence of nonoccluding thrombus. In this situation, the adjacent artery may be seen to deform as the probe pressure is increased to confirm partial obstruction in the vein.

A   B

Figure 13.3   A: A transverse image of the right common femoral vein (CFV) and femoral artery (CFA). B: Patency of the CFV is demonstrated by complete collapse of the vein (arrow) during transducer pressure.

Transducer compression should be applied in the transverse imaging plane rather than the longitudinal plane. This is because it is easy to slip to one side of the vein as pressure is applied in the longitudinal plane, and this may mimic compression of the vein when observed on the B-mode image. Unfortunately, in some areas the veins lie too deep for compression to be used, such as in the pelvis and sometimes at the adductor canal or calf. Color flow imaging is useful for demonstrating patency in this situation.

The following guidelines can be used in any sequence, depending upon the areas that require assessing. It is sometimes easier to locate a specific vein by looking for the adjacent artery, especially in the calf. The reader should also refer to Chapter 9 for more details on the probe positions for imaging the calf vessels and the main vessels in the thigh and pelvis.

1. Starting at the level of the groin, the common femoral vein is imaged in transverse section and will be seen to lie medial to the common femoral artery (Figs 13.3A and 9.6). The common femoral vein should be compressed to

A   B

Figure 13.4   A: Transverse image of the calf demonstrating the posterior tibial (PT) veins (V) and arteries (A) and peroneal (PER) veins (V) and arteries (A). B: There is complete collapse of the veins with transducer compression, but the arteries are still visible. Note that it can sometimes be very difficult to differentiate the image of the veins from the surrounding tissue.

demonstrate patency and is followed distally beyond the saphenofemoral junction, to the junction of the superficial femoral vein and profunda femoris vein. The proximal segment of the profunda femoris vein should also be assessed for patency if possible. With the transducer turned into the longitudinal plane, the flow pattern in the common femoral vein should be assessed with color flow imaging and spectral Doppler. Flow should appear spontaneous and phasic at this level if there is no outflow obstruction. A calf squeeze can provide evidence of good flow augmentation in the proximal superficial femoral vein, which is a useful indirect indicator of probable superficial femoral and popliteal vein patency. Alternatively, strong foot flexion will also normally augment flow.

2. The superficial femoral vein is then followed in transverse section along the medial aspect of the thigh to the knee, using compression to confirm patency. The vein normally lies deep to the superficial femoral artery. In the adductor canal the vein may be difficult to compress. It is sometimes helpful to place a hand behind the back of the lower thigh and push the flesh toward the transducer, which will bring the vein and artery more superficial to the transducer. Color flow imaging can also be used to confirm patency in this segment, but areas of nonoccluding thrombus could be missed. Remember that duplication of the superficial femoral vein is relatively common, and both trunks should be examined.

3. The popliteal vein is examined by scanning the popliteal fossa in a transverse plane. Starting in the middle of the popliteal fossa, the vein is followed proximally as far as possible to overlap the area scanned from the medial lower thigh. The popliteal vein will be seen lying above the popliteal artery when imaged from the popliteal fossa. The below-knee popliteal vein and gastrocnemius branches are then examined in the transverse plane. The popliteal vein can also be duplicated.

4. The calf veins are often easier to identify distally. They are then followed proximally to the top of the calf. The posterior tibial and peroneal veins can be imaged in a transverse plane from the medial aspect of the calf (Fig. 13.4A). From this imaging plane the peroneal veins will lie

Figure 13.5 Color flow imaging from the medial calf demonstrates patency of the posterior tibial veins (PTV), which are seen lying on either side of the posterior tibial artery (PTA). Color filling is seen to the vein walls. The peroneal veins (PER V) and artery (PER A) are seen lying deep to the posterior tibial vessels. The peroneal vessels may not always be seen in the same scan plane.

deep to the posterior tibial veins. It can sometimes be difficult to compress the peroneal veins from this position. Color flow imaging in the longitudinal plane may be useful for demonstrating patency (Fig. 13.5). The peroneal veins can frequently be examined from the posterolateral aspect of the calf (Fig. 9.11). The common trunks of the posterior tibial and peroneal veins can also be very difficult to image, and medial and posterolateral transducer positions may be needed to examine this region at the top of the calf.

5. Examination of the anterior tibial veins is often not requested, as isolated thrombosis of these veins is rare (Mattos et al 1996). However, assessment of the anterior tibial veins is usually easier with color flow imaging, in the longitudinal plane, as the veins are small and frequently difficult to identify with B-mode imaging.

6. When requested, the examination of the calf is completed with an assessment of the soleal veins

Figure 13.6 A transverse B-mode image of the posterior aspect of the mid upper calf to demonstrate the position of the soleus muscle (SM) and a soleal vein (SV). The gastrocnemius muscle (GM) lies above the soleus muscle and is separated by a band of echogenic muscular fascia (MF). A gastrocnemius vein (GV) is seen within the muscle. The short saphenous vein (SSV) is also visible in the superficial compartment lying above the muscular fascia (F).

Figure 13.7 A: A transverse image of the common femoral vein (V) and common femoral artery (A). The common femoral vein appears distended and contains some low-level echoes. B: The common femoral vein is seen to deform but not collapse during firm transducer pressure, confirming DVT.

and sinuses located in the soleus muscle. These veins are imaged from the posterior calf (Fig. 13.6). In practice, they can be very difficult to identify, especially in the normal subject.

7. The iliac veins are examined with the patient lying supine, as the iliac veins lie behind the bowel. The iliac veins lie slightly deeper and medial to the iliac arteries. Compression of these veins is not possible, and patency should be confirmed using color flow imaging. In addition, spectral Doppler can be used to examine flow patterns with flow augmentation maneuvers. The main limitation of examining this area is incomplete visualization due to overlying bowel gas and the potential to miss partially occluding thrombus.

8. In some cases the vena cava may need to be examined. This vessel lies to the right of the aorta when imaged in transverse section (see Fig. 11.2). Color flow imaging can be used in the transverse plane to look for filling defects, but some transverse tilt may have to be applied to the transducer to produce a reasonable Doppler angle. Flow should also be assessed in longitudinal section with color flow and spectral Doppler ultrasound. Examination of this area should be undertaken by a sonographer with a

considerable degree of experience. Other imaging modalities are generally preferable.

SCAN APPEARANCES FOR THE ASSESSMENT OF ACUTE DVT

B-mode images

Normal appearance

The vein should appear clear and contain no echoes. In practice, there are often speckle and reverberation artifacts in the image, but the experienced sonographer should have little difficulty in identifying these. Smaller veins can be difficult to distinguish from tissue planes. It is sometimes possible to image static or slowly moving blood as a speckle pattern within the lumen, owing to aggregation of blood cells, but the vein should collapse under transducer pressure (Figs 13.3 and 13.4). The deep calf veins can sometimes be difficult to identify without the help of color flow imaging. The common femoral vein should normally distend with a Valsalva maneuver if the venous outflow through the iliac veins is patent.

Abnormal appearance

In the presence of thrombus the vein will not compress (Fig. 13.7). In the very early stages of thrombosis, the clot often has a degree of echogenicity due to the aggregation of red blood cells in the thrombus. Within 1 or 2 days, the clot becomes more anechoic, owing to changes occurring in the

Figure 13.8 A transverse B-mode image of a peroneal vein thrombosis (arrow). The image is taken from the posterolateral aspect of the calf. One trunk of the vein is grossly dilated, whereas the other is difficult to distinguish on the image. The veins are lying adjacent to the fibula (F).

Figure 13.9 The proximal end of a free-floating thrombus (arrow) is seen in the superficial femoral vein. The thrombus is relatively anechoic and the thrombus tip is touching a valve cusp (curved arrow).

thrombus, and it can be difficult to define on the B-mode image. However, in practice, with advanced transducer technology, it is often possible to see subtle echoes. If the vein is totally occluded in the acute phase, it may appear distended (Fig. 13.8). The thrombus can be free-floating, with large areas being non-adherent to the vein wall. It is usually possible to identify the upper limit of the thrombosis, and the thrombus tip often demonstrates slightly increased echogenicity (Fig. 13.9). The tip is much easier to identify if it extends to the popliteal or femoral veins. Prudence should be exercised with transducer compression if free-floating thrombus is present, to avoid dislodging the thrombus. Smaller areas of nonocclusive thrombus may not cause the vein to distend, but they can be demonstrated by incomplete collapse of the vein during compression. Older thrombus, beyond two weeks in age, becomes more echogenic.

Color flow images

Normal appearance

Spontaneous phasic flow is usually seen in the larger proximal veins. There should be complete color filling of the lumen in both longitudinal and transverse planes during a calf squeeze. Color aliasing is sometimes observed if the distal augmentation causes a significant transient increase in venous flow. If it is difficult to squeeze the calf, owing to size or tenderness, it can be possible to augment flow by asking the patient to flex the ankle backward and forward, activating the calf muscle pump. The posterior tibial veins and peroneal veins are usually paired, which should be clearly demonstrated on the color flow image (Fig. 13.5). However, anatomical variations can occur. Color flow imaging of the gastrocnemius and soleal veins can be difficult, as blood flow velocities following augmentation can be low, especially if a degree of venous stasis is present.

Abnormal appearance

There is an absence of color filling in occluded veins, even with distal augmentation. Collateral veins may also be seen in the region of the occluded vein. The color flow pattern around free-floating thrombus is very characteristic, with flow seen between the thrombus and vein wall. This can be demonstrated in both longitudinal and transverse sections. Color flow imaging can be useful for demonstrating the position of the proximal thrombus tip as full color filling of the lumen will be seen just proximal to the

Figure 13.10   A color flow image of Figure 13.9. Flow is seen between the thrombus and vein wall (arrows). The superficial femoral artery (A) is lying superficial to the vein.

Figure 13.11   The Doppler waveform in the femoral vein distal to an iliac vein occlusion often demonstrates continuous low-velocity flow with a loss of phasicity.

tip (Fig. 13.10). Smaller areas of nonoccluding thrombus will be demonstrated as flow voids within the lumen. However, some care should be used in interpreting partially occluding thrombosis on the basis of color flow imaging alone, and probe compression should be used for confirmation if possible.

Spectral Doppler

Normal appearance

Spectral Doppler is the least used modality in the assessment of venous thrombosis and should not be used as the only method of investigation. However, patent veins should demonstrate normal venous flow patterns. In our experience, it should be possible to augment flow velocity in the main trunks by at least 100% with a squeeze distal to the point of measurement. For example, there should be augmentation of flow in the superficial femoral vein with a distal calf squeeze (see Ch. 12); however, this may not exclude small areas of nonoccluding thrombus. The Doppler signal at the level of the common femoral vein should exhibit a spontaneous phasic flow pattern, which temporarily ceases when the patient takes a deep inspiration or performs a Valsalva maneuver. This would suggest that there is no outflow obstruction through the

iliac veins to the vena cava. However, the presence of small amounts of nonoccluding thrombus cannot be excluded on the basis of spectral Doppler alone.

Abnormal appearance

There is an absence of a spectral Doppler signal when the vein is completely occluded. When the vein contains a significant amount of partially occluding or free-floating thrombus, there is normally a reduced flow pattern, which demonstrates little or no augmentation following distal compression. However, there are potential pitfalls when using this criterion, as there may be good collateral circulation between the point of distal calf compression and the position of the probe. An occlusive thrombosis in the iliac vein system usually results in a low-volume continuous flow pattern in the common femoral vein, with little or no response to a Valsalva maneuver (Fig. 13.11).

Diagnostic problems

The investigation of DVT can be very difficult, and it is important to use a logical protocol when performing the examination. There can be considerable variation in the anatomy of the venous system, as outlined in Chapter 12. Duplication of the superficial femoral vein and popliteal vein is not uncommon. A study by Gordon et al (1996) reported duplication of the superficial femoral vein in 25% of healthy volunteers. This could lead to potential diagnostic errors if one half of the system is occluded and the other is patent, as it is possible to miss the occluded system during the examination. Careful scrutiny of the transverse sectional image should demonstrate any bifid vein systems. The sonographer should also be highly suspicious of veins that appear small in caliber or that are located in abnormal positions with respect to their corresponding arteries. Another potentially difficult situation occurs when there is a large deep femoral vein running between the popliteal vein and profunda femoris vein, as the superficial femoral vein may be unusually small. Both the superficial femoral vein and the deeper vein should be carefully examined for defects. In addition, it is possible to misidentify veins in the deep venous system and even confuse them with superficial veins. This occurs most commonly in the popliteal fossa and upper calf. The gastrocnemius vein can be mistaken for the popliteal vein or for the short saphenous vein. It is important to be able to identify the fascial layer that separates the superficial and deep venous systems to avoid this type of error (see Figs 12.1 and 12.2).

Investigation of the iliac veins can be extremely difficult, especially in situations in which the vein may be under compression by structures in the pelvis, or by tumors, as this can be misinterpreted as a partially occluding thrombus. Compression of the iliac vein can also occur during pregnancy and is observed more frequently on the left side. This may lead to unilateral limb swelling and a reduction in the normal venous flow pattern in the femoral vein.

ACCURACY OF DUPLEX SCANNING FOR THE DETECTION OF DVT

Many studies have been performed to compare the accuracy of duplex scanning with venography. The results of these studies are variable. Baxter et al (1992) reported 100% sensitivity and specificity for the femoropopliteal veins and 95% specificity and 100% sensitivity for calf veins. Miller et al (1996) achieved sensitivities and specificities of 98.7% and 100%, respectively, at above-knee level, and corresponding values of 85.2% and 99.2% at below-knee level. In contrast, a study by Jongbloets et al (1994) that involved the screening

of asymptomatic postoperative patients at high risk of developing DVT demonstrated sensitivities as low as 38% and 50% for thigh and calf veins, respectively.

These variable results may reflect factors such as patient population, operator experience or equipment availability. To implement a high-quality service, it is essential that staff are properly trained and a patient management protocol defined. In-house comparisons, or audit of ultrasound against other imaging techniques and outcomes, should also be performed to ensure the accuracy of the service.

NATURAL HISTORY OF DVT

The natural history of a DVT is variable and is dependent on the position and extent of the thrombi (O'Shaughnessy & Fitzgerald 2001). In addition, the patient's age and physical condition will have a significant bearing on the final outcome. The thrombus can:

- spontaneously lyse
- propagate or embolize
- recanalize over time
- permanently occlude the vein.

Complete lysis of smaller thrombi can occur over a relatively short period of time due to fibrinolytic activity. Full recanalization of the vein will be seen, and the lumen will appear normal on the ultrasound image. Valve function can be preserved in these circumstances. If there is a large thrombus load, the process of recanalization can take several weeks. The thrombus becomes more echogenic over time as it becomes organized (Fig. 13.12A). The vein frequently diminishes in size due to retraction of the thrombus. As the process of recanalization begins, the developing venous flow channel within the vein lumen may be tortuous due to irregularity of lysis in the thrombus. It is even possible to see multiple flow channels within the vessel. In cases of partial recanalization, old residual thrombus can be seen along the vein wall, producing a scarred appearance (Fig. 13.12B). It is sometimes possible to see fibrosed valve cusps, which appear immobile and echogenic on the B-mode image. Deep venous insufficiency is frequently the long-term outcome of slow or partial recanalization.

Figure 13.12 Two longitudinal B-mode images of the superficial femoral vein showing different stages of organization. A: The thrombus in this image is over 10 days old and has become echogenic. Areas of lysis (arrows) are seen within the thrombus. B: Partial recanalization of the vein is demonstrated with old thrombus (T), which appears fibrosed and attached to the anterior wall.

If the vein remains permanently occluded, the thrombus becomes echogenic due to fibrosis. The thrombus retracts over time, leading to shrinkage of the vein. It may even appear as a small cord adjacent to its corresponding artery, and in some cases the vein is difficult to differentiate from surrounding tissue planes. Color flow imaging frequently demonstrates the development of collateral veins in the region of the occlusion. In the case of chronic common femoral and iliac vein occlusion, visible distended superficial veins, which act as collateral pathways, are often seen across the pelvis and lower abdominal wall. The long saphenous vein can act as a collateral pathway in the presence of a superficial femoral or popliteal vein occlusion. High-volume continuous flow recorded in the long saphenous vein should always be treated with suspicion (see Fig. 12.9).

There is considerable debate about the accuracy of duplex scanning for determining the age of thrombus, but it is generally accepted that it is possible to differentiate the acute phase, within the first week or two, from the subacute and chronic phases of venous thrombosis. However, there is much less certainty about differentiating subacute and chronic thrombus. This is due to the fact that the process of formation may not have been synchronous, and there are also irregularities in the process of lysis and fibrosis within the thrombus, producing a heterogeneous appearance. Many sonographers will not use the term 'subacute' in their reporting terminology because of this problem.

Recurrent thrombosis

Recurrent thrombotic events are common after acute DVT (Meissner et al 1995). There are considerable diagnostic problems in attempting to detect fresh thrombus in a vein that has been damaged by a prior DVT. If the patient has had a previous scan or venogram, it is possible to check the extent of the thrombosis on the last report and compare it with the current scan. However, old reports may not be available, or the patient may not have had any previous investigations. In these situations, the vein should be examined carefully with B-mode and color flow imaging to look for areas of fresh thrombus. These will appear as anechoic areas on the B-mode image, and color flow imaging will demonstrate filling defects. In practice, this can be an extremely difficult examination to undertake. If there is a high degree of suspicion, a repeat scan can be performed a couple of days later to look for changes in the appearance of the vein or possible extension of thrombus.

OTHER PATHOLOGIC CONDITIONS THAT CAN MIMIC DVT

There are a number of pathologic conditions that produce symptoms similar to DVT, and the sonographer should be able to identify these disorders.

Figure 13.13 A transverse image of the long saphenous vein demonstrates evidence of thrombophlebitis. The vein is distended and contains thrombus (arrow).

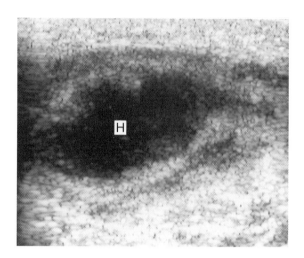

Figure 13.14 An area of hematoma (H) is seen in the calf muscle following injury. Hematomas can be mistaken for DVT.

Thrombophlebitis

Thrombophlebitis occurs due to inflammation of the superficial veins, with thrombus forming in the long saphenous vein or short saphenous vein system (Fig. 13.13). It can be felt as a hard cord in the superficial tissues, often associated with localized heat, pain and tenderness. Superficial thrombosis is generally not a serious condition compared with DVT. However, there are occasions when the thrombus tip extends along the proximal long saphenous vein and protrudes through the saphenofemoral junction into the common femoral vein. This situation can also occur in the short saphenous vein, with propagation across the saphenopopliteal junction. There is a reported risk of proximal embolization from the thrombus tip, and care should be used when examining any thrombus in this position (Blumenberg et al 1998). It is essential to report this type of presentation as soon as possible, as surgical intervention is sometimes required to remove the thrombus.

Hematoma

Hematomas are accumulations of blood within the tissues that can clot to form a solid swelling. They can be caused by external trauma, or other mechanisms such as muscle tears, can be extremely painful and can lead to limb swelling, especially in the calf. Blood in the hematoma may also track extensively along the fascial planes. The sonographic appearance of a hematoma is of a reasonably well defined anechoic area in the soft tissues or muscles (Fig. 13.14). Hematomas can be very variable in size and shape. It is sometimes impossible to image the veins in the immediate vicinity, owing to the size of the hematoma or the pain the patient experiences. The hematoma may also compress the deep veins in the local vicinity.

Lymphedema

Lymphedema is observed as chronic limb swelling due to reduced efficiency or failure of the lymphatic drainage system. This may be due to a primary abnormality of the lymphatic system or to secondary causes that lead to damage of the lymph nodes and drainage system in the groin. These include damage following surgery, trauma, malignancy and radiotherapy in the groin region. Lymphedema is usually most prominent in the calf but can extend throughout the leg, and two thirds of cases are unilateral. Other sites can be affected by lymphedema, including the arms. The B-mode appearance of lymphedema demonstrates the subcutaneous layer to be thickened, and a fine B-mode speckle is observed in this region, making the image appear grainy (Fig. 13.15). The ultrasound image of lymphedema is usually different from that caused by simple fluid edema. Ultrasound can be used to confirm the patency of the deep veins, but unfortunately

Figure 13.15 Lymphedema produces a grainy appearance in the subcutaneous tissues, as demonstrated on this transverse B-mode image. The superficial tissue is relatively thick. The muscular fascia is demonstrated by the arrow. Note the degraded image quality, typical of this disorder.

Figure 13.16 Fluid edema is demonstrated in the subcutaneous tissues as numerous anechoic channels (arrows) splaying the tissue.

Figure 13.17 The venous flow signals recorded from the common femoral vein of a patient with congestive cardiac failure demonstrate a pulsatile flow pattern.

the presence of lymphedema degrades the ultrasound image, making many deep vein scans technically challenging.

Cellulitis

Cellulitis is caused by infection of the subcutaneous tissues and skin; it produces diffuse swelling in the lower limb, often associated with pain, tenderness and redness. There is usually evidence of edema in the region of swelling. A duplex examination can confirm patency of the deep veins. In addition, there may be hyperemic flow in the veins and arteries of the limb due to the infection.

Edema

Patients can develop edema in the calf due to infection, leg ulceration, local trauma, or as a result of significant venous insufficiency. This is characterized as fluid or edema in the superficial tissues. The ultrasound appearance of edema demonstrates tissue splaying by numerous interstitial channels (Fig. 13.16). Patients with congestive heart failure often develop edema in the legs due to the increased pressure in the venous system and the right side of the heart. Another characteristic of congestive heart failure is the pulsatile flow pattern that is often observed in the proximal deep veins, which can be

mistaken for arterial flow (Fig. 13.17). Careful attention to the color display will confirm the direction of flow.

Baker's cysts

Baker's cysts are bursal dilations that normally originate on the medial side of the knee between the medial head of the gastrocnemius muscle and semimembranosus tendons. A bursa is essentially a small sac of synovial fluid that prevents friction between a bone joint or tendon. The bursa can extend out of this region and into the tissue planes in the upper calf, causing swelling, pain and discomfort. Such bursae are caused by a number of conditions, including arthritis and trauma to the knee. Baker's cysts can rupture, causing severe pain and symptoms similar to those of acute vein thrombosis. Large Baker's cysts can compress the popliteal vein or deep veins of the popliteal fossa, causing a DVT. It is always necessary to identify and confirm

Figure 13.18 A Baker's cyst (BC) is demonstrated in this transverse image of the popliteal fossa. The popliteal artery (A) and vein (V) are also seen in the image.

Figure 13.19 An enlarged lymph node (arrow) is demonstrated in this transverse image at the top of the groin. Flow is demonstrated in the lymph node. The common femoral artery (A) and vein (V) are seen below the node.

the patency of the deep veins in the popliteal fossa, even when a Baker's cyst has been diagnosed, as the Baker's cyst may be an incidental finding secondary to venous thrombosis. Baker's cysts can also be misdiagnosed as popliteal aneurysms.

Baker's cysts are easiest to define in a transverse scan plane from the popliteal fossa. They are normally anechoic due to the fluid in the cyst, but some may contain debris and osteocartilaginous fragments, which are echogenic. Many Baker's cysts have a typical oval or crescent shape, with the tail trailing away from the main bulk of the cyst to the joint space (Fig. 13.18). If the cyst is excessively large, it may distort the anatomy in the popliteal fossa. It is difficult to define a ruptured Baker's cyst with ultrasound.

Enlarged lymph nodes

Enlargement of the lymph nodes can cause limb swelling due to reduction in lymphatic drainage. Enlargement occurs as a result of pathologic conditions, including infection or malignancy. The main sites for enlargement are at the groin or axilla, and the nodes can become so large that they compress the adjacent vein. Enlarged nodes may be tender, and localized redness and heat (erythema) may be present. They can also be clinically misdiagnosed as femoral artery aneurysms if the pulsation of the

artery is amplified to the skin surface by the enlarged node.

Enlarged lymph nodes are imaged as oval or spherical masses that are found in groups (Fig. 13.19). They are mainly hypoechoic in appearance but may contain stronger echoes within the center of the node and can be mistaken for a thrombosed vein. Color flow Doppler usually demonstrates blood flow in larger nodes, especially if infection is present.

Other pathologic lesions

Other pathologic conditions that can clinically mimic DVT are abscesses, arteriovenous fistulas, muscle tears and hyperperfusion syndrome following arterial bypass surgery for lower limb ischemia.

UPPER LIMB VEINS
Anatomy of the deep upper limb veins

The upper limb veins can also be divided into the deep and superficial veins (Fig. 13.20), and there are a number of anatomical variations. Usually, paired veins are associated with the radial and ulnar arteries. They normally join at the elbow to form the brachial vein but can run separately to form the brachial vein higher in the upper arm. The brachial

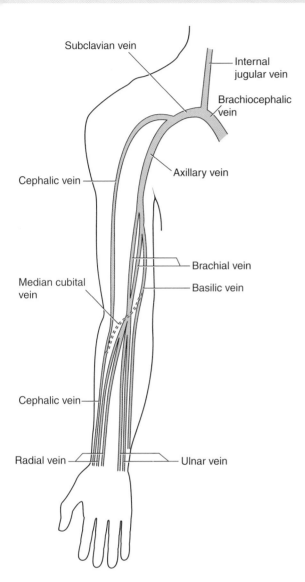

Figure 13.20   The venous anatomy of the arm.

vein is usually paired and associated with the brachial artery. At the top of the arm, the brachial vein becomes the axillary vein, which is usually a single trunk. The axillary vein becomes the subclavian vein as it crosses the border of the first rib. The subclavian vein enters the thoracic outlet but runs separately from the artery in front of the anterior scalene muscle. The internal jugular vein, from the neck, joins the proximal subclavian vein, which then drains via the brachiocephalic vein to the superior vena cava. The left brachiocephalic vein is longer than the right brachiocephalic vein. It is very difficult to image the brachiocephalic veins clearly with ultrasound.

Anatomy of the superficial upper limb veins

The cephalic vein and the basilic vein are the two major superficial veins in the arms (Fig. 13.20). The cephalic vein drains the dorsal surface of the hand and runs up the lateral aspect of the forearm to the antecubital fossa at the elbow and then continues in a subcutaneous path along the lateral aspect of the biceps muscle. Toward the shoulder, it runs in the deltopectoral groove between the deltoid and pectoralis muscles and then pierces the clavipectoral fascia to join the axillary vein in the infraclavicular region. The basilic vein drains blood from the palm and ventral aspects of the hand and runs along the medial side of the forearm to the medial aspect of the antecubital fossa. The basilic vein then penetrates the fascia in the lower aspect of the upper arm to join the brachial vein. However, its origin can be variable, and sometimes the basilic vein may run directly into the distal axillary vein.

Thrombosis of the upper limbs

DVT is the main pathology that affects the upper limb venous system. The subclavian and axillary veins are the commonest sites for thrombosis. This can lead to upper limb swelling with distension of the superficial veins. The causes of upper limb thrombosis are similar to many of those that lead to lower limb DVT. In addition, long-term catheter access for feeding and drug administration can damage the axillary and subclavian veins. Venous thoracic outlet syndrome can also cause thrombosis of the subclavian vein. Effort-induced thrombosis of the subclavian vein, referred to as Paget-Schroetter syndrome, is associated with strenuous upper body exercise or repetitive movements and is often seen in younger patients.

The appearance of thrombosis in the upper extremities is similar to that seen in the lower extremities. A combination of compression, color flow imaging and spectral Doppler is required to confirm patency, as it is sometimes difficult to apply satisfactory probe compression, particularly in the supraclavicular fossa. However, duplex scanning provides good results when compared to contrast venography in areas where compression can be applied, but caution should be used when attempting to diagnose DVT on the basis of Doppler flow patterns (Baarslag et al 2002). Upper limb swelling can also be caused by lymphedema, following mastectomy with removal of lymph nodes in the axilla and the effects of radiotherapy.

TECHNIQUE FOR ASSESSING THE BRACHIAL, AXILLARY AND SUBCLAVIAN VEINS

The patient should lie supine so that the subclavian and axillary veins are distended. The scan normally takes 10–15 min for each arm. Remember, it can be useful to compare the scan appearance from both sides in cases of suspected unilateral thrombosis. It should also be noted that the color flow image of the proximal subclavian vein can look rather confusing and 'cluttered' because of the proximity of other vessels and the often pulsatile appearance superimposed on the venous flow pattern, due to atrial contractions.

1. The arm should be abducted and placed on a comfortable support. It is easier to start the examination distally in the brachial vein, which will be seen lying adjacent to the brachial artery in the upper arm.
2. The brachial vein is imaged in transverse section and should be compressible with relatively light transducer pressure. Color and spectral Doppler recordings should demonstrate flow augmentation with manual compression of the forearm.
3. The axillary vein can be imaged by using a combination of transaxillary and infraclavicular transducer positions (see Ch. 10). The vein will be seen lying adjacent to the artery, but color flow imaging can aid identification, particularly if B-mode imaging is poor. A combination of compression and color flow imaging may be needed to confirm patency in this region. The cephalic vein may act as a collateral pathway to the subclavian vein in the presence of a distal axillary vein thrombosis.
4. The distal end of the subclavian vein is initially imaged from the infraclavicular fossa in transverse section, where it will be seen lying inferior to the subclavian artery. The midsubclavian vein is imaged from the supraclavicular fossa. A large acoustic shadow will be seen as the subclavian vein runs under the clavicle. Compression of the subclavian vein is extremely difficult, owing to the contour of the neck and the presence of the clavicle, and color flow imaging in transverse and longitudinal planes is used to confirm patency. In addition, spectral Doppler should demonstrate spontaneous phasic flow with respiration if there is no outflow obstruction. It is also usual to observe a pulsatile flow pattern superimposed on the phasic flow pattern due to atrial contractions of the heart (see Ch. 5). It should be noted that it is extremely easy to miss a proximal thrombosis in the subclavian vein, owing to poor visualization of this area, especially if it is a partially occluding thrombus. It is possible to image indwelling catheters, such as Hickman lines, in the subclavian vein. Always state any limitations or doubts about the scan in this region, as other imaging tests, such as venography, may be required.
5. Two breathing maneuvers can be used for assessing flow in the subclavian vein. The first is a Valsalva maneuver, in which there should be cessation of flow or flow reversal during Valsalva. This is followed by an enhancement in flow toward the heart during expiration. The second involves multiple sniffing through the nose. During continued sniffing the subclavian vein will be seen to contract. Neither of these maneuvers can exclude DVT, as there may be nonoccluding thrombus present. However, if an abnormal flow pattern or response is recorded, it may indicate a potential abnormality.
6. Occasionally, a thrombosis may involve the internal jugular vein in the neck. This can be imaged in cross section.
7. It is usually impossible to image the brachiocephalic veins, but a thrombosis may be indirectly suggested if there is an abnormality in the subclavian and axillary vein flow patterns.

Other upper limb venous disorders

Phlebitis of the superficial veins can occur due to repeated catheter access or intravenous drug abuse. Arteriovenous malformations are sometimes found in the arms and hands, and in some cases can be very extensive, leading to upper limb swelling.

REPORTING

The report should indicate the scan to be normal or abnormal, and, if it is abnormal, the level and extent of the thrombosis should be stated. The report should also clearly specify which veins were examined and which were omitted due to technical limitations. This avoids any confusion or assumption that veins not mentioned on the report are normal. Other pathologic conditions that may mimic the symptoms of DVT should also be reported. The report of a positive DVT should be brought to the attention of the appropriate medical staff as soon as possible, in order that the appropriate management can be implemented.

References

Aschwanden M, Labs K H, Jeanneret C, et al 1999 The value of rapid D-dimer testing combined with structured clinical evaluation for the diagnosis of deep vein thrombosis. Journal of Vascular Surgery 30(5):929–935

Baarslag H J, Van Beek E J, Koopman M M, et al 2002 Prospective study of color duplex ultrasonography compared with contrast venography in patients suspected of having deep venous thrombosis of the upper extremities. Annals of Internal Medicine 136(12):865–872

Baxter G M, Duffy P, Partridge E 1992 Color flow imaging of calf vein thrombosis. Clinical Radiology 46(3):198–201

Bjorgell O, Nilsson P E, Jarenros H 2000 Isolated nonfilling of contrast in deep leg vein segments seen on phlebography, and a comparison with color Doppler ultrasound, to assess the incidence of deep leg vein thrombosis. Angiology 51(6):451–461

Blumenberg R M, Barton E, Gelfand M L, et al 1998 Occult deep venous thrombosis complicating superficial thrombophlebitis. Journal of Vascular Surgery 27(2):338–343

Bradley M, Bladon J, Barker H 2000 D-dimer assay for deep vein thrombosis: its role with color Doppler sonography. Clinical Radiology 55(7):525–527

Cogo A, Lensing A W, Koopman M M, et al 1998 Compression ultrasonography for diagnostic management of patients with clinically suspected deep vein thrombosis: prospective cohort study. British Medical Journal 316:17–20

Cranley J J, Canos A J, Sull W J 1976 The diagnosis of deep vein thrombosis: fallibility of clinical symptoms and signs. Archives of Surgery 111(1):34–36

Fowkes F G, Evans C J, Lee A J 2001 Prevalence and risk factors of chronic venous insufficiency. Angiology Suppl 1:S5–S15

Fowkes F J, Price J F, Fowkes F G 2003 Incidence of diagnosed deep vein thrombosis in the general population: systematic review. European Journal of Vascular and Endovascular Surgery 25(1):1–5

Gordon A C, Wright I, Pugh N D 1996 Duplication of the superficial femoral vein: recognition with duplex ultrasonography. Clinical Radiology 51(9):622–624

Haenen J H, Janssen M C, Wollersheim H, et al 2002 The development of postthrombotic syndrome in relationship to venous reflux and calf muscle pump dysfunction at 2 years after the onset of deep venous thrombosis. Journal of Vascular Surgery 35(6):1184–1189

Jongbloets L M, Lensing A W, Koopman M M, et al 1994 Limitations of compression ultrasound for the detection of symptomless postoperative deep vein thrombosis. Lancet 343:1142–1144

Khaw K 2002 The diagnosis of deep vein thrombosis. In: Beard J D, Murray S (eds) Pathways of care in vascular surgery. TFM publishing, Shrewsbury, p 161–169

Labropoulos N, Kang S S, Mansour M A, et al 2002 Early thrombus remodelling of isolated calf deep vein thrombosis. European Journal of Vascular and Endovascular Surgery 23(4):344–348

Lohr J M, Kerr T M, Lutter K S, et al 1991 Lower extremity calf thrombosis: to treat or not to treat? Journal of Vascular Surgery 14(5):618–623

Mattos M A, Melendres G, Sumner D S, et al 1996 Prevalence and distribution of calf vein thrombosis in patients with symptomatic deep venous thrombosis: a color-flow duplex study. Journal of Vascular Surgery 24(5):738–744

Meissner M H, Caps M T, Bergelin R O, et al 1995 Propagation, rethrombosis and new thrombus formation after acute deep vein thrombosis. Journal of Vascular Surgery 22(5):558–567

Meissner M H, Caps M T, Bergelin R O, et al 1997 Early outcome after isolated deep vein thrombosis. Journal of Vascular Surgery 26(5):749–756

Miller N, Satin R, Tousignant L, et al 1996 A prospective study comparing duplex scan and venography for the diagnosis of lower-extremity deep vein thrombosis. Cardiovascular Surgery 4(4):505–508

Nicolaides A N, Belcaro G, Bergqvist D, et al 1994 Prevention of thromboembolism: European consensus statement. In: Bergvist D, Comerota A J, Nicolaides A N, Scurr J H (eds) Prevention of venous thromboembolism. Med-orion, London, pp 445–446

O'Shaughnessy A M, Fitzgerald D E 2001 The patterns and distribution of residual abnormalities between the individual proximal venous segments after an acute deep vein thrombosis. Journal of Vascular Surgery 33(2):379–384

White R H 2003 The epidemiology of venous thromboembolism. Circulation 107(23 Suppl 1):I4–I8

Chapter **14**

Graft surveillance and preoperative vein mapping for bypass surgery

CHAPTER CONTENTS

Introduction 208
Anatomy 208
  Vein grafts 208
  Synthetic grafts 209
Purpose of graft surveillance 209
  Vein grafts 209
  Synthetic grafts 210
Symptoms and treatment of graft stenosis or
  failure 210
Practical considerations for scanning bypass
  grafts 211
Scanning techniques 211
  In situ vein graft 211
  Reversed vein grafts 213
  Synthetic grafts 213
B-mode images 213
  Normal appearance 213
  Abnormal appearance 214
Color Doppler images 214
  Normal appearance of vein grafts 214
  Normal appearance of synthetic grafts 215
  Abnormal appearance of vein grafts 215
Spectral Doppler waveforms 215
  Normal appearance 215
  Abnormal appearance 216
Graft failure and occlusion 217
Commonly encountered problems 218
True and false aneurysms 218
Entrapments of grafts 219
Arteriovenous fistulas 219

Seromas, fluid collections and graft
  infections 220
Reporting 220
Superficial vein mapping for arterial bypass
  surgery 221
  Technique for assessing the long saphenous
    vein 221
  Arm vein mapping 222
  Technique of marking the vein 222
  Problems encountered during vein
    mapping 223

INTRODUCTION

Patients with significant lower limb ischemia or threatened limb loss usually require arterial bypass surgery if no other option is available to improve blood flow in the leg. Vascular surgeons are able to perform an extensive range of arterial bypass procedures to restore circulation to the extremities. Bypass grafts can be made of synthetic materials, such as polytetrafluoroethylene (PTFE), or constructed from native vein, which can be assessed and marked preoperatively as described at the end of this chapter. Failure of a bypass graft due to the development of a graft stenosis is a serious complication that can result in amputation if it is not possible to unblock the graft. It is therefore common practice for vascular laboratories to perform regular graft surveillance scans to detect the development of graft defects. The majority of surveillance scans are performed for native vein bypass grafts below the groin (infrainguinal grafts). The surveillance of synthetic grafts is still widely practiced, but there is evidence to suggest that the benefits are less clear-cut (Lundell et al 1995). Ultrasound can also be used to image areas of potential infection following graft surgery, to see if the region of infection is in contact with the graft. The emphasis of this chapter will be on infrainguinal vein graft surveillance.

ANATOMY

The routes of grafts vary considerably and depend on the level and extent of the native arterial disease that has been bypassed. Synthetic grafts are mainly used to bypass inflow disease, whereas vein grafts are frequently used for distal procedures below the inguinal ligament. The different types of graft frequently encountered in the graft surveillance clinic are shown in Figure 14.1.

Vein grafts

Whenever possible, native vein is used for femoral distal bypass surgery, as it offers good long-term patency rates. The long saphenous vein is the vein of choice for infrainguinal bypass surgery, although an arm vein and the short saphenous vein can also be used if the long saphenous vein is unsuitable in part or all of its length. Vein grafts composed of

Figure 14.1 Examples of bypass grafts. A: Above-knee femoropopliteal graft. B: Femoro-posterior tibial artery graft. C: Aortobifemoral graft. D: Iliofemoral cross-over graft. E: Superficial femoral artery to peroneal artery graft. F: Popliteal artery bypass graft for a thrombosed popliteal aneurysm.

more than one segment of vein are known as composite vein grafts. Femoral distal bypass surgery is performed using two common types of surgical procedure.

The first is the in situ technique, in which the long saphenous vein is exposed but left in its native position and side branches ligated to prevent blood shunting from the graft to the venous system. As the vein contains valves which would prevent blood flow toward the foot, they have to be removed or disrupted using a device called a valvulotome. The main body of an in situ vein graft lies superficially along the medial aspect of the thigh. The proximal

Figure 14.2 An example of a composite PTFE and vein graft.

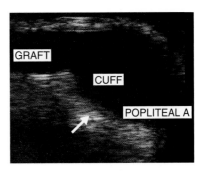

Figure 14.3 A vein cuff (arrow) at the distal anastomosis between a PTFE graft and popliteal artery.

anastomosis of a femoral distal graft is frequently located at the common femoral artery, although the position can vary. The position of the distal anastomosis is variable and depends on the distal extent of the native arterial disease. The distal anastomosis may lie very deep in the leg, particularly if the graft is anastomosed to the tibioperoneal trunk or peroneal artery. The natural taper of the vein along the leg matches the naturally decreasing diameter of the arteries as they run to the periphery.

In the second type of procedure, the long saphenous vein is completely removed and turned through 180° so that the distal end of the vein will form the proximal anastomosis. This is called a reversed vein graft. One particular advantage of this technique is that, in this orientation, the valves will not prevent blood flow toward the foot and do not need to be removed. Reversed vein grafts are often tunnelled deep in the thigh beneath the sartorius muscle, which can make imaging difficult. As the vein is reversed, the diameter of the proximal segment of the graft is usually smaller than the distal segment. This can result in a size mismatch between the proximal inflow artery and proximal graft, which is evident on the scan. When there is insufficient length of native vein available, a combination of synthetic material and vein may be used to form a composite graft (Fig. 14.2).

Synthetic grafts

Synthetic grafts are used for aortobifemoral, iliofemoral, axillofemoral and femorofemoral cross-over grafts. Synthetic PTFE grafts are also used for femoropopliteal bypass, but the long-term patency rates are not as good as grafts constructed from native vein (Klinkert et al 2003). Vein cuffs or collars are sometimes used to join the distal end of a synthetic femoral distal graft to the native artery. They produce a localized dilation at the anastomosis, which is thought to reduce the risk that a stenosis will occur (Fig. 14.3).

PURPOSE OF GRAFT SURVEILLANCE

Vein grafts

The development of an intrinsic vein graft stenosis is a major source of vein graft failure. An angiogram demonstrating a graft stenosis is shown in Figure 14.4. Research has demonstrated that a significant proportion of vein grafts develop a stenosis or defect (Grigg et al 1988, Caps et al 1995). Early graft failure, within the first month, is attributed to technical defects or poor patient selection. Such an example would be a patient with very poor run-off below the graft, resulting in increased resistance to flow and eventual graft thrombosis. Graft failure beyond 1 month is attributed to the development of intimal hyperplasia, which can occur when there is damage to the endothelium of the vessel wall. This causes smooth muscle proliferation into the vessel lumen and subsequent narrowing. Stenoses can occur at any point along the graft and can sometimes be extremely short, web-like lesions. Incomplete removal of valve cusps during in situ bypass surgery can also cause localized flow disturbance and narrowing. Late graft failure, beyond 12 months, can also be due to progression of atherosclerotic disease in the native inflow or outflow arteries, above and below the graft.

Figure 14.4 A: An angiogram demonstrating a significant graft stenosis (arrow) at the distal anastomosis of a vein graft. B: The stenosis has been successfully dilated by balloon angioplasty.

Box 14.1   Suggested program for graft surveillance following discharge from hospital; time intervals are shown in months (M)

Program if no significant abnormality is detected, peak systolic velocity (PSV) ratio <2
1M, 3M, 6M, 9M,12M, program ends at 12M or continues every 6M

Program if stenosis is detected:
PSV ratio 2–2.5, reduce follow up to 2 months
PSV ratio 2.6–2.9, reduce follow up to 4–6 weeks
PSV ratio ≥3, angioplasty or graft revision

Patients are normally scanned at 1, 3, 6, 9 and 12 months following bypass surgery (Box 14.1). Many vascular units also continue to scan patients indefinitely beyond the first year at 6-month intervals to detect late graft problems (Erikson et al 1996). The time interval between scans is shortened to 1–2 months if a patient shows signs of developing a moderate stenosis. Patients requiring angioplasty or surgical revision of a significant graft defect recommence the surveillance program from the beginning. It can be seen that graft surveillance programs require considerable commitment from the vascular laboratory, and there has been some debate as to the benefit and cost-effectiveness of surveillance programs. There is, however, some evidence to suggest that they are effective in maintaining patency rates and are less costly than surgical revision after a graft thrombosis, or rehabilitation following amputation (Lundell et al 1995, Wixon et al 2000).

Synthetic grafts

The surveillance of synthetic grafts remains debatable, as many synthetic graft occlusions occur due to spontaneous graft thrombosis. Some vascular centers perform surveillance of iliofemoral crossover grafts and aortobifemoral grafts, particularly if there have been problems with disease in the inflow or outflow arteries. Synthetic grafts are more likely to become infected, and fluid collections or pus are sometimes found surrounding the graft at the site of infection, which frequently occurs at the groin. Graft infection is a serious complication and can cause the breakdown of the graft anastomosis, leading to uncontrollable hemorrhage. Duplex scanning has proved a useful technique for detecting and monitoring potential graft infections.

SYMPTOMS AND TREATMENT OF GRAFT STENOSIS OR FAILURE

Many patients experience no symptoms in the presence of a developing graft stenosis, and grafts may fail without any prior warning. However, symptoms that can be attributable to imminent graft failure are the sudden onset of severe claudication or a sensation of coldness involving the foot. Urgent intervention is required in this situation to prevent graft occlusion. Graft surveillance programs will detect the development of most graft defects, but it may be helpful to issue patients with a card providing them with information regarding their treatment and useful contact numbers should problems be suspected. Most graft stenoses are treated successfully by balloon angioplasty (see Ch. 1). However, recurrent stenoses sometimes require surgical revision involving local patching of a defect or partial graft replacement using a new segment of vein. Early graft occlusion can be treated by thrombolysis or graft thrombectomy. There is often an underlying cause for the occlusion that requires correcting, such as a graft stenosis, inflow stenosis or run-off occlusion. Conversely, some grafts develop a local aneurysm that may become so large that a segment of graft has to be replaced.

PRACTICAL CONSIDERATIONS FOR SCANNING BYPASS GRAFTS

The objective of the scan is to detect any possible graft defects that could compromise flow and lead to graft occlusion. This usually involves some assessment of the inflow and outflow arteries above and below the graft. No special preparation is required for the examination, and the vast majority of graft scans can be completed within half an hour. The majority of bypass scans are performed with the patient lying supine or semi-supine. When scanning vein grafts, the leg should be externally rotated and the knee gently flexed and supported. It is sometimes necessary to roll the patient over to one side in order to scan the posterior lower thigh, popliteal fossa or upper posterior calf if the graft is anastomosed to the popliteal artery. Positions for scanning the tibial arteries are discussed in Chapter 9. The scanner should be configured for a graft scan, or in the absence of a specific preset, a lower limb arterial investigation. Adjustment of the controls is frequently necessary, especially if there is low-volume flow in the graft (see Ch. 7).

Before beginning the scan, it is important to know the position and type of graft that is to be examined. The examination request card or operation notes should indicate this information. A potentially confusing situation can occur if a previous graft has been performed, which has since occluded. An old thrombosed graft might be mistakenly identified as the new graft, which would then be reported as occluded. A combination of 5 and 10 MHz, or broad-band equivalent, flat linear array transducers are most suited for graft surveillance in the thigh and calf. A 3.5 MHz probe is required for imaging grafts above the inguinal ligament or for grafts that have been tunnelled very deep in the thigh.

SCANNING TECHNIQUES

In situ vein graft

The main body of an in situ vein graft remains superficial in the leg and runs along the medial aspect of the thigh (Fig. 14.5). It is often easier to locate the graft in the upper medial thigh using a transverse imaging plane and then to follow the graft up to the proximal anastomosis (Fig. 14.5A).

The transducer is rotated into a longitudinal scan plane at the proximal anastomosis (Fig. 14.5B). Ideally, a minimum 5 cm length of the inflow artery above the graft origin should be examined to exclude any disease. For instance, damped waveforms at this level are likely to indicate significant inflow disease. The proximal anastomosis should be carefully interrogated using color flow imaging and spectral Doppler for any signs of stenosis.

The graft is then carefully followed in longitudinal section along the thigh (Fig. 14.5C) with the color pulse repetition frequency (PRF) optimized to use the full color scale to demonstrate any flow disturbances. A 10 MHz (or broad-band equivalent) transducer provides the best image of the main body of the graft. Frequent spectral Doppler measurements should be made along the length of the graft, looking for waveform changes. It is often difficult to obtain good Doppler angles when scanning superficial vein grafts, and gentle 'heel-toeing' of the transducer may be required. However, it is important not to apply too much pressure with the transducer, as this can cause compression of superficial in situ vein grafts, giving the impression of a stenosis, especially if the graft passes over a bony surface. A wedge of ultrasound gel can help if there is a specific region that needs close examination.

The distal portion of many in situ vein grafts runs deep to join a native artery at the distal anastomosis (Fig. 14.5D). This is especially true for grafts joined to the popliteal or peroneal arteries. It is often necessary to use a 5 MHz transducer in this region. The distal anastomosis should be scrutinized very closely with color flow imaging and spectral Doppler. Grafts that are anastomosed to the anterior tibial artery are commonly tunnelled through the interosseous membrane (Fig. 14.6). The graft is imaged on the medial or posteromedial aspect of the calf, where it is seen to drop away very sharply and disappear through the membrane. The graft can then be relocated by scanning over the anterolateral aspect of the calf, where it will be seen to rise toward the transducer, and followed distally to locate the anastomosis. There should be a

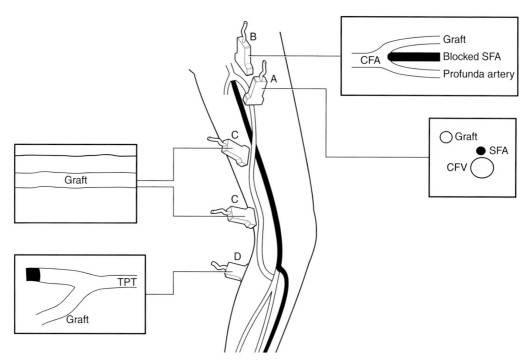

Figure 14.5   Transducer positions for assessing a femoral to tibioperoneal trunk (TPT) in situ vein graft. A: Proximal graft, transverse section. B: Proximal anastomosis, longitudinal section. C: Main body of the graft, longitudinal section. D: Distal anastomosis below the popliteal fossa, longitudinal section. Scanning from a medial position below the knee may also provide a good image of the distal anastomosis.

Figure 14.6   Grafts to the anterior tibial artery are usually tunnelled through the interosseous membrane between the tibia and fibula.

Table 14.1   Common transducer positions for imaging the distal anastomosis of an infrainguinal graft

Level of anastomosis	Transducer position
Above-knee popliteal artery	Medial aspect of lower thigh or posterior lower thigh just above popliteal fossa
Below-knee popliteal artery and tibio-peroneal trunk	Popliteal fossa or posterior and medial aspects of upper calf
Posterior tibial artery	Medial aspect of calf
Peroneal artery	Medial aspect of calf or from a lateral posterior position
Anterior tibial artery	Anterolateral aspect of calf

longitudinal scar on the anterior aspect of the calf in the region of the anastomosis. Transducer positions for locating the distal anastomosis are shown in Table 14.1.

Reversed vein grafts

The imaging techniques are similar to those for in situ grafts, but reversed vein grafts are frequently tunnelled deep in the thigh and, consequently, are more difficult to image. A 5 MHz transducer is usually required for imaging such grafts. The graft is best located in transverse section as it divides from the native artery. The graft may drop away deeply from the proximal anastomosis. If the proximal anastomosis is located at the common femoral artery, the graft can be mistaken for the profunda femoris artery, or vice versa. If the graft lies deep, it may be very difficult to follow from the medial aspect of the thigh, and it can be easier to image from a posterior thigh position. If the graft is proving very difficult to locate in the thigh, attempt to find a more distal segment around the level of the knee in the popliteal fossa and work upward. In extreme cases, it may be necessary to use a 3.5 MHz transducer to locate a deep segment of graft in the thigh.

Synthetic grafts

The majority of problems occurring in synthetic grafts are located at the proximal or distal anastomosis. It is rare for problems to develop in the main body of the graft, and a surveillance scan can often take the form of a spot check for patency combined with a more detailed assessment of the anastomoses. It is necessary to perform a detailed assessment of the inflow and outflow of the graft when abnormal graft flow is recorded in the absence of any obvious graft defect.

Femoropopliteal PTFE grafts   These are scanned in a similar fashion to vein grafts. The graft is often tunnelled deep in the leg.

Aortobifemoral grafts   These are imaged by locating the graft at the level of the groin and following it proximally to the aorta. A combination of 5 and 3.5 MHz transducers is required for this examination.

Femorofemoral cross-over grafts   These can be imaged by starting at either groin and following the graft across the pubic region to the opposite side. This can normally be achieved with a 5 MHz transducer.

Iliofemoral cross-over grafts   These grafts are easier to scan by starting at the distal anastomosis at the level of the femoral artery and following the graft back to the proximal anastomosis in the contralateral iliac artery. A combination of 5 and 3.5 MHz transducers is needed for this assessment. It is usually worth scanning the iliac artery above the proximal anastomosis to identify any inflow disease.

Axillobifemoral grafts   These usually remain relatively superficial along their length. The cross-over section of the graft can be scanned from the distal anastomosis at the femoral artery to its bifurcation from the main segment of the graft on the opposite side of the body. The remainder of the graft is then imaged from the ipsilateral groin, along the lateral wall of the abdomen and chest, to the infraclavicular fossa, where the anastomosis to the axillary artery can be imaged.

B-MODE IMAGES

Normal appearance

Vein grafts

The graft lumen should be clear and of a reasonably even caliber. Some gentle tapering is often seen in the lower portion of an in situ vein graft, as the native long saphenous vein is smaller in the lower leg. In contrast, the proximal lumen of a reversed vein graft may be smaller in caliber than the distal graft. It is common to see slight areas of dilation along a vein graft at points corresponding to valve sites (Fig. 14.7). The proximal and distal anastomoses are sometimes difficult to image clearly, due to surrounding scar tissue or depth. It may be

Figure 14.7   Normal B-mode image of an in situ vein graft. Note the slightly dilated area corresponding to a valve site (arrow).

difficult to image a deep reversed vein graft without color flow imaging.

Synthetic grafts

Synthetic grafts made of PTFE produce a characteristic image, with the anterior and posterior walls displaying a 'double line' appearance due to the strong reflection of ultrasound (Fig. 14.2). Some PTFE grafts are externally supported by rings that can be seen on the image (see Fig. 7.3). The corrugated structure of Dacron grafts, used mainly for aortobifemoral bypass surgery, is usually easy to see (see Fig. 14.16). Vein cuffs or collars are sometimes used to join the graft to the distal native

artery, and these are often seen as a short dilation at the anastomosis (Fig. 14.3).

Abnormal appearance

Many vein graft stenoses are difficult to identify with B-mode imaging alone, as they can be short or web-like and poorly echogenic. Larger areas of hyperplasia can appear as moderately echogenic regions in the vessel lumen (Fig. 14.8). It is sometimes possible to see remnant valve cusps flapping in the lumen of in situ vein grafts due to inadequate stripping with the valvulotome. Areas of vein grafts may become tortuous and dilated over time, and changes in graft diameter should be recorded. In some cases large areas of thrombus or hyperplasia can be seen in aneurysmal segments, and the B-mode image may show partial stagnation or stasis of blood flow in these areas. This will be visualized as strong specular reflections in the dilated region, swirling in time with arterial pulsation. True and false aneurysms of vein or synthetic grafts can be easily seen and are discussed later in this chapter.

COLOR DOPPLER IMAGES

Normal appearance of vein grafts

An ultrasound montage of an in situ vein graft is shown in Figure 14.9. The color flow image often

Figure 14.8 In this magnified B-mode image, a large area of intimal hyperplasia (arrow) is seen in a vein graft.

Figure 14.9 A color montage of an in situ vein graft. Areas of color flow aliasing and flow disturbance within the body of the graft may indicate a graft stenosis (arrow). These areas should be closely checked with spectral Doppler. There is retrograde filling of a short segment of the popliteal artery (curved arrow) above the distal anastomosis.

demonstrates areas of marked flow disturbance and flow reversal at the proximal anastomosis due to the size, geometry and orientation of the graft origin from the native artery. This may also be seen at the level of the distal anastomosis and should not be considered abnormal unless spectral Doppler recordings demonstrate significant velocity changes. Beyond the proximal anastomosis, the color flow image should demonstrate an undisturbed flow pattern. Grafts with well-established biphasic or triphasic flow will display normal reversal of flow (from red to blue or vice versa) during the diastolic phase. New grafts may demonstrate hyperemic flow due to peripheral dilation and the flow requirements of healing tissue, exhibited as constant forward flow throughout the cardiac cycle. If the graft has a large lumen, the flow velocity may be very low, and the PRF may have to be significantly lowered to demonstrate color filling. Some areas of flow reversal may be seen in areas of vein grafts corresponding to valve sites. In rare instances in which the vein is found to be bifid for a short segment, it is possible to see two flow lumens. The distal anastomosis of a femoral distal graft is usually easier to identify with color flow imaging than with B-mode imaging. It is common to see the graft supplying a patent segment of the native artery above the anastomosis as well as distally, and retrograde flow will be seen in the native vessel above the anastomosis, producing a Y-shaped junction (Fig. 14.9). There is often a considerable size discrepancy between the distal end of a vein graft, which can be quite large, and the outflow artery, which may be a smaller tibial vessel. This will cause a natural velocity increase due to the change in vessel diameter, possibly producing color aliasing at the position of the anastomosis and proximal run-off vessel, but this should not be assumed to indicate a significant stenosis without close interrogation with spectral Doppler.

Normal appearance of synthetic grafts

Flow in synthetic grafts can sometimes be difficult to demonstrate using color flow imaging, as the graft material attenuates the Doppler signal, requiring an increase in the color gain. Significant flow disturbance can be seen at the origins and ends of synthetic iliofemoral or femorofemoral cross-over

grafts, as the graft is often joined at a 90° angle to the native artery.

Abnormal appearance of vein grafts

A significant graft stenosis will produce marked flow disturbance, which is usually associated with aliasing on the color flow image (Fig. 14.9; see Fig. 14.12), and there may be considerable flow disturbance beyond the stenosis. Failing grafts may demonstrate very low volume flow, which can sometimes be difficult to demonstrate with color flow imaging, and the graft may be mistakenly reported as occluded. If no flow is detected in the graft, the color PRF and high-pass filter setting should be reduced to confirm the occlusion, which should also be checked with spectral Doppler. Arteriovenous fistulas and aneurysms are other graft abnormalities that are visible with color flow imaging, as discussed below.

SPECTRAL DOPPLER WAVEFORMS
Normal appearance

The waveform shapes in normal vein grafts can vary considerably depending on the age of the graft. New grafts may demonstrate a hyperemic monophasic flow profile because of sustained peripheral vasodilation, which can be due to a combination of the previous ischemia and healing tissue (Fig. 14.10A). Over time, the flow pattern should become pulsatile, and biphasic or triphasic waveforms are usually recorded (Fig. 14.10B). It is good practice to take spectral Doppler measurements at regular intervals along a graft, even in the presence of a normal color flow display, as changes in the waveform shape can indicate an approaching problem. Disturbed flow, including areas of flow reversal, is usually encountered around the proximal anastomosis, but there should be no significant increase in systolic velocity. Natural changes in the diameter of the graft will produce changes in the peak systolic velocity (PSV), which should not automatically be assumed to represent a stenosis. In this situation, velocities should be compared in adjacent areas of similar vessel diameter. Perhaps the most difficult assessment to make during graft surveillance is the estimation of the degree of narrowing at the distal anastomosis, where there is often a

Figure 14.10   A: Hyperemic flow is often seen in the early postoperative period. B: Over time, the flow normally assumes a pulsatile flow pattern.

Figure 14.11   Problems in interpreting flow velocities in a vein graft anastomosed to the posterior tibial artery. At point A, the PSV in the distal graft is 65 cm/s. At point B the PSV in the posterior tibial artery, just distal to the anastomosis, is 120 cm/s. This represents a near doubling in velocity, suggesting a stenosis. However, the diameter of the posterior tibial artery is significantly smaller than that of the distal graft, leading to a natural increase in systolic velocity, as flow velocity is inversely related to cross-sectional area, and in this example no narrowing is indicated. Unfortunately, at point C, a significant stenosis is demonstrated in the posterior tibial artery, 2 cm distal to the anastomosis, by color flow aliasing and a significant increase in the PSV, >400 cm/s. In this image there is some retrograde filling of the native vessel above the anastomosis (curved arrow).

large-diameter vein graft joined to a smaller outflow artery, producing a natural velocity increase. In this situation, it is possible to see a significant increase in the PSV in the absence of a stenosis (Fig. 14.11). However, flow velocities just below the distal anastomosis should be similar to those several centimeters downstream, provided that the vessel diameter is the same. A significant stenosis would be indicated if the velocities at the anastomosis were found to be substantially higher (i.e., 3–4 times) than distal velocities. It is also important to ensure that the spectral Doppler angle is set correctly at the distal anastomosis, as flow is not always parallel to the vessel walls, and this can lead to errors in velocity measurements.

Abnormal appearance

Graft stenoses are categorized using a similar method to that for grading lower limb arterial disease. The PSV across the stenosis is divided by the PSV in a normal segment of graft just proximal to the stenosis (Fig. 14.12). The criteria for grading graft stenoses are shown in Table 14.2. Intervention by angioplasty or surgical revision is usually performed when the PSV ratio is equal to or greater than 3 (London et al 1993, Olojugba et al 1998, Landry et al 2002). Stenoses producing a PSV ratio of 2–2.9 are kept under close surveillance. In addition, a PSV of less than 45 cm/s within the graft has been suggested to indicate a graft defect (Mills et al 1990). Care must be exercised in the use of this criterion as patients with large-diameter grafts may have relatively low velocity flow within the graft, because velocity is inversely related to cross-sectional area. In our experience, many normal grafts with velocities below this level do not occlude. Poor spectral Doppler angles may produce considerable errors in one-spot velocity measurements, and it is therefore important to select an area of the graft where a good Doppler angle can be obtained for accurate velocity measurement.

Figure 14.12   The PSV ratio is used to estimate the degree of narrowing across a graft stenosis. A: Color flow imaging demonstrates a severe graft stenosis. B: The PSV just proximal to the stenosis is 16.4 cm/s. C: The PSV across the stenosis is 319 cm/s, associated with marked spectral broadening. This represents a 19 times velocity ratio, indicating a critical stenosis.

Figure 14.13   A color flow image of the distal end of a vein graft demonstrates occlusion of the posterior tibial artery (arrows) at the distal anastomosis. However, the graft remains patent due to retrograde flow (R), filling a segment of native vessel above the anastomosis.

grafts remain patent for years, despite occlusion of the run-off vessel. This is due to retrograde flow into a patent segment of artery above the anastomosis, filling collateral vessels (Fig. 14.13).

GRAFT FAILURE AND OCCLUSION

Despite the most aggressive surveillance programs, some grafts will occlude for a variety of reasons. Occluded vein grafts can be difficult to identify by B-mode imaging, especially if the graft lies deep, as it may merge into the tissue planes. When it is possible to identify the graft, there is usually thrombus seen within the lumen. An occluded graft is usually easiest to identify by scanning at the level of the proximal anastomosis. The most obvious signs of graft occlusion are an absence of color flow and spectral Doppler signals. Ankle–brachial pressures will also be reduced. A thrombosing graft may contain clot at the distal end, and spectral Doppler will demonstrate a characteristic low-volume, high-resistance flow pattern in the patent lumen above this area with no net forward flow (Fig. 14.14). In this situation the B-mode image may demonstrate slight backward and forward pulsation of the blood, exhibited as a speckle pattern. This indicates imminent graft occlusion and should be reported immediately. Conversely, a low-volume damped waveform in the proximal graft would indicate an inflow stenosis.

Table 14.2   Spectral Doppler criteria for grading a graft stenosis

Diameter reduction	Spectral Doppler criteria
<50%	PSV ratio < 2
50–70%	PSV ratio 2–3; increased spectral broadening and turbulence just beyond the stenosis; waveform becomes more monophasic
70–99%	PSV ratio > 3; marked turbulence distal to the stenosis; waveform may be monophasic
Occlusion	No flow signal present

Damped flow in the artery proximal to the proximal anastomosis often indicates an inflow stenosis, and this should be examined with duplex, as poor inflow can lead to graft occlusion. A stenosis of the outflow artery below the distal anastomosis can also dramatically reduce flow in the graft by increasing distal resistance. For this reason, it is important to scan the run-off artery below the graft. However, it is interesting to note that some

Figure 14.14 Extremely low volume flow recorded from an in situ vein graft indicates imminent graft occlusion. In this example the distal end of the graft had already thrombosed and the Doppler waveform demonstrates no net forward flow.

COMMONLY ENCOUNTERED PROBLEMS

Large and obese patients can be difficult to examine, and it may be necessary to use a lower frequency transducer. Early postoperative scans can be difficult if the wounds are still healing, and scanning over a sterile transparent plastic dressing is useful in this situation. Having no prior knowledge of the type and position of graft can lead to considerable problems. For example, a popliteal to tibial vein bypass graft may require the long saphenous vein to be harvested from the thigh, as it is larger at this level. Therefore, a large scar will be seen in the thigh, but the graft will not be located at this level; however, the sonographer may automatically assume that this corresponds to the position of the proximal graft. A copy of the operation notes is a useful aid to locating the graft.

It is also possible for grafts to be routed in unusual directions, such as across the anterolateral thigh to join the anterior tibial artery in the calf. Some patients may have had a previous graft that has since occluded, and this could be mistaken for the new graft, which may still be patent. It is also possible for segments of native vessels to be patent, such as the superficial femoral artery, and this may cause some confusion or may even be mistaken for the graft.

TRUE AND FALSE ANEURYSMS

Vein grafts can develop true aneurysmal dilations over time, particularly at valve sites or at the anastomoses (Fig. 14.15). This can occur if the vein

Figure 14.15 An aneurysmal area in a vein graft corresponding to a valve site. Note the area of hyperplasia or thrombus (arrow) in the area of dilation.

Figure 14.16 A false aneurysm (FA) has occurred at the distal end of a femorofemoral cross-over graft (G) due to failure of the anastomosis. Note the corrugated appearance of the dacron material.

wall becomes structurally weak. A localized doubling in the graft diameter indicates the development of an aneurysm, and this should be reported and kept under regular surveillance to monitor progression. It is not uncommon to see thrombus in aneurysmal areas. Color flow imaging and spectral Doppler usually demonstrate areas of flow reversal in the aneurysmal regions. Large true aneurysms are repaired surgically by replacing the aneurysmal area with a new segment of vein.

False aneurysms are caused by blood flowing into and out of a defect in the vessel wall (see Ch. 11). They are typified as swirling areas of flow in a contained cavity outside the true flow lumen and may contain thrombus. They can occur if the suture line at the anastomosis fails or as a complication of balloon angioplasty, due to splitting of the graft wall following high-pressure balloon inflation (Fig. 14.16). False aneurysms also occur at catheter puncture sites (see Ch. 11).

A   B

Figure 14.17   An example of graft entrapment. A: A vein graft is running between two muscles in the lower thigh, and a moderate stenosis is seen (arrow). B: During leg flexion the graft is compressed between the muscles, causing a virtual occlusion (arrow).

ENTRAPMENTS OF GRAFTS

Entrapment of grafts can occur around the knee level, especially where in situ vein grafts run from superficial to deep, through a tunnel in the muscles. In this situation, normal flow may be recorded with the leg extended, but mild to moderate flexion of the knee joint produces pinching of the graft between muscle groups, causing a temporary stenosis (Fig. 14.17). Conversely, some grafts become temporarily obstructed during full knee extension. This is a relatively rare problem, but it will be seen from time to time in a busy laboratory. If the problem is significant, the muscle can be divided or the graft re-routed.

ARTERIOVENOUS FISTULAS

Arteriovenous fistulas occur in in situ vein grafts where there has been incomplete ligation of a long saphenous vein side branch, allowing blood to short-circuit from the graft directly into the venous system (Fig. 14.18). Arteriovenous fistulas are characterized by hyperemic or high-volume flow in the graft proximal to the fistula, with an area of marked color flow disturbance at the site of the fistula (Fig. 14.19). Spectral Doppler also demonstrates turbulent high-volume flow with a low-resistance waveform at this site. The veins leading from the fistula also demonstrate a high-volume flow pattern. Flow in the graft distal to the fistula

Figure 14.18   An arteriogram demonstrates an arteriovenous fistula (arrow) between a vein graft (G) and the venous system (V).

is usually lower in volume and more pulsatile. In some circumstances, the graft below the site of the fistula may be totally occluded. Arteriovenous fistulas can be ligated or embolized. It is useful to

Figure 14.19 A transverse color flow image of a vein graft demonstrating an arteriovenous fistula (arrow). The Doppler waveform displays low–resistance, high–volume flow across the fistula.

Figure 14.20 A fluid-filled seroma (S) adjacent to a vein graft (VG).

mark the level of the defect using duplex so that the surgeon can easily locate the fistula.

SEROMAS, FLUID COLLECTIONS AND GRAFT INFECTIONS

Seromas are fluid-filled collections that are occasionally seen adjacent to vein grafts, particularly at the level of the groin. They can be mistaken for false aneurysms on B-mode imaging, but color flow imaging will demonstrate an absence of flow (Fig. 14.20). Fluid collections around synthetic grafts can be due to local reaction of the surrounding tissues, but they can also be due to graft infection. Graft infections are a serious complication and are more frequently associated with synthetic grafts. The outcome for patients with synthetic graft infections is often poor (Mertens et al 1995). Infections at the level of the groin are common due to the rich source of bacteria in this region, and aortobifemoral, iliofemoral and axillobifemoral grafts are especially at risk. Complications of infection can lead to the disintegration of a graft anastomosis, resulting in severe hemorrhage. Failure of wound healing is also a frequent complication. Ultrasound imaging can be useful for investigating wound infections, as the B-mode image can show whether the graft is in direct contact with suspected areas of infection, especially if the suspected region tracks to discharging wounds or openings on the skin surface (Fig. 14.21). It is essential to image any suspected area of graft infection in cross-section to see how it relates to the graft and surrounding structures. It can be difficult to differentiate areas of infection from simple hematomas, and bacterial cultures are often required to isolate infective organisms. Ultrasound can be used to guide the needle puncture during the sampling of fluid collections to avoid accidentally puncturing the graft. CT and MRI are also commonly used for investigating graft infections, especially in the abdomen. Methicillin-resistant *Staphylococcus aureus* (MRSA) is now endemic in most hospitals. Graft infections caused by MRSA are difficult to treat, requiring prolonged use of powerful antibiotics. In some cases, graft removal is necessary to remove the focus of infection, but this may lead to inevitable amputation of the limb, owing to poor blood flow. In extreme situations, the patient may be overwhelmed by the infection and die.

REPORTING

The easiest method of reporting the scan results is by the use of diagrams. The graft position can be drawn onto the diagram with velocity measurements and other relevant information recorded (Fig. 14.22). It is also useful to keep a file for each patient in the graft surveillance program in the

A

B

Figure 14.21   A: A transverse image of a PTFE graft (G) demonstrating an echo region (I) tracking to the skin surface that is in contact with the graft. There was pus discharging from the skin surface at this point, indicating a potential graft infection. B: A longitudinal image of the same graft, indicating a suspicious area (I) lying over the graft (G). Note that the ring supports of the graft can be seen in this image.

vascular laboratory, as this makes comparison of serial follow-up scans easier. Any significant graft problems must be reported to the appropriate medical staff immediately. In addition, many vascular units combine the duplex assessment with a measurement of the ankle–brachial pressure index (ABPI). An ABPI <1 can indicate a problem. A serial reduction >0.1 in ABPI readings is indicative of a significant problem (Brennan et al 1991). Some vascular units combine ABPI measurements with a walking test to unmask a less significant stenosis.

Figure 14.22   Diagrams are the simplest method of reporting the results of graft surveillance scans.

SUPERFICIAL VEIN MAPPING FOR ARTERIAL BYPASS SURGERY

A preoperative duplex scan can determine the suitability of a superficial vein for use as a bypass graft (Bagi et al 1989). Careful marking of its path avoids undermining of skin flaps during surgery and possible wound necrosis. The long saphenous vein is the most commonly used vein for arterial bypass surgery, due to its length. Arm veins and the short saphenous vein can also be used for bypass grafts, provided that their lumens are of sufficient diameter.

Technique for assessing the long saphenous vein

The patient should be positioned with the feet tilted down to distend the veins. A high-frequency 10 MHz, or broad-band equivalent, flat linear array transducer should be used to image the veins. Starting at the top of the leg, the long saphenous vein should be identified in transverse section at the level of the saphenofemoral junction and followed distally down the thigh and into the calf. Scanning the vein in transverse section is important, because it is easier to assess its diameter and to identify any large branches dividing from the vein, or duplicated or bifid systems. The diameter of the vein should be recorded at frequent intervals throughout its length. Ideally, the diameter should be greater than 3 mm to be suitable as a graft. Veins of less than 2 mm in diameter are regarded as too small to be used for femoral distal bypass grafting. Veins that become excessively large (>0.8 cm diameter) or grossly varicose may also be unsuitable, and this should be drawn to the attention of the surgeon. The common femoral vein, superficial femoral vein and popliteal vein should always be examined when vein mapping to ensure deep venous patency, as the long saphenous vein can act as an important collateral pathway if the deep veins have been obstructed and, in such circumstances, should not be harvested for a graft. In this situation, other sources of vein can be assessed.

Arm vein mapping

It is not uncommon to find that part or all of the long saphenous vein is unsuitable for use as a graft because it is too small, because it is varicose or because the deep veins are obstructed. In addition, the long saphenous vein may have already been removed for coronary artery bypass surgery. The cephalic or basilic veins of the arm can be harvested for bypass grafts provided they are of adequate diameter. The cephalic vein is the vein of choice, as it is longer than the basilic vein, and the anatomy of the basilic vein is more variable in its proximal segment. To image the veins, the arm should be in a comfortable dependent position with the palm facing upward. The cephalic vein can be located in transverse section along the outer aspect of the forearm 2–3 cm above the wrist, lateral to the radial artery and followed proximally. Alternatively, it can be located in the anterior aspect of the upper arm, lying superficial to the biceps muscle and then followed proximally toward the shoulder and then distally into the forearm. The vein can be difficult

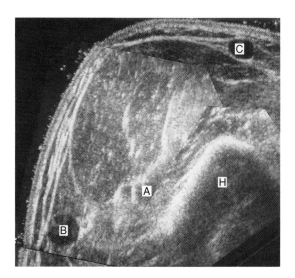

Figure 14.23   A transverse B-mode montage of the left upper arm demonstrating the position of the basilic vein (B), cephalic vein (C) and brachial artery and veins (A). The arm was positioned with the palm up so that the cephalic vein lies on the anterior aspect of the arm and the basilic vein and brachial vessels on the medial aspect. The humerus is also seen (H).

to follow as it crosses the antecubital fossa, as there are a number of superficial veins crossing this area. The basilic vein is easiest to locate with the arm extended outward (abducted) and the palm facing upward. The probe is placed on the medial aspect of the arm 2–3 cm above the elbow joint. Imaging in cross-section, the basilic vein should be seen as separate from the brachial artery (Fig. 14.23). The vein can then be followed proximally, where it is usually seen to course toward the proximal brachial vein or the axillary vein, although there can be anatomical variation of the veins in this region. Following the basilic vein distally into the forearm can be confusing, as it sometimes joins the cephalic vein in the forearm via the median cubital vein, but it usually runs toward the medial (ulnar) aspect of the wrist. One potential pitfall of mapping the basilic vein is accidentally confusing it with the brachial artery, but use of probe compression to collapse the vein and color flow imaging should avoid this error.

Technique of marking the vein

There are two techniques for marking leg or arm veins (Fig. 14.24). Using the first method, the vein

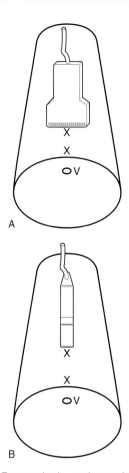

Figure 14.24 Two methods can be used for vein mapping. A: The vein (V) can be marked (X) in the transverse plane. B: The vein can also be marked in a longitudinal plane.

removed and the dots joined up with a continuous line using a permanent felt-tipped marker pen.

The second technique involves assessing the vein in transverse section for its size and position, and then marking the vein with the transducer turned into a longitudinal plane and the vein imaged in this direction. A dot is placed against the end of the transducer to correspond to the position and direction of the vein. This technique is more difficult in terms of imaging, as it is easy to 'slip off' the image of the vein and follow a tissue plane, but it does seem to produce a more accurate map of the vein. Once the position of the vein has been marked using this technique, it is wise to run down the length of marking with the transducer in transverse section to ensure that the dots follow the main trunk, in case a smaller side branch in the lower leg has been accidentally followed using this method.

Problems encountered during vein mapping

One major practical problem of vein mapping is trying to mark the position of the vein with a felt-tipped pen through the ultrasound gel, as the pen quickly becomes clogged with gel and no longer works. Many vascular units have their own personal preferences for overcoming this problem. A charcoal pencil can be useful for dotting in the position of the vein and the dots joined up later with a felt-tipped pen once the gel has been removed. Alternatively, using small amounts of gel and frequently wiping the gel away from the probe edge before marking prevent the pen tip from becoming saturated in ultrasound gel. It is also useful to place a non-sterile probe cover over the transducer when vein mapping, as this prevents the probe from becoming covered in ink from the marker pen.

If the patient has very poor muscle volume and the superficial tissues are baggy, it can be very difficult to ensure that the marking is accurate. If in any doubt, tell the surgeon. In obese patients, the vein may be very deep, and it can be difficult to mark it in the correct incision plane.

is imaged in transverse section with the vein appearing in the center of the image. Using a marker pen, a dot is then placed on the skin surface against the middle of the probe. It is easier to start by marking the vein in the upper thigh, rather than at the level of the saphenofemoral junction and then to work toward the saphenofemoral junction. The vein should be marked with a dot at frequent intervals along the thigh and calf. Finally the gel is completely

References

Bagi P, Schroeder T, Sillesen H, et al 1989 Real time B-mode mapping of the greater saphenous vein. European Journal of Vascular Surgery 3(2):103–105

Brennan J A, Walsh A K, Beard J D, et al 1991 The role of simple non-invasive testing in infrainguinal graft surveillance. European Journal of Vascular Surgery 5(1):13–17

Caps M T, Cantwell-Gab K, Bergelin R O, et al 1995 Vein graft lesions: time of onset and rate of progression. Journal of Vascular Surgery 22(4):466–475

Erickson C A, Towne J B, Seabrook G R, et al 1996 Ongoing vascular laboratory surveillance is essential to maximize long-term in situ saphenous vein bypass patency. Journal of Vascular Surgery 23(1):18–27

Grigg M J, Nicolaides A N, Wolfe J H 1988 Femorodistal vein bypass graft stenoses. British Journal of Surgery 75(8):737–740

Klinkert P, Schepers A, Burger D H C, et al 2003 Vein versus polytetrafluoroethylene in above-knee femoropopliteal bypass grafting: five-year results of a randomized controlled trial. Journal of Vascular Surgery 37(1):149–155

Landry G J, Moneta G L, Taylor L M, et al 2002 Long-term outcome of revised lower-extremity bypass grafts. Journal of Vascular Surgery 35(1):56–63

London N J M, Sayers R D, Thompson M M, et al 1993 Interventional radiology in the maintenance of infrainguinal vein graft patency. British Journal of Surgery 80(2):187–193

Lundell A, Lindblad B, Bergqvist D, et al 1995 Femoropopliteal-crural graft patency is improved by an intensive surveillance program: a prospective randomized study. Journal of Vascular Surgery 21(1):26–34

Mertens R A, O'Hara P J, Hertzer N R, et al 1995 Surgical management of infrainguinal arterial prosthetic graft infections: review of a thirty-five-year experience. Journal of Vascular Surgery 21(5):782–791

Mills J L, Harris E J, Taylor L M Jr, et al 1990 The importance of routine surveillance of distal bypass grafts with duplex scanning: a study of 379 reversed vein grafts. Journal of Vascular Surgery 12(4):379–389

Olojugba D H, McCarthy M J, Naylor A R, et al 1998 At what peak velocity ratio should duplex-detected infrainguinal vein graft stenoses be revised? European Journal of Vascular and Endovascular Surgery 15(3):258–260

Wixon C L, Mills J L, Westerband A, et al 2000 An economic appraisal of lower extremity bypass graft maintenance. Journal of Vascular Surgery 32(1):1–12

Appendix A

Decibel scale

The decibel scale allows the large range of values of ultrasound intensities, or signal voltages, to be expressed by a smaller range of numbers, as shown in Table A.1. The decibel scale expresses the ratios of intensities, or voltages, using a logarithmic scale. The decibel scale is used to describe ultrasound attenuation and amplifier gain.

Table A.1 Decibel scale applied to intensity and voltage (or echo amplitude)

Intensity ratio (I/I_0)	Decibel (dB)	Amplitude ratio (V/V_0)
1 000 000	60	1000
10 000	40	100
100	20	10
10	10	3
2	3	1.4
0.5	−3	0.7
0.1	−10	0.3
0.01	−20	0.1
0.0001	−40	0.01
0.000001	−60	0.001

Intensity I (relative to I_0) in dB $= 10 \log_{10} (I/I_0)$.
Gain in dB $= 20 \log_{10}(V/V_0)$.

Appendix B

Sensitivity and specificity

When a new test is developed, a threshold at which the results are considered to indicate the presence or absence of the disease has to be selected. To do this the results of the test are compared to another method of detecting the disease, often known as 'the gold standard'. Unfortunately, there is usually an overlap between the results obtained in the presence of the disease with the results obtained in the absence of disease. This means that some patients will be falsely diagnosed as having the disease whereas others will be falsely diagnosed as not having the disease. Selecting the best threshold for the test depends partly on the prevalence of the disease within the group tested and also on the consequence of a false classification (i.e., missing the disease or incorrectly diagnosing disease in a normal patient). The performance of a diagnostic test can be measured by its sensitivity and specificity, which are defined as follows:

$$\text{Sensitivity} = \frac{\text{Number of patients with the disease correctly diagnosed}}{\text{Number of patients with the disease}}$$

$$\text{Specificity} = \frac{\text{Number of patients without the disease correctly diagnosed}}{\text{Number of patients without the disease}}$$

The value of the sensitivity and specificity will vary as the threshold of the test is altered. For example, if the threshold is changed to improve sensitivity, the specificity will fall. Altering the threshold and calculating the specificity and sensitivity can permit the selection of the optimal threshold and allow the value of the diagnostic test to be assessed. Other closely related qualities of a test often quoted in the literature are the positive predictive value, the negative predictive value and the accuracy. The positive predictive value is the probability that a subject who has a positive test (i.e., disease is detected) will be correctly classified. The negative predictive value is the probability that a subject who has a negative test (i.e., no disease is detected) is correctly classified.

Further reading

Bland M 1995 An introduction to medical statistics. Oxford University Press, Oxford

Index

Page numbers in *italic* print refer to illustrations.

A

Abdominal aorta
 anatomy 146
 aneurysms *see* Aneurysms
Abdominal aortic aneurysm (AAA)
  145, 146
Absorption 11
Acoustic impedance 9
Acute ischemia 117–18, 135
Adventitia 50
Aliasing
 color flow imaging 41–2
 pulsed Doppler 31–3
 velocity measurement 71
Amaurosis fugax 88
Ambulatory venous pressure 61–2
Amplification 13–14
Aneurysms
 aortic
  distance from renal arteries 154
  endovascular repair 1, 148–9,
   154–7
  measurements 152–4
  scanning 149–50, 154
  shapes and types 149
  symptoms 146–7
  ultrasound appearance 150–2
 carotid 105
 definition 145–6
 dissecting 146, 149, 151
 false *see* False aneurysms
 femoral artery 158
 grafts 218
 iliac 157
 inflammatory 151

leakage 147
open repair 147–8
pathology 146
popliteal 157–8
reporting 160
rupture 147
saccular 149
subclavian artery 140
upper limbs 142
Angiography, carotid artery disease
  1, 85, 97, 98, 107
Angioplasty 2–3, 98, 117, 135, 210
Angle of insonation
 color flow image 39–41, 79
 Doppler shift 25, 33
 velocity measurements
  errors in 67–8
  for estimating 69–70
Ankle–brachial pressure index (ABPI)
  113–16
 venous ulceration 171
Anterior cerebral artery (ACA) 86
Anterior tibial (AT) artery 113
 grafts *212*
 scanning 122–3
Anterior tibial (AT) vein 164
 scanning 194
Anterolateral vein 167
Anticoagulation 191
Aorta
 anatomy 111–12, 146
 aneurysms *see* Aneurysms
 diameter measurement 152–4
Aortic bifurcation
 anatomy 111–12
 obstruction 117

scanning 120
Aortobifemoral grafts *208*, 209
 scanning 213
 surveillance 210
Aortoiliac arteries, assessment
  119–20
Arm vein mapping 222
Artefacts
 color imaging 80–1
 imaging 76–8
 refraction 10, 77
 spectral Doppler 81
Arteries
 see also individual arteries
 bifurcating *13*
 disease 2–3
 emboli *see* Emboli
 flow profiles 53–8
 stents 98, 116, 129, 157
 structure 50
 thrombosis 117
 variable vessel diameter 71
Arteriography *see* Angiography
Arterioles 50, 52
Arteriovenous fistulas (AVF) 142–3,
  219–20
Arteriovenous malformations 139,
  205
Asymptomatic Carotid
  Atherosclerosis Study (ACAS)
  98
Atheroma 93, *94*, 100, 103–4, 124
Atherosclerosis 2, 116
Attachment site endoleaks 156
Attenuation 11–12
Autocorrelation detection 37

Axial resolution 19, 45
Axillary artery
    anatomy 134
    aneurysms 135
    dissection 138
    false aneurysms 142
    obstruction 133
    scanning 136–7
Axillary vein 203
    assessing 204
    thrombosis 203
Axillobifemoral grafts 209, 213

B

B-mode imaging 12–13
    controls 76
Back-scatter 26, 35–6
    contrast agents 46, 47
    power Doppler imaging 45–6
Baker's cysts 158, 201–2
Basilar artery 86
Basilic vein
    anatomy 203
    assessment for bypass graft 222
Beam
    angle 10, 17
    focusing 18–19
    shape 9, 16–17
    steering 17, 39, *40*
Bernoulli's law 50–1, 52
Bicuspid valves 60
Blood 26
Blood flow 49–62
    Doppler effect 24–5
    enhanced imaging 46–7
    mechanism 50–1
    profiles 53–8
        around curves in a vessel 57–9
        blunt 53, 58, 64
        disturbed 53
        Doppler spectrum 63–4
        hyperemic 55, 103, 125, *186*
        laminar 53, 59
        monophasic 55–6
        parabolic 53, 57, 64
        pulsatile 54–6
        through stenosis 58–60
        turbulent 53, 59–60, 64
        venous 60–2
    resistance to 51–2
    reversal 54–5, 113
        at bifurcations and branches 56–7
        true 41, *42*
        venous 60
        vertebral arteries 103
    velocity *see* Velocity
    vertebral arteries 103
    volume flow measurement 70–2
Blood vessels
    see also Arteries; Veins
    diameter measurement 70–2
    imaging tortuous 40
    structure of walls 49–50
Blood–tissue discrimination 38
Boyd's perforator 166
Brachial artery
    anatomy 134
    dissection 138
    false aneurysms 142
    obstruction 133
    scanning 137
Brachial vein
    anatomy 202–3
    assessing 204
Brachiocephalic bifurcation, pulsatile swelling 105
Brachiocephalic (innominate) artery 86
British Medical Ultrasound Society (BMUS) 82
Buerger's disease 129
Bursa 201
Bypass grafts *see* Grafts

C

Calcified atheroma 103–4, 124
Calf compression 172
Calf muscle pump 61–2
Calf perforators 184
Calf veins
    scanning 194
    thrombosis 191
Calliper velocity calibration 71
Capillaries 50
Cardiac cycle, blood flow 60
Carotid arteries
    anatomy 86
    diseases *see* Carotid artery disease
    dissection *78*, 105, 106
    postoperative and post-angioplasty appearance 105
    scanning 79, *80*
    tortuous *41*, 104
Carotid artery disease
    angiography 85, 97, 98, 107
    asymptomatic 88
    atheroma 93, *94*, 100, 103–4, 124
    B-mode imaging 93–5
    collateral pathways 86–7
    color imaging 95–6
    compound imaging *18*
    grading 97–8
        combining scan information 102–3
        imaging 98–100
        spectral Doppler 100–2
    non-atheromatous 105–6
    problems encountered in imaging 103–4
    reporting 107
    resistance to flow 52
    scanning
        objectives and preparation 88–9
        techniques 89–93
    spectral Doppler 96–7
    stroke 85
    surgery *see* Carotid endarterectomy
    symptoms 88
    treatment 98
Carotid artery stenosis
    aliasing and flow reversal *42*
    color imaging 95–6
    grading 97–102
    spectral Doppler waveforms 96–7
    symptoms 88
    ultrasound scan *2*
Carotid bifurcation 105
    blood flow profile 56
    calcified plaque 103
    color image *91*
    longitudinal B-mode image *90*
    pulsatile swelling 105
Carotid body tumours 105–6
Carotid bruit 88
Carotid bulb 41, 86
Carotid endarterectomy 3, 85, 98, 106
    atheroma 93, *94*
    postoperative appearance 105
Carotid siphon 86
Cavitation 82, 83
Celiac axis 146
Cellulitis 201
Cephalic vein 203
    assessment for bypass graft 222
Cervical ribs 139, *140*
Circle of Willis
    anatomy 86
    collateral pathways 86–7
Claudication 116, 210
Clutter filter 39, 43
Collateral endoleaks 155
Color box angle/size 79–80
Color Doppler controls 78–80
Color flow imaging 2, 35–47
    aliasing 41–2
    angle of insonation 39–41

artefacts 80–1
blood–tissue discrimination 38
color coding 38–9
frame rate 43–4
hue 38
low velocity flow 42–3
luminosity 38
noise 79
resolution and sensitivity 44–5
saturation 38–9
scanner elements 37–9
transcranial 106
two-dimensional maps 35–6
Color scales 39
Color write enable/priority control 38, 80
Common carotid artery (CCA)
anatomy 86
B-mode imaging 89–90
color flow imaging 90–1
spectral Doppler 91
velocity profiles 55
waveform showing reverse diastolic flow *97*
Common femoral artery (CFA)
anatomy 112–13, *118*
assessment 119–20
velocity profiles 55
waveforms 129
Common femoral vein
anatomy *118*, 165, 168
assessment 177
respiration effects *61*
scanning 193–4
transverse image *193*
Common iliac artery
anatomy 111–12
emboli 117
scanning 120
stenosis *2*
Common iliac vein 60, *165*, 168
Common interosseous artery 134
Compartment syndrome 117
Composite vein grafts 208
Compound imaging 17, *18*
Compression bandaging 171
Compression curves 14–15
Computed tomography (CT) 1, 192
Congestive heart failure
abnormal venous flow 62
edema 201
Continuous wave Doppler *27*, 29
limitations 33
Contrast agents 46–7
Costoclavicular maneuver 140
Critical lower limb ischemia (CLI) 116–17

Crocket's perforators 166
Cystic adventitial disease, popliteal artery 130

D

D-dimers 191–2
Decibel scale 14, 225
Deep femoral (profunda femoris) artery 112–13, *118*, 120
Deep femoral (profunda femoris) vein *118*, 164, 168
Deep inspiration maneuver 140–1
Deep venous reflux, grading 173–6
Deep venous system, lower limbs 164–5
Deep venous thrombosis (DVT)
B-mode-images 195–6
collateral veins 199
color flow images 196–7
conditions mimicking 199–202
diagnostic problems 197–8
epidemiology 189–90
free-floating thrombi 190, 196
investigations for diagnosing 191–2
natural history 198–9
pathology 189–90
recanalization 198
recurrent 199
reporting 205
risk factors *190*
scanning 189, 192–8
spectral Doppler 197
symptoms 190–1
treatment 191
upper limbs 203–4
Demodulation 26
Depth gain compensation (DGC) 14
optimizing 76
Diabetes 115, 124
Digital arteries, scanning 138
Dodd's perforator 166
Doppler effect 23–4
applied to vascular ultrasound 24–6
Doppler shift 23–4
Doppler spectrum, factors influencing 63–6
Doppler ultrasound 2, 23–33
aliasing *see* Aliasing
color *see* Color flow imaging
continuous wave *see* Continuous wave Doppler
pulsed *see* Pulsed Doppler
signal analysis 27–33
signal extraction 26–7

Dorsalis pedis artery
anatomy 113
flow profiles 55, *56*
scanning 123
Duplex ultrasound 1, 33
Dwell time 42
Dynamic focusing 18–19
Dynamic range 14–15
Dysphasia 88

E

Ectasia 145
Edema 201
Elastic arteries 50
Emboli
acute ischemia 117–18
aneurysms 140
arterial disease 88, 133
pulmonary 189, 190
Endoleaks 149, 156–7
Endotension 157
Endothelium 50
Endovascular aneurysm repair 1, 148–9, 154–7
Endovenous saphenous obliteration 170
Ensemble length 44
Entrance effect 53
European Carotid Plaque Study Group 93
European Carotid Surgery Trialist's Collaborative Group (ECST) 97, 98, 100
European Federation of Societies for Ultrasound in Medicine and Biology (EFSUMB) 82
European Working Group on Critical Limb Ischemia 117
Exercise testing 115–16
External carotid artery (ECA)
anatomy 86
carotid body tumour 105–6
color image *91*
spectral Doppler 91–2
transverse B-mode image 89–90
External iliac artery
anatomy 112
occlusion *126*
scanning 120
External iliac vein 165, 168

F

False aneurysms 142, 146, 158–60
grafts 218

Fasciotomy 117
Fast Fourier transforms (FFTs) 28, 36
Femoral artery
    see also Common femoral artery;
        Superficial femoral artery
    false aneurysms 146
        scanning 159–60
        treatment 160
    idealized pressure waveforms *54*
    scanning 120–2
    transverse image *193*
    true aneurysms 158
Femoral bifurcation
    B-mode image 124
    color flow image *126*
    obstruction 117
Femorodistal bypass graft
    color image *214*
    preoperative assessment 123
    stenoses *216, 217*
    vein grafts 208
Femorofemoral cross-over grafts
    209, 213
Femoropopliteal grafts *208*, 213
Flash filter 38
Fluid collections, around grafts 220
Fluid energy 50–1
Focal zone settings 76
Focusing 18–19
Frame rate 13, 43–4
Frame-averaging 38, 46
Frequency 6
    color imaging 41
    harmonic 47
    pulsed ultrasound 8–9
    resonant 7
    spectrum 8–9

G

Gain control 13–14, 65
    optimizing 76
Ganglions 142
Gangrene 116
Gastrocnemius vein 164
Ghost images 77, 80, *81*
Giacomini vein 167
    incompetent 185
    scanning 181
Grafts
    anatomy 208–9
    aneurysms 218
    aortobifemoral *see* Aortobifemoral
        grafts
    arteriovenous fistulas 219–20
    axillobifemoral 209, 213

B-mode images 213–14
color doppler images 214–15
commonly encountered problems
    218
endovascular 148, *156*
entrapments 219
failure 210–11, 217–18
femorodistal *see* Femorodistal
    bypass graft
femorofemoral cross-over 209,
    213
femoropopliteal *208*, 213
fluid collections 220
hemodialysis access grafts
    142–3
iliofemoral cross-over *208*, 209,
    210, 213
infection 210, 220
occlusions 210–11, 217–18
reporting 220–1
scanning
    practical considerations 211
    techniques 211–13
seromas 220
spectral Doppler waveforms
    215–17
stenoses
    grading 216–17
    symptoms and treatment
        210–11
surveillance, purpose of 209–11
vein grafts *see* Vein grafts
vein mapping 221–3
Grating lobes 77
Gravitational potential energy 50–1
Gray-scale maps 15

H

Harmonic imaging 46–7, 76
Hematomas 151, 200
Hemiparesis 88
Hemodialysis access grafts 142–3
Heparin 191
Hertz 6
High-pass filters 27, 39, 43
    settings 65, 71
Hydrostatic pressure 61, 113
Hyperabduction test 140

I

Iliac artery
    see also Common iliac artery;
        Internal iliac artery
    aneurysms 157

bifurcation 111–12
disease *126*, 129
Iliac veins
    compression during pregnancy
        198
    investigation 198
    scanning 195
Iliofemoral cross-over grafts *208*,
    209, 210, 213
Image processing curves 14–15
Image resolution 19–21, 71
In situ technique 208–9, 211–12,
    213
Infection
    control 83
    grafts 210, 220
Innominate artery 86
Insonation
    angle of *see* Angle of insonation
    non-uniform 64
Intensity, of ultrasound 82
Internal carotid artery (ICA)
    anatomy 86
    carotid body tumour 105–6
    color image *96*
    Doppler frequency detection 40
    high resistance waveform *97*
    peak systolic velocity 100
    power Doppler image *45*
    reverse flow *56*
    spectral Doppler 91–2
    tortuous *58, 104*
    transverse B-mode image 89–90
Internal iliac artery 112, 113
Internal iliac vein 165
Internal jugular vein 203
Intima 50
Intrinsic spectral broadening (ISB)
    65–6, 100
Ipsilateral carotid artery 88
Ipsilateral vertebral artery 138
Ischemia
    lower limbs 116–18
    upper limbs 135

J

Jugular vein
    Doppler waveform *60*
    transverse B-mode image *90*

K

Kinetic energy 50, 51
Klippel-Trenaunay syndrome (KTS)
    186–7

L

Lateral resolution 19, 45
Left heart agents 47
Line density
  B-mode imaging 13
  color flow imaging 43
Lipodermatosclerosis 170–1
Long saphenous vein (LSV)
  anatomy 165, 166
  assessment
    for bypass graft 221–2
    for reflux 177–8
  duplicated 168
  grafts 208
  high-volume spontaneous flow
    169
  ligation 170
  thrombophlebitis 200
  varicose veins 169, 182–4, 185
Low velocity flow 42–3, 78–9
Lower limbs
  arterial disease
    ankle–brachial pressure index
      113–16
    arterial stents 129
    B-mode images 124–5
    collateral pathways 113
    diabetes 115, 124
    duplex scanning 118–24
    intermittent claudication
      116
    ischemia 116–18
    other abnormalities and
      syndromes 129–30
    reporting 130
    spectral Doppler 126–9
  arterial system 111–13
  color flow images 125–6
  deep venous system 164–5
  edema 201
  hematomas 200
  venous disorders 164
    Klippel-Trenaunay syndrome
      186–7
    reporting *186*, 187
    skin changes 170–1
    superficial thrombophlebitis
      186
    treatment of superficial 170
    ulcers *see* Venous ulceration
    varicose veins *see* Varicose veins
    venous hemangioma 187
  venous reflux 173–6
  venous system 164–9
    anatomical variations 168
    flow patterns 169
    scanning 171–2
    scanning protocol 176–82
    valves *see* Valves
Lymph nodes, enlargement 202
Lymphedema 200–1

M

M-mode (motion mode) 12
Magnetic resonance angiography
  (MRA) 1, 85
Magnetic resonance imaging (MRI)
  1, 192
Maximum peak systolic velocity 67
Mean velocity, measuring 67
Mechanical index 82–3
Media 50
Methicillin-resistant *Staphylococcus
  aureus* (MRSA) 220
Microemboli 117–18
Microvascular disorders 143
Middle cerebral artery (MCA) 86
Mirror image artefacts 77, 80, *81*
Monoparesis 88
Moving string test object 66
Multiple zone focusing 18
Muscular arteries 50

N

Neck injury 88
Neovascularization 184
Neurogenic thoracic outlet syndrome
  139–40
Noise 71–2
North American Symptomatic
  Carotid Endarterectomy Trial
  Collaborators (NASCET) 97,
  98, 100
Nyquist frequency 32

O

Occupational hazards 82
Ophthalmic artery 86

P

Palmar arch 134
  scanning 138
Parallel beam forming 19
Patients, examination of 76, 185–6
Peak systolic velocity (PSV) ratio
  100, 127–8
Penetration depth 14, 19, 21
Percutaneous balloon angioplasty
  2–3, 98, 117, 135, 210
Perforators 166
  B-mode appearance 181–2
  incompetent 185
  recurrent varicose veins 184
Peroneal artery 113, 123
Peroneal vein
  anatomy 164
  scanning *193*, 194
Persistence 44
Phase shift 37
Phlebitis 204–5
Piezoelectric effect 7
Plantar arch, preoperative assessment
  123
Plantar arteries 113
Poiseuille's law 51–2
Polytetrafluorethylene (PTFE) grafts
  148, *209*, 213, 214
Popliteal aneurysms 146, 157–8
Popliteal artery
  anatomy 113
  cystic adventitial disease 130
  occlusions 125
  scanning 120–2
Popliteal entrapment syndrome
  129–30
Popliteal fossa 113, 167
  diffuse varicosities 185
Popliteal vein
  anatomy 164, 167
  assessment 178
  duplicated 168
  incompetence 173
  scanning 194
  thrombi *190*
Post-processing 38
Posterior tibial (PT) artery 113
  scanning *79*, 123
Posterior tibial vein
  anatomy 164
  scanning *193*, 194
Posteromedial vein 167
Posture 61–2
Pourcelot's resistance index 72
Power Doppler imaging 45–6
Pressure energy 50, 51
Profunda femoris artery 112–13,
  118, 120
Profunda femoris vein *118*, 164, 168
Pulmonary embolism (PE) 189, 190
Pulsatile swelling 105, 142
Pulsatility index (PI) 72
Pulse repetition frequency (PRF) 30,
  32, 33, 41, 42–3, 44, 49, 65
  optimizing 78–9
Pulse wave velocity 72–3

Pulsed Doppler ultrasound 7–8, 29–31
   frequency content of pulses 8–9
   limitations 33

R

Radial artery
   anatomy 134
   dissection 138
   false aneurysms 142
   scanning 137
Range ambiguity 77
Range gate 30
Raynaud's phenomenon 143
Reflections, multiple 77, 80
Reflex sympathetic dystrophy (RDS) 143
Refraction 10, 77
Region of interest (ROI) 35, 43, 44
Renal arteries 146, 154
Repetitive strain injury 82
Resistance index (RI) 72
Resolution 19–21, 71
   color flow imaging 44–5
Respiration, venous flow 60–1
Reverberation artefacts 77
Reversed vein grafts 209, 213
Reynolds number 59
Right heart agents 45–6

S

Saddle embolus 117
Safety 82–3
Sample volume (sensitive region) 30
   size 64–5, 81
Saphenofemoral junction *118, 166*
   assessment 172, 177
   incompetence 173, 174
   incomplete ligation of 182–3
Saphenopopliteal junction
   color flow image *173*
   incomplete ligation 184–5
   scanning 180, 181
Saphenous compartment 165–6
Scanners
   color flow imaging 37–9
   volume flow measurement 70
Scattering 11
Secondary varicose veins 184
Sensitive region *see* Sample volume
Sensitivity, color flow imaging 44–5
Sensitivity of diagnostic test 227–8
Seromas 220

Short saphenous vein (SSV)
   anatomy 165, 166, 167
   assessment 178–81
   incompetence 169, 173, 184
   ligation 170
   recurrences 184–5
   thrombophlebitis 200
Slice thickness 19
Soleal veins
   anatomy 164
   scanning 194–5
Sound
   speed of 6–7
   waves 5–7
Spatial pulse average intensity 82
Specificity 227–8
Spectral broadening 64, 72
   intrinsic 65–6, 100
Spectral Doppler analysis 2, 27–9
   optimization 81
Spectrum analyser 26, *27*
Specular reflection 9, 11
Spider veins 169
Stenoses
   blood flow profiles 58–60
   carotid artery *see* Carotid artery stenoses
   common iliac artery *2*
   hemodynamically significant 52
   trickle flow 53
   velocity changes 52–3
   velocity ratios 67
Sternocleidomastoid muscle 89
Stroke 85, 88, 98
Subclavian artery (SA)
   anatomy 86, 133–4
   aneurysms 135, 140
   color flow image *142*
   compression (thoracic outlet syndrome) 139–42
   mirror image 80, *81*
   occlusions 138, 142
   scanning 136–7, 141
Subclavian steal syndrome 87, 88
Subclavian vein 203
   assessing 204
   compression 204
   thrombosis 203
Superficial femoral artery (SFA)
   anatomy 113, *118*
   assessment 121
   atheroma 124
   color flow images
      forward and reverse flow *55*
      high velocity *54*
   hyperemic flow *186*
   occlusions 121, 125, *126*
   stenosis *125*

   velocity waveform *54*
Superficial femoral vein
   anatomy *118*, 164
   B-mode images *199*
   competence 172–3
   duplicated (bifid) 168
   hyperemic flow *186*
   scanning 194
Superficial venous reflux, grading 173–6
Superior mesenteric artery (SMA) 146
Surgery
   see also Carotid endarterectomy
   aortic aneurysm repair 147–9
Synthetic grafts 209
   B-mode images 214
   color Doppler images 215
   scanning 213
   surveillance 210

T

Test objects 20, 66
Thermal index (TI) 82–3
Thigh perforators 184
Thoracic outlet
   anatomy 139, *140*
   assessment 136
Thoracic outlet syndrome (TOS) 139–40
   duplex assessment 141–2
   maneuvers for assessing 140–1
Thread veins 170
Thrombophlebitis 186, 200
Tibial arteries, assessment 122–3
Tibioperoneal trunk 113, *212*
Time averaged velocity 71–2
Time gain compensation (TGC) 14
Time-domain processing 37
Tissue harmonic imaging (THI) 21–2
Tissue heating 83
Transcranial Doppler ultrasound 106–7
Transducers 7
   broad-band 7, 22, 47, 89
   curvilinear array 16, 40, 79
   designs and beam forming 15–17
   infection control 83
   linear array 15–16, 33, 39, 65–6, 68, 79, 89
   phased array 17, 33, 40
Transient ischemic attack (TIA) 88
Transverse wave 5
Treadmills 115–16
'Trickle flow' 53

U

UK Small Aneurysm Trial
    Participants 147
Ulceration 116
Ulnar artery
    anatomy 134
    scanning 137
Ultrasound
    amplification 13–14
    developments in technology 1
    energy loss (attenuation) 11–12
    generation of ultrasound waves
        7–9
    image production 12–13
    intensity 82
    interaction with surfaces 9–11
    nature of 5–7
    safety 82–3
    speed of 6–7
Upper limbs
    arterial disease
        aneurysms 142
        arteriovenous fistulas 142–3
        collateral pathways *135*
        duplex assessment 135–6
        hemodialysis access grafts 142–3
        other disorders 143
        reporting 143
        scanning techniques 136–8
        symptoms and treatment
            135
        thoracic outlet syndrome
            139–42
        ultrasound appearance 138–9
    arterial system 133–5
    venous disorders 204–5
        thrombosis 203–4
    venous system 202–3

V

Valsalva maneuver 172–3
Valves 168–9
    abnormal venous flow 62
    assessing 172–3
    congenital valve aplasia 169
Valvulotome 208
Variance 39
Varicose ulcers 171
Varicose veins 164
    B-mode appearance 181–2
    causes 169–70
    duplex scanning 171–2
    investigation of recurrent 182–5
    treatment 170
Vein cuffs 214
Vein grafts 208–9
    B-mode images 213–14
    color Doppler images 214–15
    failure 209
    scanning 211–13
    stenosis 209, *210*, 214
    surveillance 209–10
    waveform shapes 215–16
Veins
    see also individual veins
    blood flow 60–2
    mapping for bypass surgery
        221–3
    structure 50
    varicose *see* Varicose veins
Velocity 27–8
    changes within stenoses 52–3
    low velocity flow 42–3
    measurements
        color flow imaging 36–7
        conversion from Doppler
            frequencies 66–7

optimizing angle of insonation
            69–70
        sources of errors 67–9, 70
        using duplex ultrasound 33
    ratio measurements 67, 69,
        127–8
Velocity estimator 39
Vena cava 60, *165*, 168
    scanning 195
Vena caval filters 191
Venography 191
Venous hemangioma 187
Venous hypertension 170
Venous reflux, grading 173–6
Venous ulceration 170–1
    assessment of patients 185–6
Vertebral arteries
    anatomy 86
    blood flow 103
    collateral flow 87
    color flow image *93*
    disease
        reverse flow 103
        symptoms 88
    subclavian steal syndrome 87
Vibration white finger disease 143
Visuospatial neglect 88
Volume flow measurement 70–2

W

Wall thumps 27, 71
Warfarin 191
Waveform analysis 72–3
Wavelength 6
World Federation of Ultrasound in
    Medicine and Biology
    (WFUMB) 82